Medical care, humanitarianism and intimacy in
the long Second World War, 1931–1953

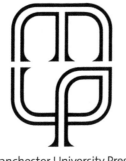

Manchester University Press

Cultural History of Modern War

Series editors

Ana Carden-Coyne, Max Jones, Jo Laycock and Bertrand Taithe

To buy or to find out more about the books currently available in this series, please go to: https://manchesteruniversitypress.co.uk/series/cultural-history-of-modern-war/

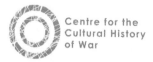

https://www.alc.manchester.ac.uk/history/research/centres/cultural-history-of-war//

# Medical care, humanitarianism and intimacy in the long Second World War, 1931–1953

*Edited by*

Marie-Luce Desgrandchamps, Laure Humbert,
Bertrand Taithe and Raphaële Balu

MANCHESTER UNIVERSITY PRESS

Copyright © Manchester University Press 2025

While copyright in the volume as a whole is vested in Manchester University Press, copyright in individual chapters belongs to their respective authors, and no chapter may be reproduced wholly or in part without the express permission in writing of both author and publisher.

An electronic version of this book has been made freely available under a Creative Commons (CC BY-NC-ND) licence, thanks to the support of the Arts and Humanities Research Council [grant number AH/T006382/1], which permits non-commercial use, distribution and reproduction provided the author(s) and Manchester University Press are fully cited and no modifications or adaptations are made. Details of the licence can be viewed at https://creativecommons.org/licenses/by-nc-nd/4.0/

Published by Manchester University Press
Oxford Road, Manchester, M13 9PL

www.manchesteruniversitypress.co.uk

British Library Cataloguing-in-Publication Data
A catalogue record for this book is available from the British Library

ISBN 978 1 5261 8347 7 hardback

First published 2025

The publisher has no responsibility for the persistence or accuracy of URLs for any external or third-party internet websites referred to in this book, and does not guarantee that any content on such websites is, or will remain, accurate or appropriate.

EU authorised representative for GPSR:
Easy Access System Europe, Mustamäe tee 50, 10621 Tallinn, Estonia.
gpsr.requests@easproject.com

Typeset by Newgen Publishing UK

# Contents

| | |
|---|---|
| List of figures | vii |
| List of contributors | ix |

Introduction: humanitarianism and medical care during the long Second World War, 1931–1953 – Marie-Luce Desgrandchamps, Laure Humbert, Bertrand Taithe and Raphaële Balu 1

1 Humanitarianism, estrangement and intimacies during the long Second World War: new historiographical perspectives – Laure Humbert 30

2 Colonial medicine and 'Black strength' in the French colonies of Africa during the long Second World War – Delphine Peiretti-Courtis 58

3 Africa, the Africans and the Red Cross: assessing the impact of the long Second World War – Marie-Luce Desgrandchamps 84

4 (Un)Settling intimacies: boundaries of aid in a North African refugee camp, 1944–1946 – Esther Möller and Katharina Stornig 109

5 'National Defense Medicine': Chinese-style physicians and medical relief during the war against Japan – Jean Corbi 131

6 'There is no enemy here!' Humanitarian rhetoric in South America during the Second World War: Peru/Ecuador – François Bignon 154

vi                          *Contents*

7 Unitarian Service Committee's activities with refugee
  populations and the Resistance in France during and
  after the Second World War – Jon Arrizabalaga and
  Àlvar Martínez-Vidal                                              178
8 Cultural actors in rehabilitation: Second World War
  craft therapy and white, ableist, heteronormative
  masculinity – Jennifer Way                                        202
9 Trauma of warfare: maxillofacial surgery and medical
  relief in wartime China, 1948–1956 – Jinghong Zhang               235
10 Dying on enemy ground: the ICRC and the German
   soldiers killed in France during the Second
   World War – Taline Garibian                                      256

Index                                                               277

# Figures

8.1 'Craftsmen and the War', *Craft Horizons,*
2:2 (May 1943), p. 12 (American Craft Council)                208

8.2 Mildred G. Burrage, 'Craftsmen Can Help:
An Account of the Arts and Skills Unit of the
New York Chapter of the American Red Cross at
Halloran Hospital', *Craft Horizons,* 3:6 (August 1944),
p. 18 (American Craft Council)                                210

8.3 War Department, *Technical Manual for Occupational
Therapy,* TM-8291 (Washington, DC: U.S. Government
Printing Office, 1944), p. 65 (US Government)                 211

8.4 'Tuskegee Veteran Hospital Exhibit at Exposition
Shows How Patients Are Cured', *The Chicago Defender,*
August 24, 1940, p. 4                                        213

8.5 'Creative Work for Veterans', *Design Magazine*
(March 1945), p. 14                                          214

8.6 Occupational therapy, Lawson General Hospital,
Atlanta, Georgia, 1944 (Newberry Library)                    215

8.7 War Department, *Technical Manual for Occupational
Therapy,* TM-8291 (Washington, DC: U.S. Government
Printing Office, 1944), p. 72                                216

8.8 Helen S. Willard and Clare S. Spackman, *Principles
of Occupational Therapy* (Philadelphia, PA:
J. B. Lippincott Company, 1947) (Wolters, Kluwe
Health Inc.)                                                 217

viii                          *List of figures*

8.9   'Ex-Marine Claire Moore, the school's first trainee,
      shapes a bowl in the metal class, under direction
      of Aiden Wood', *Dartmouth Alumni Magazine*
      (March 1945), p. 12                                    220
8.10  Poster, War Veterans' Art Center, 1942, Early
      Museum History: Administrative Records, I.3.o.
      (The Museum of Modern Art Archives, New York).
      © The Museum of Modern Art/Licensed by
      SCALA/Art Resource, NY                                 223
8.11  Kenneth Chorley, Chairman of the War Veterans' Art
      Center, and Admiral Monroe Kelly (right) watch veteran
      at potter's wheel at the opening of the exhibition Art
      for War Veterans, September 26, 1945 to November 25,
      1945 (Photographic Archive, The Museum of Modern
      Art Archives, New York. Photograph by Henry Mallon).
      © The Museum of Modern Art/Licensed by SCALA/Art
      Resource, NY                                           225
8.12  *How to Make Objects of Wood* (New York:
      Museum of Modern Art with Simon & Schuster,
      1951) (Simon & Schuster)                               227
9.1   The Huaxi plastic surgery team, 1952, Chengdu.
      Photograph reproduced with kind permission of
      Mr. Deng Changchun, the son of Deng Xianzhao           245

# Contributors

**Jon Arrizabalaga** is Research Professor in the History of Science at the Spanish National Council for Scientific Research (CSIC-IMF), Barcelona. During the last fifteen years, his research has been mainly focused on humanitarian action and war medicine in modern Spain, with particular attention to the Third Carlist War (1872–1876) and the Spanish Civil War and its aftermath (1936–1950). Among his publications are 'Medicine, Religion, and the Humanitarian Ethos: Walter B. Cannon, the Unitarian Church, and the Care of Spanish Republican Refugees in France' (co-authored with Àlvar Martínez-Vidal), *Journal of the History of Medicine and Allied Sciences*, 77:2 2022, 158–185; and *John Furley. Entre carlistas. Edición, estudio introductorio y notas* (co-authored with Guillermo Sánchez) (Pamplona: Pamiela, 2023).

**Raphaële Balu** is a postdoctoral fellow at Sorbonne University, and an associate researcher at the University of Caen-Normandie ('Histemé'). She was a research associate on the AHRC-funded project (AH/T006382/1) 'Colonial and Transnational Intimacies: Medical Humanitarianism in the French External Resistance, 1940–1945' from 2021 to 2022. Her latest articles include 'Médecine clandestine en France occupée: soignantes et soignants de la Résistance (1943–1945)' (*Le Mouvement Social*, 2024/3 288,75–94) and 'Des soignants parachutés en France occupée: la résistance médicale au-delà des frontières' (*European Review of History: Revue Européenne d'histoire*, 31(1), 129–156).

**François Bignon** teaches modern and contemporary history at the University of the French West Indies, Martinique. He has a PhD from the University of Rennes 2, France, and has lived and worked x *List of contributors*

in several Latin American and Caribbean countries. His research focuses on international armed conflicts and the creation of borders and national identities in contemporary Andean America and the Amazon region.

**Jean Corbi** is a PhD candidate in history at Sciences Po where he held the position of Research and Teaching Assistant (ATER). He was awarded a Doctoral Dissertation Fellowship from the Chiang Ching-kuo Foundation in 2022. His research interests focus on the social history of medicine in China, with an emphasis on the province of Sichuan during the first half of the twentieth century.

**Marie-Luce Desgrandchamps** is a lecturer at the University of Geneva and senior researcher at the University of Fribourg on the SNSF Research Project 'The Red Cross and the Red Star: Humanitarianism and Communism during the XXth Century'. She was one of the co-investigators of the AHRC-funded project 'Colonial and Transnational Intimacies: Medical Humanitarianism in the French External Resistance' (2021–2023), from which this book originated. She is the author of various publications on the history of humanitarianism and the Red Cross in Africa, including *L'humanitaire en guerre civile: La crise du Biafra (1967–1970)* (Rennes: PUR, 2018).

**Taline Garibian** is a lecturer at the Maison de l'Histoire of the University of Geneva. She is also an associate researcher at the Institute of Humanities in Medicine (Unil/CHUV) and a visiting fellow at the Wellcome Centre for Ethics and Humanities (University of Oxford). Specialising in modern history, her areas of interest include the history of medicine and science; the history of wars, violence and genocide; and the history of gender and sexualities. In 2017, she completed a dual PhD at the University of Lausanne and the University Jean Jaurès of Toulouse. Her dissertation focused on the history of sexology in French-speaking Switzerland. From 2017 to 2021, she was a research associate and then British Academy Postdoctoral Fellow at the University of Oxford, where she conducted a research project on the history of war violence and forensics and taught in the master's programme in Modern European History. She is the Principal Investigator of the new FNS-funded

## List of contributors

project 'Mass Death, Science and Medicine: Handling the Corpses of War in Modern Europe (1850–1960)'.

**Laure Humbert** is a senior lecturer at the University of Manchester. She is the author of *Reinventing French Aid: The Politics of Humanitarian Relief in French-Occupied Germany, 1945–1952* (Cambridge: Cambridge University Press, 2021), which examines the everyday encounters between Allies, Displaced Persons and Germans in the French zone. From 2021 to 2023, she led an AHRC-funded project on the history of medical care in the French Resistance (AH/T006382/1). This co-edited volume is the result of an online seminar series that was organised by the project team.

**Àlvar Martínez-Vidal** has been a lecturer in the history of science at the Spanish universities of Zaragoza, Cantabria, Barcelona (UAB) and Valencia, where he is an honorary researcher at the Instituto Interuniversitario López Piñero. His research has mostly focused on Catalan and Spanish Republican medical exiles and the humanitarian medical action in France (1936–1950). Among his publications are *L'Hôpital Varsovie: Exil, médecine et résistance (1944–1950)* (Toulouse: Loubatières, 2011); 'La ayuda médica humanitaria a los refugiados republicanos españoles en Francia (1939–1950)' (special issue co-edited with Jon Arrizabalaga), *Dynamis*, 40:1 (2020), 13–21; and *El metge Josep Torrubia Zea. Lliurepensador, maçó i socialista* (co-authored with Rosa Toran) (Valencia: Afers, 2021) (French version in preparation).

**Esther Möller** is currently the German vice-director of Centre Marc Bloch, a Franco-German research centre in social sciences and humanities in Berlin, and a visiting professor of history at Humboldt University Berlin. She is a historian of the modern Middle East and its multiple connections to Europe in the fields of humanitarianism, forced migration, and cultural and educational politics. Among her recent publications are, together with Shaimaa Esmail El-Neklawy, 'Between Local Philanthropic Traditions and State Politics: Endowments and Charitable Associations in 19th- and 20th-Century Egypt', *Endowment Studies*, 6(2022), 192–220. She also edited, together with Katharina Stornig and Johannes Paulmann, xii *List of contributors*

*Gendering Global Humanitarianism: Practice, Politics and the Power of Representation* (London: Palgrave Macmillan, 2020).

**Delphine Peiretti-Courtis** is an associate professor at the University of Aix-Marseille and a member of the Telemme laboratory. She was a guest professor of history at the University of Montreal in 2023–2024. She works on the history of racial representations in French medicine in the nineteenth and twentieth centuries and the construction of racial and sexual stereotypes about Black bodies. She published a book in French entitled *Black Bodies and White Doctors: The Making of Racial Prejudice* (La Découverte, 2021). She is currently working on medical violence during colonisation and is co-writing a book on the international circulation of scientific racism.

**Katharina Stornig** is a lecturer in modern history at the University of Giessen. Her research interests include women's and gender history, the history of child welfare, mission history, the history of colonialism and decolonisation and the history of mobility. She has recently published *Spenden, Retten, Helfen: Das 'ferne Kind' und die Transnationalisierung der Wohltätigkeit, 1830–1930* (Göttingen: Wallstein, 2024) and edited, together with Esther Möller and Johannes Paulmann, *Gendering Global Humanitarianism: Practice, Politics and the Power of Representation* (London: Palgrave Macmillan, 2020).

**Bertrand Taithe** is a professor of cultural history at the University of Manchester and a founder member of the Humanitarian and Conflict Response Institute. He works on the history of humanitarian aid and of its representations, the history of war and medicine and contemporary humanitarian practices. His most recent articles and books include *L'Humanitaire s'exhibe – The Humanitarian Exhibition* (Geneva: Georg, 2022); 'The Politics of Catholic Humanitarian Aid: Missionaries and American Relief in Algeria 1942–1947', *French History*, 37:2 (2023), 160–176; 'Living Humanitarian Dreams: The Oneiric and Spiritual Life and Activism of Elizabeth Wilson (1909–2000)', *Cultural and Social History*, 20:3 (2023), 429–445, and 'Dossier: History Writing and Attacks on Healthcare', *Humanity* (Winter 2023). He is a co-investigator of the

## List of contributors

'Researching the Impact of Attacks on Healthcare' (FCDO funded) and 'Colonial and Transnational Intimacies' projects (AHRC: AH/ T006382/1), and Principal Investigator of the Wellcome Discovery Award project 'Developing Humanitarian Medicine: From Alma Ata to Bio-Tech, a History of Norms, Knowledge Production and care (1978–2020)' (Wellcome: 226515/Z/22/Z). See the full list of publications at: https://research.manchester.ac.uk/en/persons/bertrand. taithe

**Jennifer Way** is a professor of art history at the University of North Texas, where she teaches craft and conflict, and American art and healing. Her book *The Politics of Vietnamese Craft: American Diplomacy and Domestication* (London: Bloomsbury Visual Arts, 2019) explores how Americans appropriated a foreign art form in programmes that intersected their diplomatic agendas and domestic lives with South Vietnam on questions of Vietnamese belonging in the Free World, 1955 to 1961. Among her forthcoming publications are an anthology, *Craft and War: Makers, Objects and Armed Conflicts since the mid 19th Century* (Bloomsbury), and a monograph, *Craft, Wellness, and Healing in Contexts of War* (Routledge). She is the author of 'The Museum of Modern Art's Craft-Based Occupational Therapy', published in the volume *Modernism, Art, Therapy* (New Haven, CT: Yale University Press, 2024).

**Jinghong Zhang** is an assistant professor of history at the University of Maryland, Baltimore County, United States. Her research focuses on the social and cultural history of modern China and the history of medicine and public health. She is currently working on a book manuscript that examines the history of dentistry and the discourse of oral hygiene in modern China.

# Introduction: humanitarianism and medical care during the long Second World War, 1931–1953

*Marie-Luce Desgrandchamps, Laure Humbert, Bertrand Taithe and Raphaële Balu*

In 1943, the Quaker social worker Hertha Kraus compiled a humanitarian manual drawing lessons from previous conflicts that she considered relevant to her trainee humanitarians about to leave for Europe with the Mennonites and Quakers' relief services.[1] Ten years later, back in the United States, she reflected on her experiences in recent decades, noting: 'World War II and the preceding period, beginning with persecution and displacement in central Europe in the middle 30s, challenged us anew to contribute.'[2] In her account, she preached the new remit of American social work methods, without acknowledging her previous and personal experiences in Europe. She omitted that she was herself one of those who had to flee. According to her, there was a continuum between social work in times of economic strife, war-work and international humanitarianism.[3] This circulation of expertise reaching out across national borders had deep roots at the international level,[4] but field practitioners, such as Kraus, experienced it in a very practical and everyday manner. For them, humanitarian aid took the form of a continuum of needs assessments and provision of specialist expertise, all processes that transcended war declarations and peace treaties.[5] For many humanitarian actors across the world, like Hertha Kraus, it was impossible to draw clear boundaries between wartime and peacetime work during the decades spanning from the 1930s to the 1950s.[6]

From the perspective of the Cameroonian nurse Marcel Eyidi Bebey, who joined the medical corps of the Free French Forces in 1940 and only returned to Cameroon in the mid-1950s after

2  *Introduction*

completing a medical thesis in Paris, the 'long' Second World War was also a period of slow, but significant, professional and political transformation.[7] Trained in the 1930s in the nursing school of Ayos, a colonial medical infrastructure to combat sleeping sickness, Eyidi Bebey started his war as a nurse in 1940. In 1943, he was granted the status of auxiliary medical doctor (*médecin auxiliaire*). Following Free French troops through Libya, Tunisia and Europe, he acquired new knowledge of frontline nursing and medical care, before being offered the opportunity to study medicine in Paris after the war. He then played an important role in the Cameroonian independence movement.[8] Whether for Hertha Kraus or for Marcel Eyidi Bebey, the traditional periodisation of the Second World War, as starting in 1939 and ending in May 1945, did not fit in with their wartime experiences or their professional and, in Eyidi Bebey's case, political careers. For many medical and humanitarian actors like them, the beginning and the end of the war were not events but processes, with different temporalities, some actors 'entering into' and 'getting out of the war' earlier than others. Thus, their histories – and other like it told in this book – point to the necessity to rethink the war's chronology. They also invite us to reconsider the relationships between individual grassroots experiences of the conflict and the global framework in which these experiences occurred.

Adopting a broad chronological and decentred approach to the war, this book explores this continuum of experiences from the 1930s to 1950s from a multiplicity of perspectives. The histories of the Swiss ICRC delegates, French colonial doctors, Egyptian relief workers, Chinese physicians, Peruvian and Ecuadorian nurses, and American Quakers at the heart of this book reveal underexamined sites of interactions among humanitarians and medical workers, both national and international. Focusing on the Second World War as both a global war and a collection of local conflicts, this book revisits well-established questions, central to historiographical debate about humanitarianism during this crucial period. It asks: Did the war *really* constitute an important moment of reckoning with race inequality in the humanitarian and medical realm, or did it, instead, reinforce racial boundaries? Did the many and various connections between people from a variety of backgrounds, forced or made temporarily possible by the war, lead to more *intimate* and collective bonds or, on the contrary, more estrangements?

*Introduction* 3

And finally, how can we access this hidden circulation of knowledge and practices, unaccounted for in the existing historiography of medicine and humanitarianism?

Drawing on separate strands of historiography (including the literature on aid during the Italo-Ethiopian War, the Spanish Civil War, the Peruvian-Ecuadorian conflict, the Sino-Japanese War and irregular warfare in occupied Europe), we offer situated and micro-global histories of humanitarianism and medical care during the long Second World War, which challenge the traditional chronology of 1939/1945 marking sharp historical divides. These approaches allow us to bring the field of 'global' histories of the Second World War and humanitarianism together, integrating current historiographical re-evaluations of the global dimension of the conflict with local histories of aid. Acknowledging the potential of global approaches to shed light on underexamined connections, Jean-Paul Zuniga underlines the necessity to study these points of contact through a situated approach, so as not to downplay 'the weight of the forces that determine the quality, direction and density of the connections that make up a social space'.[9] As John-Paul A Ghobrial and others have demonstrated more recently, a 'micro-global' history enables the study of global historical processes to be combined with a focus on close analysis and contextualization of primary sources.[10]

This book is thus neither structured around breaks and ruptures nor linear shifts from what Michael Barnett called 'imperial humanitarianism' to 'neo-humanitarianism', or from what other scholars have identified as a shift from 'amateurism' to 'professionalism'.[11] Instead of creating a metanarrative and an 'overarching story' of humanitarianism during the long Second World War, we consider the slow, messy and ambivalent transformation of humanitarian actors' relations to the suffering 'distant other' during this period and the co-existence of old and new ideas about the sexed, gendered, racialised and wounded body. The history of humanitarian aid and humanitarianism, as the practice of succouring others and upholding ideals of humanity, precisely offers a way of engaging with sources closest to human suffering. Humanitarian work occurred at the most intimate level, while campaigning for humanitarianism called for global solutions. As such this history contributes to weaving together the history of medicine and ideas and gendered

# 4                                    *Introduction*

studies of the conflict, enabling us to reassess how social and political transformation reverberate through people's lives.

## Global histories of the Second World War and humanitarianism

For decades, national and bilateral analysis of the Second World War strongly shaped memories of the events, whether it was in the USSR's 'Great Patriotic War', the 'Thirty Years War' between France and Germany or the 'Battle of Britain' in the United Kingdom.[12] These vivid national memories born out of the conflict, the outbreak of the Cold War and subsequent difficulties in accessing archives prevented the study of transnational circulations of actors, practices and ideas for a long time. However, since the beginning of the twenty-first century, historians have called for more global and transnational approaches to the history of the Second World War, contesting this long-held hegemony of national historiography. While one could argue that forms of transnational history have existed for a long time, transnational historians have insisted more vigorously since the 1990s on the necessity to go beyond spatially and geographically defined history. Transnational histories have documented contacts between communities, organisations and individuals that lived in between and through self-contained entities (such as states) and uncovered how experts disseminated their knowledge and practice often outside the direct control of national government.[13] These historians have also challenged established periodisation that previously shaped national historiographies in order to better understand these processes of change over different timescales.[14] Global historians have shared with transnational scholars an interest in connectivity and scales above and below those of the nation or region.[15] The historiography of the Second World War has adopted these methodologies, shifting to the global level and re-emphasising the original American definition of the conflict as a 'world' war.[16]

In recent years, these global histories of the Second World War have reassessed the interactions between different military fronts and geographical spaces, highlighting, for instance, the importance of the Mediterranean Sea and the African continent.[17] They have also paid increased attention to the history of international organisations

## Introduction                                                    5

during the conflict and the 'internationalism of war'.[18] In globalising the history of the conflict, they have adopted various periodisations. For Alya Aglan and Robert Frank, the 'world-war' covers the years 1937–1947. It spanned from the Japanese invasion of China to the peace treaty of February 1947 – ending with the alleged 'paradigm shift' that accompanied the beginning of the Cold War,[19] and the wars of national liberations against colonial domination. Andrew Buchanan chose instead the 1931 Japanese invasion of Manchuria as a starting point, which inaugurated a decade of renewed imperial expansion and the partition of Korea as an end.[20] For him, this periodisation highlights the 'volcanic eruption of the United States' and the imposition of its world system (calibrated to American interests).[21] Sharif Gemie and colleagues have structured their histories of the Second World War around the great transformative journeys undertaken by large sections of the population of Europe and linked countries, starting with refugees leaving Spain in 1936 and ending with Palestinian Arabs fleeing Israeli forces in 1948.[22] These periodisations have enabled historians to highlight strong continuities from one war to another, either at a European scale[23] or at a global one,[24] and to consider the connections between a number of different kinds of war (interstate wars, civil wars, insurgencies, partisan wars).[25] Others have favoured a broader timeframe running from 1870 to 1945 in order to characterise the sequence of conflicts by their combination of imperial and industrial features.[26] Focusing on the European continent, Mark Mazower considers 1950 as a possible turning point, marking the end of the post-war reconstruction and long-lasting period of 'violent peace'.[27] These different perspectives are not merely about chronology but reflect broader questions of scale and subject matter, subjectivities and political narratives.

Despite these important historiographical developments, the long Second World War remains an uneasy object for historians of humanitarianism. It sits awkwardly in broad periodisation of global humanitarianism. The conflict is either regarded as a moment of acceleration, a rupture, or a catalyst for the development of new international organisations, which for a brief period included both communist and capitalist visions of internationalism.[28] Kevin O'Sullivan, Matthew Hilton and Juliano Fiori have argued that 'moments of acceleration' were periods which 'saw a burst of activity that refreshed the sector while carrying with them the baggage of

6                        *Introduction*

what had come before'.[29] For Enrico Dal Lago and Kevin O'Sullivan, the long Second World War saw two moments of acceleration. First, the Great Depression in the 1930s represented a key turning point in global capitalism, which in turn led to an acceleration in global humanitarian activity beginning in the United States.[30] Second, the aftermath of the Second World War saw the development of new economic and financial structures initiated at Bretton Woods in 1944, which greatly impacted global humanitarian activity and made states more central to the funding, regulation and organisation of humanitarian action.[31] For Michael Barnett, this represented in fact an important rupture, signalling the end of 'imperial humanitarianism' and the start of 'neo-humanitarianism', marked by increased centralisation, bureaucratisation and rationalisation. For him, while prior to the Second World War, voluntary agencies looked for funding from parishioners and households, after the conflict, governments began to provide more funding because 'they now imagined a relationship between security and foreign aid'.[32] Michael Barnett's argument has been nuanced in many ways, notably by historians highlighting the importance of the 'mixed economy' of voluntary and state aid in the aftermath of the First World War.[33]

Other historians have insisted instead on continuities between the provision of humanitarian aid in the era of the First and Second World Wars, highlighting how many humanitarian and medical actors envisaged aid through the lessons learned from the previous conflict. Continuity is encapsulated in Johannes Paulmann's notion of 'conjunctures': for Paulmann the epochs of humanitarian aid, rather than consecutive, are best understood as overlapping. The Second World War is part of Paulmann's first 'historical conjuncture', which coincided with the establishment of the League of Nations in the aftermath of the First World War and the development of Save the Children and the American Relief Administration. According to him, 'World War Two can be seen as a sort of extension of the experience gained after World War I rather than the beginning of a new period.'[34] This insistence on continuities is also clear in Silvia Salvatici's *A History of Humanitarianism* or Sebastien Farré's work on humanitarian aid parcels.[35] For Salvatici, the period after the First World War saw the emergence of a 'transnational humanitarian regime', which was 'not occasional' and was 'entrusted to international institutions'.[36] According to her, it represented a

*Introduction* 7

crucial phase in the process of humanitarianism's institutionalisation, largely driven by women's international associations.[37] This period of the long Second World War was also characterised by a redefinition of activities delivered by the Vatican.[38] Drawing on the transformations undertaken a generation earlier by Catholic social workers and campaigners who wanted to counter-influence communism, the Vatican sought to affirm more clearly its humanitarian mandate in under-privileged settings and expand its influence in the humanitarian realm while depoliticising its agenda.[39]

Building on but also departing from these two strands of scholarship (global histories of the Second World War and global histories of humanitarianism), this book considers the long Second World War as a distinct period in histories of humanitarianism and examines its numerous fronts, rears and aftermaths, from the 1930s to the 1950s. The war involved civilians on an unprecedented scale, blurring the lines between state and civil society humanitarian initiatives, between civil and military organisations. To assess its impact on humanitarian practices, the book adopts a broad definition of humanitarian and medical actors, including but also going beyond what some scholars have called 'traditional' humanitarian activities and actors, namely Red Cross societies, international organisations (League of Nations, United Nations), voluntary associations (such as Save the Children and the American Friends Service Committee) or the private Swiss organisation the International Committee of the Red Cross. As recent studies have demonstrated, this focus on international and institutionalised actors overlooks important dimensions of the aid provided by local actors, trade unionists (notably during the Spanish Civil War), missionaries, and so on.[40] By paying attention to a variety of actors instead, we do not wish to erase the important differences that existed between disparate actors, such as the Chinese physician (Chapter 5) who contributed to wartime medical efforts through non-state organisations, the Egyptian guard (Chapter 4) employed by UN agencies to control refugee camps or the American member of the Unitarian Service Committee (Chapter 7) who helped Jewish refugees getting out of Europe. However, adopting new categorisations about who was or was not a 'humanitarian' negates a more holistic story of humanitarianism: crucially, one which recognises its complexity and the intensification of circulations from one conflict to another, one front to another.

8                                      *Introduction*

The humanitarians evoked in this book include nurses, both professional and improvised, who belong to a well-known nursing historiography harking back to Florence Nightingale, such as the Peruvian nurse and First Lady Enriqueta Garland de Prado (Chapter 6), Chinese war and plastic surgeons such as Song Ruyao and Wang Hanzhang who learned both from American and Soviet medicine (Chapter 9), but also civilian networks of helpers, artists and craft workers, and art museums which became actors of veterans' rehabilitation (Chapter 8). Rethinking the global history of the Second World War from their perspective troubles the clear waters of war distance and the enmities of warring by recentring on sufferings and bodies in pain, of close bodily contact between enemy bodies in the context of hospitals, on intimate acts of care and symbolic governing of bodies, even if they were never free of racialised, gendered or ableist prejudices and perspectives (Chapter 1).[41] This approach enables us to reassess the boundaries of humanitarian governance, its traditional activities (Chapters 8, 10) and geography. As the chapter on Peruvian and Ecuadorian medical care reminds us (Chapter 6), for instance, the Second World War was not only a global war but also a collection of local conflicts with important consequences for the development of humanitarianism. For Peru and Ecuador, humanitarian aid was considered as a moral duty essential to gain international respectability, influenced by European traditions of aid but also a practice, fundamentally rooted in the historical and cultural ties that bound the countries that had emerged from the former Spanish Empire together.

In doing so, this book makes four key contributions to the existing scholarship. First, this book offers a productive way of rethinking the role of the United States during this period and its rise as a 'humanitarian superpower'. To be sure, American involvement in the war left it unrivalled in its command of humanitarian logistics, and humanitarianism served multiple American diplomatic, strategic and economic objectives.[42] Yet, many territories were left unaffected by American aid, while other international actors developed and diversified their range of activities. The book thus complicates the standard narrative of a linear rise of the United States as a humanitarian superpower. Second, this book reconsiders the issue of medical modernisation, disturbing the well-told stories of Western 'charity' simply giving way to 'professionalisation'. It shows that

*Introduction*                                                    9

the long Second World War implied competing notions of professionalisation, a process which operated differently in China, for example (Chapter 5). It also questions the transformation of medical categories of alterities (Chapter 2), nuancing the view of a linear shift from medical and humanitarian racism to more equal relationships (Chapters 2 and 3). In French colonial medicine, for instance, the pseudo-racial science of the late nineteenth century continued to exist, and a new focus on hereditary and blood characteristics breathed fresh life into raciology (Chapter 2). Third, the book revisits the long-established historiographical question concerning the use of humanitarianism as a diplomatic tool and instrument of soft power from the vantage point of South America.[43] Chapter 6 uncovers, in particular, the specificities of Latin American rhetoric and highlights the need to consider circulations from the 'centre' (Europe, the US) to the 'periphery' (Latin America), but also from Latin America back to Europe. Fourth, the book challenges the traditional dichotomy between civilian and military cultures of rehabilitation and provision of aid (Chapters 2, 8, 9).

## The humanitarian reconfigurations of the 1930s to the 1950s

Studying the interconnections between spaces at war on a global scale,[44] and the ways in which humanitarians circulated between these sites, this book takes as a starting point the war in China in 1931, which led to the progressive dislocation of the League of Nations, with Japanese, German and Soviet departures in the 1930s. Historians have shown that Japanese aggression in 1931 led to a gradual incorporation of the Red Cross into the Chinese Nationalist government's plans for national defence, while other organisations (such as the Daoyuan and Red Swastika Society) developed more complex relationships with the Nationalist government, occasionally supporting Japanese imperialism in Manchuria.[45] After the Japanese attacks on Shanghai in 1932, Red Cross activism served more clearly patriotic and anti-Japanese defence aims, even if this was not without local conflicts.[46] The Italo-Ethiopian War (1935–1936), the Spanish Civil War (1936–1939) and the Second Sino-Japanese War (1937–1945) were also decisive, as they gave rise to important transnational humanitarian mobilisations

10　　　　　　　　　　　　*Introduction*

and the formation of new anti-fascist solidarity networks focusing on health, care and the provision of relief. They also had a significant impact on the ways in which humanitarian questions were framed. For example, it was during the Italo-Ethiopian War that humanitarian campaigners in Africa started replacing anti-slavery rhetoric by mobilising the issue of refugees and images of displaced Africans.[47] In this volume, Chapter 3 argues that this conflict marked the beginning of a new interest in Africa within the Red Cross Movement, even if the scope and nature of aid remained limited by the imperial and racial framework in which Red Cross actors were evolving at the time. Indeed, situated at the intersection between the imperial and the international realm, the Italo-Ethiopian War forced humanitarian actors to position themselves in regard to the violation of international laws, notably around the use of chemical warfare and the bombing of medical structures. They were caught in a political context, marked by fascist propaganda and racial discrimination, which impacted their actions in the subsequent years.[48] Crucially, there were international efforts at reckoning with war crimes committed in Ethiopia after 1945. Crimes committed in Ethiopia were fully part of the war crimes for which the Italians were supposed to be judged, even if this process did not succeed.[49] The Sino-Japanese War raised the issue of how combatants might ensure the protection of civilians in wartime with the perhaps illusory humanitarian proposition of guaranteed civilian sanctuaries.[50]

These conflicts functioned also as forerunners for further humanitarian engagements. The well-known ICRC delegate Marcel Junod started his career in Ethiopia, before going to Spain during the Spanish Civil War, travelling through different places in Europe between 1939 and 1945 and Hiroshima after the nuclear bomb.[51] Part of the medical personnel dispatched with the Norwegian Red Cross ambulance during the Italo-Ethiopian War, he took part in Norwegian humanitarian activities during the First Soviet-Finnish War (1939–1940) and then the Korean War (1950–1953).[52] In a more political vein, the Second Sino-Japanese War opened up new opportunities for Indian humanitarianism. Until 1937, Indian humanitarians abroad mainly aligned with the interests of the British Empire. Their work in the Sino-Japanese War led them to become more closely associated with global leftist solidarity networks, established during the Spanish Civil War. Indian humanitarian

*Introduction*                                                          11

initiatives in China became intrinsically linked with their broader nationalist claims for sovereignty from British colonial rule.[53] During this decade, humanitarian work was often shaped and transformed by prevailing political and ideological motivations which contested the liberal understanding of humanity underpinning humanitarian work. As the American sociologist of Czechoslovak origins Joseph Slabey Roucek put it in 1938:

> Today bolsheviks and fascists are laughing at humanitarianism. Most parts of the European Continent are proclaiming loudly that they have no respect for human life and its attributes. Every bourgeois, who dresses himself up in a coloured shirt gains thereby the right to speak with disgust about humanitarianism in the phrases of Nietzsche.[54]

While often indifferent to the politics and compromises of classical humanitarian politics or to the structural violence of humanitarianism in an international order dominated by colonial powers, humanitarians were timid when faced with vehement violence. In Ethiopia, while the ICRC was concerned about preserving neutrality and afraid of angering the Italian government, the ICRC delegate Sydney Brown was accused of taking a more radical political stance in favour of Ethiopians.[55] In the continuity of the Italo-Ethiopian War, the Spanish Civil War represented an important moment for further anti-fascist humanitarian engagement.[56] For example, in the segregated United States, the Afro-American nurse Salaria Kea O'Reilly led fundraising campaigns for Ethiopia in Harlem before 'having the chance' to directly help the Spanish Loyalist government by volunteering in Spain.[57] This experience gained in Spain, often shaped by transnational solidarities, was reinjected in other theatres of operation, such as in the Second Sino-Japanese War (1937–1945) or Yugoslavia partisan warfare.[58] In this book, the humanitarian actors studied in Chapter 7 engaged in an ideological struggle against fascism in Nazi-occupied France, redefining the boundaries of what constituted resistance to the occupiers. Carrying on humanitarian tasks that were neglected by the Vichy collaborationist regime was in itself a challenge to the state and a form of resistance, even before the action became illegal. Beyond that, Arrizabalaga and Martínez-Vidal show that the humanitarian responses to the Spanish Civil War on French soil were much more than a 'prelude' to those of the Second World War: they were a matrix for transnational solidarities involving American, French and Swiss organisations and volunteers, well beyond 1945.

12                         *Introduction*

Stretching the chronological boundaries of the Second World War until the beginning of the 1950s is thus methodologically productive to capture these transnational solidarities, shaped in the late 1930s and transformed throughout the 1940s. It also enables historians to place the upheavals of population movement at the centre of the historical analysis. The end of the military operations of the Second World War was followed by what Peter Gatrell has called the period of 'violent peacetime' and continuation of involuntary migration on a mass scale.[59] During the late 1940s, more people were displaced than at any other time in modern history. Outside of Europe, mass displacement was caused by state formation in the context of decolonisation and social revolution. In Europe, it was the result of population expulsions, state-sanctioned deportations and internecine warfare in Eastern and southeastern Europe.

This approach enables historians of humanitarianism to engage critically with the notion of 'sortie de guerre' [getting out of the war], a concept developed to better understand how wartime attitudes were gradually dismantled and how societies came to terms with the war.[60] Initially developed by historians of the First World War,[61] the concept of 'sortie de guerre' has now been used by historians of the Second World War, in part because it allows for a more nuanced understanding of the distinction between the wartime and post-war periods.[62] As Chapter 10 shows in this book, wartime had certainly not faded away in 1945 for those researching their dead ones. Relief continued long after the end of military operations: the aftermath is a time for redeployment and reorganisation of aid, often 'remobilising' military actors for 'humanitarian purposes'.[63] Further, this deployment of aid was planned well before the cessation of military operations, when the conflict was at its height. As Jessica Reinisch, Mark Mazower, and others have demonstrated, during the war itself, reconstruction and humanitarian aid were considered as an international problem, which required collaboration between state and non-state actors to avoid what were perceived as the 'errors' of Versailles. For a brief period, from 1942 to 1946–1947, US humanitarian workers even cooperated (not without issues) with Soviet and Chinese actors.[64]

The concept of 'sortie de guerre' also enables scholars to highlight continuities of experiences beyond the conclusion of hostilities and the diplomatic agreements that often define the end of warfare in the historical consciousness.[65] To some extent, caring for displaced

*Introduction* 13

persons and healing injured bodies and minds appears as a continuation of the war. Establishing precise and meaningful chronological boundaries is even more difficult when it comes to the individual consequences of the war: studying wartime humanitarianism from the perspective of those who provided and received care suggest that there are as many chronologies as individual experiences of the war.[66] Focusing on intimacies (Chapters 1 and 4) underlines how disruptive war was for those who survived, depriving them of their loved ones, turning their lives upside down, leaving them with lifelong scars – and in many cases inter-generational trauma. Chapter 9 recalls the long-lasting trauma of disfigured people, showing that injured soldiers and civilians had another fight to go through after the war. For dozens of millions of families, the aftermath was a period of mourning which was made even more unbearable by the disappearance of corpses in combat zones, bombed places, deportation camps and mass massacres. Anthropological approaches have profoundly renewed our understanding of the aftermath.[67] They shed light on the multiple implications of this massification of death, on a material, psychological and symbolic level, from the grieving families[68] to the national and international policies of corpses research, identification, repatriation and commemoration.[69]

Opting for a multiplicity of points of view and scales of analysis, as we have done in this volume, makes it even more difficult to define precise chronological boundaries. However, we argue that the turn of the 1940s to 1950s can be considered the end of a sequence in terms of medical and humanitarian practices, norms as well as geopolitical relations within humanitarian networks and organisations for different reasons. First, the beginning of the 1950s saw the progressive end of some of the displacement movement generated by the long Second World War. The refugee camp of El Shatt studied in Chapter 4 of this volume closed in 1947, whereas Chapter 7 demonstrates that the beginning of the 1950s marked the end of a cycle in the solidarity practices for Republican refugees in France, for example. Second, historians have shown how different organisations such as Care or World Vision turned their attention to other part of the world.[70] As Chapter 3 of the volume shows, the end of the repatriation process of the soldiers stationed in South Africa and Rhodesia opened up spaces for ICRC delegates to reflect on the Red Cross's role in Africa

14 *Introduction*

in the event of conflict between the white minority and the local population, and to question the racial boundaries that characterised Red Cross work on the continent at the time. Similar dynamics of internationalisation of colonial problems also took place in Asia.[71] Third, at the same time, the international community tried to draw lessons from the war by strengthening the international law apparatus with the elaboration of the Convention on the Prevention and Punishment of the Crime of Genocide in 1948, the Geneva Conventions in 1949 and the elaboration of a new refugee status with the Convention of 1951. While trying to end a particularly violent sequence, the drafters of these texts also tried to shape the future of warfare.[72] However, they rapidly proved not to be well suited for application to the Cold War and decolonisation conflicts. In the same vein, the UN scheme of collective security did not resist the crystallisation of the Cold War. The termination of the Korean War in 1953 represented the end of the first (and last) United Coalition and UN Peace enforcement operation and marked the apogee of Western domination over the UN institutions.[73]

## Towards a micro-global history of humanitarianism during the long Second World War

The first part of this book provides an examination of the links between imperial and national politics and aid networks,[74] showing that the war brought about unlikely aid coalitions and intimate networks of aid. It also led to a transformation of the relationships between some European organisations and colonial peripheries, leading to the emergence of new activities and actors. Chapters 1 to 4 contribute to this history by moving across scales of analysis, reconsidering the links between the global and the local, and rethinking the geographic and racial boundaries of humanitarianism. Chapter 1 explores how the notion of intimacy provides a new way of approaching the history of humanitarianism. Drawing on the example of medical care in the French Resistance, this chapter takes 'intimacy' to mean any form and instances of relatedness, which shape people's senses of selves, their feelings, their attachments and their identifications. After reflecting on how various strands of historical scholarship on 'intimacies' offer a potential complement to

*Introduction* 15

the literature on gender, affects and humanitarian care, it argues that the notion of intimacy provides a productive methodological approach to move across scales of analysis, from the global to the local, an opportunity to rethink the boundaries between the public and the private and a way to interrogate humanitarians' relations to the norms and the normative. This chapter demonstrates that to think about humanitarianism *intimately* means to go beyond a grassroot and biographical approach to the history of humanitarianism to consider archival materials that are not usually associated with emotions, affects or bodies, such as surgical protocols and hospital logs, and to attempt to make affective connections between the past and the present.

Chapter 2 examines the impact of the long Second World War on medical networks in French colonies, considering the tensions between medical power and violence, medical utopia and failures in the French Empire. It explores the various political uses of Black bodies, highlighting how these have been 'racialised' by white European doctors since the nineteenth century and assessing the extent to which the war led to a rupture in both their representations and treatments. To do so, this chapter draws on medical literature, mainly health services in the colonies, reports from colonial doctors, medical and anthropological monographs and directives issued by public authorities in mainland France. It unpacks various racial stereotypes and 'uses' of Black bodies during and after the war, and critically reviews various health projects implemented to ensure the 'survival' of African populations by colonial doctors. It argues that the long Second World War did not fundamentally alter racial boundaries in the French Empire, even though the lexicon to talk about race changed and despite the arrival of new international actors.

Chapter 3 highlights the specific role played by the long Second World War in the progressive inclusion of Africa and Africans within the scope of the Red Cross Movement. By putting in the same analytical framework the Italo-Ethiopian War and the Second World War, it suggests that the Red Cross Movement, which sat somewhere in between the colonial order (as exemplified by the colonial sections of national Red Cross societies) and the international order with its international actors – the League and the International Committee of the Red Cross (ICRC), was significantly transformed by the upheavals of this period on the continent.

16    *Introduction*

Crucially, it revisits the old question of the links between Red Cross activism and colonialism, shedding new light on race relations within the Movement during this period. To do so, the chapter first argues that the Italo-Ethiopian War was a key moment that led to the inclusion of the first 'Black' African national Red Cross Society within the Movement. Second, it shows that the long Second World War led to the first contacts between African soldiers and their families through the Red Cross apparatus, the Central Agency for the prisoners of war of the ICRC setting up a tracing service dedicated to the prisoners from French colonies. This Central Agency offered these prisoners the same kind of services as their European counterparts. Third, the division of the French Empire, and in particular the rupture created by the split between the Vichy regime and the Gaullist movement, as well as the presence of European prisoners of war on the continent fostered the creation of an embryonic Red Cross network in sub-Saharan Africa composed of ICRC delegates and Red Cross colonial branches. This evolution carried the seeds for a new, although limited, interest in the situation and the inclusion of Black African people within the Movement.

Moving beyond the perspective of European humanitarian organisations deploying aid to 'peripheries', Chapter 4 explores the boundaries of aid in El Shatt, a refugee camp established mainly for Europeans by the Allied powers on the Sinai Peninsula in 1944 and maintained until 1947. Moving across scales of analysis, from the global to the local, and drawing on similar methodologies to those in Chapter 1 it highlights the multiple segments of population providing aid to refugees in Egypt. It argues that El Shatt's main protagonists constituted several 'circles of intimacy', which were central to the organisation of both camp life and humanitarian aid. It pays close attention to the different relations that refugees developed both with Western humanitarian organisations and with local Egyptians, who provided food and groceries and guarded the camps. By highlighting the role of Egyptians in the camp which outlived the war years, this chapter makes an important contribution towards globalising the history of the long Second World War. It also forcefully reminds us that migration and flight not only occurred from the Middle East to Europe but also from Europe to the Middle East, inviting us to rethink humanitarian organisations' (mis)perceptions of and cooperation with host societies.

*Introduction* 17

The second part of this book rethinks the complex politics of humanitarianism during the conflict by examining the contribution of humanitarians and medical workers to the development of nation state and their 'imagined communities' and by reconsidering the links between partisan warfare and aid. Chapter 5 discusses how Chinese-style physicians, at various levels and through different means, contributed to humanitarian work during the Second Sino-Japanese War, focusing on the province of Sichuan. After 1938, when the Chinese government retreated to Chongqing, the main commercial city of the province, Sichuan became the centre of free China until 1945, breaking almost two decades of instability and isolationism. The establishment of the national government in Chongqing meant the reunification of the province, the reaffirmation of the civil administration previously overshadowed by military apparatus and, more specifically, a renewed attention to health and medical questions. Participating in wartime medical relief was a way for Chinese physicians to present themselves as participants in the strengthening of the Chinese nation. Rescuing the injured or fighting epidemics – and not leaving these tasks to Western medicine alone – contributed to increasing their legitimacy in the eyes of the state and the public. It was also a function of the professionalisation of Chinese medicine, the development of a collective professional ethic of service to the people, moving away from – although integrating parts of – the discourse of charity that had prevailed until then.

Chapter 6 considers humanitarianism as a diplomatic tool during the war between Peru and Ecuador in 1941 to 1942. The peculiarity of this South American war lies in its interlocking nature in the world conflict. At its heart was a conflict for vast territories located from the Pacific coast to the heart of the Amazonian forest, which started at the beginning of the nineteenth century. The outbreak of war in July 1941 while the war was raging in Asia and Europe represented an attempt to finally settle the issue at the most opportune moment. The chapter explores why the treatment of the wounded became a matter of public concern and an important political issue. It compares how the Peruvian and Ecuadorian medical services were politicised during the war and considers how far medical aid was used to promote the status of both states in international affairs. It raises fascinating questions about the specificities

18                     *Introduction*

of Latin American humanitarian rhetoric and the crucial role of humanitarian issues in delegitimising the adversary and attracting new and powerful sympathies.

While Chapter 6 examines how small states mobilised humanitarian actors and issues as instruments of soft-power, Chapter 7 considers how transnational humanitarian actors confronted new political regimes in the 1940s in a war opposing liberal democracies, fascism and (later on) communism. Chapter 7 pays particular attention to the entanglements between humanitarian aid, the collaboration with the Resistance against fascism and Nazism, and the medical relief work with Spanish Republican refugees. Focusing more particularly on two major medical care institutions set up by the Unitarian Service Committee (USC) in France – the Marseille Clinic and the Varsovie Hospital in Toulouse – it examines the activities, actors and intervention spaces of this Committee. During the war, the frontier between the medical relief activities of the USC with European refugees fleeing from fascism, including Spanish Republican exiles, and its support to those refugees who choose to stand up to the aggressors became more and more blurred. At the end of the Second World War, the mutual political loyalties among those so far allied in the fight against the fascist Axis dramatically split between two irreconcilable blocs according to the logics of the Cold War, with important repercussions for the provision of aid for refugees in France and its long-term divide according to ideology. What this chapter shows, however, is how expertise could cross this divide and circulate more widely.

The third part of this book explores the transnational circulations of knowledge, such as maxillofacial surgical expertise and forensic intervention, between the military and civilians across conflicts and between wartime and peacetime (Chapters 8, 9, 10). It questions the role that humanitarians and medical workers played in the fabrication and transformation of normative discourses about the reconstruction of bodies and minds in the aftermath of war from different perspectives. It also traces the specific role of humanitarians in recovering dead bodies, making funeral services for former enemies possible and bringing a sense of closure. All together, these chapters show well how humanitarians and medical specialists could play a role in complex emotional processes affecting families and communities as they transitioned to peacetime.

*Introduction*                                    19

While much of the literature has focused on military and state control of bodies, particularly in the context of the mobilisation of war, very little yet has been written on how humanitarians could imprint a distinct regulatory framework on bodies which could draw on their own aspirations.

Through an examination of the production and exhibition of the Museum of Modern Art's War Veteran's Art Center, Chapter 8 explores the links between military and civilian cultures of rehabilitation in the United States. Since the nineteenth century, humanitarian actors have encouraged the production of handicrafts by wounded soldiers for the purposes of fundraising, overcoming mental strains, 're-masculinising' war victims or fostering national traditions. Chapter 8 demonstrates how American cultural actors, including museum curators and art specialists, understood the role of art in processes of healing and transitioning from war to peace. It argues that craft therapy programmes contributed to the fabrication of normative discourses centred around the white, capable and ableist men that largely fitted in with dominant conceptions of idealised white masculinity in the United States, 'normalising the image of the veteran as white'. In so doing, this chapter makes two important contributions to this book: first, it highlights the ways in which arts were used to 're-masculinise' and 'recuperate' wounded men in the aftermath of war; second, it invites us to take into consideration the role of non-traditional humanitarian and medical actors in the construction of norms about the able, fit and 'recuperable' bodies and minds, while remaining attentive to the ways in which art could also serve as a mode of agency and soft resistance for ex-soldiers.

If the war proved a turning point in terms of codification of medical ethics following the Nuremberg medical trials, it was also a stage of rethinking medical categories along ableist and optimistic lines. When the newly reinvented World Health Organization defined what being healthy might mean in its 1948 founding declaration, it described it as 'a state of complete physical, mental and social well-being and not merely the absence of disease or infirmity'. As Lars Thorup Larsen shows, the definition's genealogy was complex and drew from a League of Nations precedent drafted by Raymond Gautier, probably drawing inspiration from Henry E. Sigerist's view of Soviet medical approaches, not to mention possible Chinese inputs.[75] This definition, drawing from social

20 *Introduction*

medicine, recast care in wartime among the many social projects centred on citizenship and rights on the one hand, but also on the extraordinary internationalisation of practices and ideas which the tumult of wartime facilitated. Chapter 9 demonstrates how surgical knowledge travelled through the United States and the USSR to China, until it was ultimately reinvested to care for combatants of the Korean War. The competitive draw of expertise reflects the symbolic significance of some particular war injuries treatable only by multidisciplinary teams of experts through maxillofacial services and how training and funding could flow between countries at war. Drawing on the account of surgical teams sent to assist North Korea during the Korean War (1950–1953), Chapter 9 argues that the conflict played a pivotal role in establishing maxillofacial surgery as a formal medical specialty in the early People's Republic of China. Looking at the perspectives of both surgeons and injured men, it demonstrates how maxillofacial surgery mattered to men's reconstruction of their facial structure and later their affective experience and social identity, which was crucial to their reintegration in the newly established socialist society.

Drawing on a close reading of the ICRC's role in exploring the treatment of corpses in France in the years following 1944, Chapter 10 shows how humanitarians could take on roles which would normally fall within the remits of sovereign states in their duty of care for their fallen soldiers. In the absence of a German political entity able and willing to engage with the missing bodies of the fallen, the ICRC took on a role galvanising states to address their international commitments and people to transcend their war grievances. This was not an easy task. According to the international law in force at the time, the management of the bodies of fallen soldiers or prisoners of war was the responsibility of the state that had control of the ground. But as French authorities were slow and reluctant to address this issue, the ICRC took over this matter and acted as a 'substitute' for a negligent state. Drawing mainly on the archives of the ICRC, this chapter examines the work of the mission headed by Paul Thomas, the ICRC delegate in charge of locating the German soldiers buried in France, considering the material difficulties posed by the identification of corpses. It also considers the inconsistencies between French national priorities and the practices of a humanitarian organisation which claimed to adopt a neutral approach. Providing adequate funeral services to former

*Introduction* 21

enemies was a highly politically sensitive issue in the aftermath of the Nazi occupation of France.

It is clear that we need more comparative work to understand why medical elites across the world devoted so much effort into preserving categories of the 'other' and to what extent the war, as both a global conflict and a series of local disputes, destabilised these racial boundaries. We also still know little about the political consequences of close bodily encounters in hospitals and how far colonial intimate encounters might have fuelled anti-colonial dynamics. The history of humanitarian aid in certain regions, such as Latin America, still remains under-researched, while the research devoted to Muslim aid networks lags behind the new research on Christian, Jewish and Protestant relief during this period. Yet, collectively, by moving across scales of analysis and going beyond the traditional chronology of the war, these chapters offer new insights into old historiographical questions about the modernisation and Americanisation of aid as well as the links between colonialism and humanitarianism, and the circulation of medical knowledge and humanitarian practices. They also address new themes, such as intimacies, the role of humanitarians in the search for dead bodies and the issue of humanitarian aesthetics. Crucially, they open avenues for future research.

## Acknowledgements

This book originated in a seminar series organised at the University of Manchester in 2021 to 2022 and funded by the Arts and Humanities Research Council, grant reference: AH/T006382/1. The authors would like to thank colleagues who participated in these seminar series. They would also like to thank Andrew Buchanan, Ruth Lawlor and Davide Rodogno for providing feedback on a draft of this introduction.

## Notes

1 Hertha Kraus, *American Friends Service Committee, Brethren Service Committee and Mennonite Central Committee* (Philadelphia, PA: Brethren Service Committee and Mennonite Central Committee,

1944); Hertha Kraus, *International Relief in Action, 1914–1943: Selected Records, with Notes* (Scottdale: Herald Press, 1944); Hertha Kraus, 'Are we Ready?', *The Family*, 24:1 (1943), 16–21.

2 Hertha Kraus, 'Identifying Professional Requirements for Social Service Abroad', *Social Casework*, 35:4 (1954), 147–154, at p. 147.

3 In the historiography: Elizabeth Borgwardt, *A New Deal for the World: America's Vision for Human Rights* (Cambridge, MA: Harvard University Press, 2007); Silvia Salvatici, ' "Help the People to Help Themselves": UNRRA Relief Workers and European Displaced Persons', *Journal of Refugee Studies*, 25:3 (2012), 428–451; Jessica Reinisch, 'Internationalism in Relief: The Birth (and Death) of UNRRA', *Past and Present*, 210:6 (2011), 258–289; Jessica Reinisch, 'Auntie UNRRA at the Crossroads', *Past and Present*, Supplement 8 (2013), 70–97; Mark Mazower, Jessica Reinisch and David Feldman (eds), 'Post-War Reconstruction in Europe: International Perspectives, 1945–1949', *Past and Present*, Supplement 6 (2011); Davide Rodogno, *Night on Earth: A History of International Humanitarianism in the Near East, 1918–1930* (Cambridge: Cambridge University Press, 2021).

4 Davide Rodogno, Bernhard Struck and Jakob Vogel (eds), *Shaping the Transnational Sphere: Experts, Networks, Issues, 1850–1930* (New York: Berghahn, 2015), pp. 5–6.

5 Kraus thus resumed in 1951 work abandoned in 1932 in Germany. Roland Brake and Kerstin Faßbender, 'History and Development of Community Development in Germany', in Roland Brake and Ulrich Deller (eds), *Community Development: A European Challenge* (Obladen: Barbara Budrich, 2008), pp. 41–52, at p. 42.

6 Silvia Salvatici, *A History of Humanitarianism, 1755–1989: In the Name of Others* (Manchester: Manchester University Press, 2019), pp. 80–81.

7 Marcel Eyidi Bebey, 'Le vainqueur de la maladie du sommeil: Le Docteur Eugène Jamot' (PhD dissertation, Université de Paris, 1951); Enoh Meyomesse, *Marcel Eyidi Bebey: Un homme politique comme il n'en existe plus* (Paris: edkbooks, 2019).

8 Guillaume Lachenal, 'Célébrer le passé, construire le futur: l'indépendance et le microcosme médical au Cameroun', in Odile Georg, Jean-Luc Martineau and Didier Nativel (eds), *Les indépendances en Afrique* (Rennes: Presses universitaires de Rennes, 2013), pp. 353–376.

9 Jean-Paul Zuniga, 'L'histoire impériale à l'heure de l'histoire globale. Une perspective atlantique', *Revue d'histoire moderne et contemporaine* (2007), pp. 54–68, at p. 68.

10 Romain Bertrand and Guillaume Calafat, 'La micro-histoire globale: une affaire à suivre', *Annales. Histoire, Sciences Sociales*, 73:1 (2018),

Introduction                    23

3–17; John-Paul A. Ghobrial, 'Introduction: Seeing the World like a Microhistorian', *Past & Present*, 242, Supplement 14 (2019), 1–22.

11  Michael Barnett, *Empire of Humanity: A History of Humanitarianism* (Ithaca, NY: Cornell University Press, 2011). For the shift from 'amateurism' to 'professionalism', see, for instance, Bruno Cabanes, *The Great War and the Origins of Humanitarianism* (Cambridge: Cambridge University Press, 2014); Bertrand Taithe 'The "Making" of the Origins of Humanitarianism?', *Contemporanea*, 3 (2015), 489–496.

12  Olivier Wieviorka, *Histoire Totale de la Seconde Guerre mondiale* (Paris: Perrin, 2023), introduction.

13  Patricia Clavin, 'Defining Transnationalism', *Contemporary European History*, 14:4 (2005), 421–439; Pierre-Yves Saunier, *Transnational History* (Basingstoke: Palgrave Macmillan, 2013).

14  Clavin, 'Defining Transnationalism', p. 428.

15  Sebastian Conrad, *What is Global History?* (Princeton, NJ: Princeton University Press, 2016); Richard Drayton and David Motadel, 'Discussion: The Futures of Global History', *Journal of Global History*, 13:1 (2018), 1–21.

16  Andrew Buchanan, 'Viewpoint: Globalizing the Second World War', *Past and Present*, 258:1 (2023), 246–281, at p. 249.

17  See, for example, John Ferris and Evan Mawdsley (eds), *The Cambridge History of the Second World War, Volume I: Fighting the War* (Cambridge: Cambridge University Press, 2025); Jean-Francois Muracciole and Guillaume Piketty (eds), *Encyclopédie de la Seconde Guerre Mondiale* (Paris: Gallimard, 2015); Alya Aglan and Robert Franck (eds), *1937–1947: La guerre-monde* (Paris: Gallimard, 2015); Andrew N. Buchanan, *World War II in Global Perspective, 1931–1953: A Short History* (Newark, NJ: Wiley Blackwell, 2019).

18  Patricia Clavin, 'International Organizations', in Richard Bosworth and Joseph Maiolo (eds), *The Cambridge History of the Second World War, Volume II: Politics and Ideology* (Cambridge: Cambridge University Press, 2015), pp. 139–161.

19  Aglan and Franck, *1937–1947*.

20  Buchanan, *World War II in Global Perspective*.

21  Andrew Buchanan, 'Globalizing the Second World War', *Past and Present*, 258:1 (2023), 246–281, at p. 246.

22  Sharif Gemie, Fiona Reid, Laure Humbert with Louise Ingram, *Outcast Europe: Refugees and Relief Workers in an Era of Total War 1936–1948* (London: Bloomsbury, 2011).

23  Enzo Traverso, *1914–1945. La guerre civile européenne* (Paris: Hachette, 2009).

24 *Introduction*

24 Julie Le Gac and Nicolas Patin, *Guerres mondiales. Le désastre et le deuil* (Paris: Armand Colin, 2022).

25 Richard Overy, *Blood and Ruins: The Great Imperial War, 1931–1945* (London: Penguin, 2021), p. xi.

26 André Loez (ed.), *Mondes en guerre. Tome III: Guerres mondiales et impériales, 1870–1945* (Paris : Passés Composés/Ministère des Armées, 2020); Overy, *Blood and Ruins*.

27 Mark Mazower, *The Dark Continent: Europe's Twentieth Century* (London: Allen Lane: The Penguin Press, 1998), 'Epilogue: Making Europe'; Ian Kershaw, *To Hell and Back: Europe, 1914–1949* (New York: Vikings, 2015).

28 On the co-existence of these visions, see Jessica Reinisch, 'We Shall Rebuild Anew a Powerful Nation': UNRRA, Internationalism and National Reconstruction in Poland', *Journal of Contemporary History*, 43:3 (2008), 451–476; Reinisch, 'Auntie UNRRA at the Crossroads'.

29 Kevin O'Sullivan, Matthew Hilton and Juliano Fiori, 'Humanitarianisms in Context', *European Review of History*, 23, 1–2 (2016), 1–15, at p. 6.

30 Enrico Dal Lago and Kevin O'Sullivan, 'Introduction: Towards a New History of Humanitarianism', *Moving the Social*, 57 (2017), 5–20, at p. 13; Reinisch, 'Internationalism in Relief'.

31 Dal Lago and O'Sullivan, 'Introduction'.

32 Barnett, *Empire of Humanity*, p. 104.

33 Tehila Sasson, 'From Empire to Humanity: The Russian Famine and the Imperial Origins of International Humanitarianism', *Journal of British Studies*, 55 (2016), 519–537.

34 Johannes Paulmann, 'Conjunctures in the History of International Humanitarian Aid during the Twentieth Century', *Humanity: An International Journal of Human Rights, Humanitarianism and Development*, 4:2 (2013), 215–238, at p. 226.

35 Sébastien Farré, *Colis de guerre* (Rennes: Presses universitaires de Rennes, 2014).

36 Salvatici, *A History of Humanitarianism*, p. 82.

37 Salvatici, *A History of Humanitarianism*, p. 83. On the role of women during this period, see also Elisabeth Piller, 'Beyond Hoover: Rewriting the History of the Commission for Relief in Belgium (CRB) through Female Involvement', *The International History Review*, 1:45 (2023), 202–224; Jo Laycock and Francesca Piana (eds), *Aid to Armenia: Relief, Humanitarianism and Intervention from the 1890s to the Present* (Manchester: Manchester University Press, 2020); Esther Möller, Johannes Paulmann and Katarina Stornig (eds), *Gendering Global*

*Introduction* 25

*Humanitarianism in the Twentieth Century: Practice, Politics and the Power of Representation* (London: Palgrave Macmillan, 2020).

38 Marie Levant, Laura Pettinaroli and Oliver Sibre 'Bilan historiographique et pistes de recherche à l'heure de l'ouverture des archives Pie XII', *Monde(s)*, 2:22 (2022), 7–33; Nina Valbousquet, 'L'ouverture des archives du Vatican pour le pontificat de Pie XII (1939–1958): controverses mémorielles, apports historiographiques et usages de l'archive', *Revue d'Histoire Moderne et Contemporaine*, 69:1 (2022), 56–70; Nina Valbousquet, 'Le Vatican, l'Église catholique et la Shoah. Renouveau historiographique autour des archives Pie XII', *Revue d'Histoire de la Shoah*, 218 (2023); Bertrand Taithe, 'The Politics of Catholic Humanitarian Aid: Missionaries and American Relief in Algeria 1942–1947', *French History*, 37:2 (2023), 160–176.

39 Matthieu Brejon de Lavergnée, 'Charité sans frontières: Les religieuses, les soins et l'aide humanitaire (1850–1920)', *Le mouvement social*, 1 (2023), 35–60; Paul Droulers, 'L'action populaire et les semaines sociales de France, 1919–1939', *Revue d'histoire de l'Église de France* 67 :179 (1981), 227–252. For example, Sœur Marie-André du Sacré-Cœur, *La Femme Noire en Afrique Occidentale* (Paris: Payot, 1939).

40 See, for example, Célia Keren, 'Quand la CGT faisait de l'humanitaire: l'accueil des enfants d'Espagne (1936–1939)', *Le mouvement social*, 264:3 (2018), 15–39; de Lavargnee, 'Charité sans frontières'.

41 We draw here on the rich literature on the history of intimate care, including Anna Carden-Coyne, *The Politics of Wounds: Military Patients and Medical Power in the First World War* (Oxford: Oxford University Press, 2014); Jane Brooks, *Negotiating Nursing British Army Sisters and Soldiers in the Second World War* (Manchester: Manchester University Press, 2018).

42 Julia Irwin, *Catastrophic Diplomacy: US Foreign Disaster Assistance in the American Century* (Chapel Hill, NC: University of North Carolina Press, 2023); see also 'Hegemonic Humanitarian Aid? Rethinking American Humanitarianism', seminar series, https://colonialandtransnationalintimacies.com/2022/03/14/hegemonic-humanitarian-aid-rethinking-american-humanitarianism/ (accessed 20 October 2023).

43 On humanitarianism as a tool of diplomacy, see for instance Matthew Hilton, Emily Baughan, Eleonor Davey, Bronwen Everill, Kevin O'Sullivan and Tehila Sasson, 'History and Humanitarianism: A Conversation', *Past and Present* 241:1 (2018), 1–38; Elisabeth Piller, *Selling Weimar: German Public Diplomacy and the United States,*

26 *Introduction*

*1918–1933* (Stuttgart: Franz Steiner Verlag, 2021); Laure Humbert, *Reinventing French Aid: The Politics of Humanitarian Relief in French-Occupied Germany, 1945–1952* (Cambridge: Cambridge University Press, 2021).

44 Buchanan, *World War II in Global Perspective*.

45 Alexandra Pfeiff, 'Two Adoptions of the Red Cross: The Chinese Red Cross and the Red Swastika Society from 1904 to 1949' (PhD dissertation, European University Institute, 2018), pp. 18–19; Jiang Sun, 'The Predicament of a Redemptive Religion: The Red Swastika Society Under the Rule of Manchukuo', *Journal of Modern Chinese History*, 7:1 (2013), 108–126.

46 Pfeiff, 'Two Adoptions of the Red Cross', p. 130.

47 Bronwen Everill, 'The Italo-Abyssinian Crisis and the Shift from Slave to Refugee', *Slavery & Abolition*, 35:2 (2014), 349–365; Brett L. Shadle, 'Reluctant Humanitarians: British Policy Toward Refugees in Kenya during the Italo-Ethiopian War, 1935–1940', *The Journal of Imperial and Commonwealth History*, 47:1 (2019), 167–186.

48 Rainer Baudendistel, *Between Bombs and Good Intentions: The Red Cross and the Italo-Ethiopian 1935–1936* (New York: Berghahn Books, 2006); Nicola Perugini and Neve Gordon, 'Between Sovereignty and Race: The Bombardment of Hospitals in the Italo-Ethiopian War and the Colonial Imprint of International Law', *State Crime Journal*, 8:1 (2019), 104–125.

49 Perugini and Gordon, 'Between Sovereignty and Race', p. 119; Filippo Focardi, 'Criminels impunis. L'absence d'un "Nuremberg italien"', in Jean-Marc Berlière, Jonas Campion, Luigi Lacchè and Xavier Rousseaux (eds), *Justices militaires et guerres mondiales* (Louvain: Presses universitaires de Louvain), pp. 363–379.

50 Marcia R. Ristaino, *The Jacquinot Safe Zone: Wartime Refugees in Shanghai* (Stanford, CA: Stanford University Press, 2008).

51 Marcel Junod, *Warrior without Weapons* (Geneva: ICRC, 1982).

52 Ian-Thore Lockersten, seminar series, https://colonialandtransnation alintimacies.com/2022/09/10/non-un-end-to-the-war-humanitarian-aid-in-the-age-of-the-united-nations/ (accessed 20 October 2023).

53 Maria Framke, ' "We Must Send a Gift Worthy of India and the Congress!" War and Political Humanitarianism in Late Colonial South Asia', *Modern Asian Studies*, 51:6 (2017), 1969–1998.

54 Joseph Slabey Roucek, 'The Rattling Bones of Europe', *International Social Science Review*, 13:1 (1938), 45–51, 47.

55 Baudenstitel, *Between Bombs and Good Intentions*.

# Introduction 27

56 On humanitarianism during the Spanish Civil War, see Célia Keren, 'Préserver la nation en exil. Les enfants espagnols évacués en France pendant la guerre d'Espagne', *20 & 21. Revue d'histoire*, 154 (2022), 45–60; Sébastien Farré, *L'affaire Henny* (Geneva: Georg, 2022); Keren, 'Quand la CGT faisait de l'humanitaire'.

57 Dolorès Martín-Moruno, 'Salaria Kea's Memories from the Spanish Civil War', International Conference, Warriors without Weapons: Humanitarian Action during the Spanish Civil War and the Republican Exile (Geneva: The Louis Jeantet Auditorium Foundation, 2016). See also: Dolorès Martín-Moruno, *Beyond Compassion: Gender and Humanitarian Action* (Cambridge: Cambridge University Press, 2023), pp. 28–32.

58 Ljubica Spaskovska, 'From the Battlefields of Spain to the Balkans – the Yugoslav Partisan Medical Service and its Legacies', *Le Mouvement social*, 288:3 (2024), 17–34; Framke, 'We Must Send a Gift'.

59 Peter Gatrell, 'Trajectories of Population Displacement in the Aftermaths of Two World Wars', in Jessica Reinisch and Elizabeth White (eds), *The Disentanglement of Populations: Migration, Expulsion and Displacement in Postwar Europe, 1944–1949* (London: Palgrave Macmillan, 2011), pp. 3–26; Peter Gatrell, *The Unsettling of Europe: The Great Migration, 1945 to the Present* (London: Allen Lane, 2019).

60 Henry Rousso, 'Sorties de guerre: Introduction', in Bruno Cabanes (ed.), *Une histoire de la guerre du 19ᵉ siècle à nos jours* (Paris: Seuil, 2018), pp. 621–630.

61 Stéphane Audoin-Rouzeau and Christophe Prochasson (eds), *Sortir de la Grande Guerre. Le monde et l'après 1918* (Paris: Tallandier, 2008); Bruno Cabanes, *La victoire endeuillée. La sortie de guerre des soldats français (1918–1920)* (Paris: Seuil, 2004); John Horne, 'Démobilisations culturelles après la Grande Guerre', in *14–18, Aujourd'hui, Today, Heute* (Paris: Éditions Noésis, 2002), pp. 45–53.

62 Bruno Cabanes and Guillaume Piketty, 'Sortir de la guerre: jalons pour une histoire en chantier', *Histoire@Politique*, 3:3 (2007).

63 Cabanes, *The Great War*; Silvia Salvatici, '"Fighters without Guns": Humanitarianism and Military Action in the Aftermath of the Second World War', *European Review of History*, 25:6 (2018), 957–976.

64 Reinisch, 'Internationalism in Relief'; Silvia Salvatici, "'Help the People to Help Themselves'"; Rana Mitter, 'Imperialism, Transnationalism, and the Reconstruction of Post-War China: UNRRA in China, 1944–7', *Past & Present*, 218, Supplement 8 (2013), 51–69.

28  *Introduction*

65 Ruth Lawlor and Andrew Buchanan, 'Hopes Foreclosed and a World Remade: The Long Endings of World War II', text presented at the University of Manchester in May 2023.

66 In that respect, this book is pursuing the discussions raised by the seminar series it proceeds from, adjusting this general timeframe from one chapter to another. https://colonialandtransnation alintimacies.com/

67 For a summary, see Annette Becker, 'Le temps du deuil', in Cabanes (ed.), *Une histoire de la guerre*, pp. 692–701.

68 Stéphane Audoin-Rouzeau, 'Corps perdus, corps retrouvés: Trois exemples de deuils de guerre', *in Annales. Histoire, Sciences Sociales*, 55:1 (2000), 47–71. https://doi.org/10.3406/ahess.2000.27983

69 Élisabeth Anstett, 'Des cadavres en masse', *Techniques & Culture*, 60 (2013), https://doi.org/10.4000/tc.6909; Élisabeth Anstett and Jean-Marc Dreyfus (eds), *Human Remains and Mass Violence: Methodological Approaches* (Manchester: Manchester University Press, 2015); Luc Capdevila and Danièle Voldman, *Nos morts. Les sociétés occidentales face aux tués de la guerre* (Paris: Payot, 2002); Luc Capdevila and Danièle Voldman, 'Rituels funéraires de sociétés en guerre (1914–1945)', in Stéphane Audoin-Rouzeau, Annette Becker, Christian Ingrao and Henry Rousso (eds), *La Violence de guerre 1914–1945* (Paris: Complexe, 2002), pp. 289–312; Jean-Marc Dreyfus, 'Remettre les corps en place à la Libération: exhumations, identifications et transferts après 1944', *Guerres mondiales et conflits contemporains*, 185:1 (2022), 129–147.

70 Sébastien Farré, 'De l'économie de guerre au secours philanthropique: care et les enjeux de l'aide américaine dans l'Europe de l'après-guerre', *Relations internationales*, 146:2 (2011), 25–41; Heike Wieters, *Showered with Kindness? The NGO CARE, and Food Aid from America, 1945–1980* (Manchester: Manchester University Press, 2017); Barnett, *Empire of Humanity*, pp. 132–160.

71 Boyd van Dijk, 'Internationalizing Colonial War: On the Unintended Consequences of the Interventions of the International Committee of the Red Cross in South-East Asia, 1945–1949', *Past & Present*, 250:1 (2021), 243–283.

72 Boyd van Dijk, *Preparing for War: The Making of the Geneva Conventions* (Oxford: Oxford University Press, 2022). Timothy L. Schroer, 'The Emergence and Early Demise of Codified Racial Segregation of Prisoners of War under the Geneva Conventions of 1929 and 1949', *Journal of the History of International Law*, 15 (2013), 53–75.

# Introduction 29

73 Seminar series: https://colonialandtransnationalintimacies.com/2022/09/10/non-un-end-to-the-war-humanitarian-aid-in-the-age-of-the-united-nations/ (accessed 20 October 2023).

74 Emily Baughan, *Saving the Children: Humanitarianism, Internationalism, and Empire* (Oakland, CA: University of California Press, 2021).

75 Lars Thorup Larsen, 'Not Merely the Absence of Disease: A Genealogy of the WHO's Positive Health Definition', *History of the Human Sciences*, 35:1 (2022), 111–131.

# 1

# Humanitarianism, estrangement and intimacies during the long Second World War: new historiographical perspectives

*Laure Humbert*

In the early spring of 1942, in the military camp of Bir Hakeim situated in the Libyan desert, a small group of British conscientious objectors (COs) assisted Free French medical officers as medical orderlies.[1] As pacifists, the roots of their humanitarian commitments could not be more different from that of the Free French doctors, with whom they shared the difficulties of tending to the wounded, from bandaging wounds to cleanings tents amid sandstorms. While British COs publicly committed themselves not to take up arms to defend their country against totalitarian violence, Free French doctors rejected the defeat and capitulation of France to the Nazi occupiers. Despite their opposite stands, both groups stood up for what they believed in, sometimes against the societies from which they came, often at great personal costs. In an international mobile hospital (the Hadfield-Spears Unit), close physical and affective bonds developed between them, and more broadly the 'remarkable variety of races, colours and creeds which passed through the hospital'.[2] According to the British volunteer Michael Rowntree, medical care elicited important new physical and *intimate* relations between individuals of diverse ethnic, national, class, religious and professional backgrounds. '[D]ifferences of language were forgotten, and both English and French developed a common tongue, known as "Spears", in which English, French and occasionally Arabic words were mingled in a polyglot riot'.[3] Intimate contact brought the members of this medical community together, but also occasionally tore them apart. The British volunteer Nik

*Estrangement and intimacies: new perspectives*     31

Alderson compared British COs' relations to French officers to 'various types of bridges', 'with one of a footbridge, that you skipped merrily across, with another the Albert Bridge, used always for a slow and ponderous traffic, and with another Tower Bridge – closed altogether at certain hours of the day'.[4] These questions of intimate bonds and estrangements, of how humanitarians crossed certain bridges but not others, and how they constituted themselves as communities are central themes in this chapter. Like many other humanitarians, COs and French medical resisters were not only people moved by high principles (such as opposition to war and resisting Nazi occupiers), but also individuals that *felt* their way to humanitarian convictions through intimate ties, which shaped in turn transnational medical and humanitarian cooperation.[5]

In this chapter, I consider how the notion of intimacy provides a new way of approaching the history of humanitarianism during the long Second World War. I take 'intimacy' to mean 'any form and instances of relatedness', which shape 'people's senses of selves, their feelings, their attachments, and their identifications'.[6] After reflecting on how various strands of historical scholarship on 'intimacies' offer a potential complement to the literature on gender, affects and humanitarian care, I argue that the notion of intimacy provides a productive methodological approach to move across scales of analysis, from the global to the local, an opportunity to rethink the boundaries between the public and the private and a way to enter medical and humanitarian spaces and interrogate people's relations to the norms and normative.[7] It enables historians to consider how prevailing norms about humanitarian duties, moral behaviours, acceptable and unacceptable forms of physical and emotional proximity with 'distant others' were produced in specific spaces but, fundamentally, how they were transgressed. A focus on intimacies also allows us to depart from studies that primarily focus on elite women and men to consider the lived experiences of medical workers and humanitarians more on the historical margins, who have left fewer traces in the archival records, and to capture the complexity of their identities, perspectives and desires.

This chapter demonstrates that to think about humanitarianism *intimately* means to go beyond a grassroots and biographical approach to the history of humanitarianism and to consider archival materials that are not usually associated with emotions, affects or

32    *The long Second World War, 1931–1953*

bodies. As Saidiya Hartman demonstrates, writing 'intimate histories' implies making affective connections between the past and the present, which can be facilitated by writing in a style of close narration and using critical fabulation.[8] At the heart of this approach is the question of how we can access people's most intimate thoughts, behaviours and relationships, and how we deal with what was left unsaid and unwritten. According to Bruno Cabanes and Guillaume Piketty, the intimate is 'the space in which one's self-image and deep relationship with others are formed, through the body, bodily techniques (gestures, know-how), filiation (real or imaginary), homes, objects invested with memories, representations of the self (including private writings)'.[9] If we take the example of French medical doctors, there is a deep sense that runs through the historiography that the *intimate* lives of resisters is an aspect of the history of resistance that historians cannot (and should not) touch. This is particularly the case for those medical workers who joined the resistance within occupied France, whose experiences were radically different from those outside France and whose life in clandestinity was entirely dependent on secrecy. As Laurent Douzou puts it, many resisters believed that 'the resistance was a clandestine and elusive adventure "intimately known" only by its members'.[10] According to him, many resisters did not speak about their feelings and kept to themselves 'what belonged to a kind of intimacy'.[11] What is more, some groups, such as the medical auxiliaries of French colonies within the international hospital mentioned above, have left very little traces behind. The intimate is hard to define, and perhaps even harder to get at, as historians can only access traces of what was expressed about intimate thoughts, actions or relations.[12] As Clémentine Vidal-Naquet observes, whether used to describe a close friend, a conviction or a part of the body, *something intimate* was that which was hidden from the world, revealed in private to a chosen few.[13]

Drawing on the example of medical care in the French Resistance, this chapter interrogates how intimate relations within medical and humanitarian spaces transformed individual and collective group identities. Even though medical workers and patients working for the French Resistance formed a very small and fringe group in the 'global' Second World War, medical spaces of the French Resistance provide a paradigmatic case to study the ways in which contests over political authority among French and Allied military

*Estrangement and intimacies: new perspectives*     33

elites took place at the level of individual bodies. On the one hand, French resisters were considered as 'pariahs' on the international stage and were highly dependent on their British allies and colonies for resources and legitimacy. On the other hand, even among the French, they were regarded as a small intransigent tiny minority, whose histories remain to some extent 'perilous' to write due to a widely shared belief that only those who participated in the movement were suitably qualified to write about it.[14] These challenges are further compounded by the fact that these medical workers had radically different experiences of war, depending on whether they working for the liberation of France from within or abroad. Within occupied France, medical workers had to hide and adopt different identities to survive. As the former female resister Elisabeth Terrenoire observed, clandestine life imposed the most absolute discretion, transforming what could be said to closest ones (such as husbands, wives and trusted friends) and exposing them to constant fears and worries.[15] Those who joined the Free French movement did not face the same risk of repression and deportation, but they confronted a life in exile, often marked by a long separation from their family (often also threatened by the Nazi occupiers). Despite these difficulties, this chapter draws on Tobias Kelly's view that 'the ethical and social tensions of society are often played out most intensely through lives lived on the edges, and it is through such people that otherwise taken for granted assumptions are refracted and come to the surface'.[16] Using the history of transnational medical care in the Resistance as a case study, the chapter thus reflects on some of the promises and core difficulties in foregrounding 'intimacies' in histories of transnational medical care and humanitarianism and draws together diverse historiographical perspectives that point towards new directions of future research in the field.

## The challenges of definition

While the rise of global history has birthed a renewed interest in the intimate, few historians of humanitarianism have deployed this notion as a category of analysis, despite a flourishing interest in gendering the history of global humanitarianism and the growing use of feminist epistemology to deconstruct gender discourses and

34 *The long Second World War, 1931–1953*

stereotypes.[17] In existing historiography, notions of intimacy have for a long time revolved around familial, sexual and romantic relations in domestic settings. Yet foregrounding intimacy can help us better understand the social worlds of humanitarians, their contradictory desires and convictions, and their complex encounters with distant sufferers, which as Didier Fassin notes always 'presupposes a relation of inequality'.[18] That said, the first challenge to the use of 'intimacy' as an explanatory methodology is that of definition.[19] The *Oxford English Dictionary* provides three main definitions for the noun 'intimacy' (1. Familiar intercourse, close familiarity; 2. close connection or union; 3. the inner or inmost nature of something – *obsolete*), two for the noun 'intimate' (1. One who intimately belongs to something, a typical representative – *obsolete*; 2. a very close friend or associate) and five for the adjective 'intimate' (1. Inmost, most inward; 2. pertaining to the inmost thoughts of feelings; 3. close in acquaintance or association; 4. involving or resulting from close familiarity; 5. very close).[20] Additionally, *to intimate* is also a verb, which can mean 'to make known formally', 'to communicate by any means however indirect' and 'to familiarise'. In short, according to the *Oxford English Dictionary*, the notion of intimacy can be deployed to explore and historicise past individual actors' relations to their self or to others. It can be mobilised to document the practices and representations around caring for oneself, but also others. Crucially, it can also be used to interrogate historians' own relationship to the historical actors that they are studying.

The use of intimacy has proliferated in various strands of historical scholarship, including in gender studies and the histories of sensibilities, emotions, private life, the body, psychoanalysis, gynaecology, colonialism, sexuality, internationalism and political thought. As the use of intimacy has grown rapidly, its meaning has been stretched in different directions. These are the results of both disciplinary and language differences. In French and English, for instance, the term has different meanings. In French, the adjective *intime* still suggests something hidden and the innermost nature of something and often secret, while in English this meaning has been obsolete since the eighteenth century.[21] Further, scholars working in the French context often highlight the religious dimension of the concept, tracing its invention back to Saint Augustine, who contended that within us there was a part that was so deeply inside

*Estrangement and intimacies: new perspectives*     35

that it was only available to God.[22] It was only in the late nineteenth and early twentieth centuries that the notion of sexuality and corporality was aggregated to the concept of *intime* in French.[23] As a result, French scholars have tended to consider intimacy as an analytical category,[24] which draws on the lexical field of spaces (focusing on the secret garden, the nuptial room, the *boudoir*, the confessional, the inner self).[25] Applying such an approach to the history of humanitarianism, Bertrand Taithe has recently focused on dreams as an intimate space, exploring the oneiric and spiritual life of the founder of the Huddersfield Famine Relief Committee Elizabeth Wilson from 1942 to 1999.[26] This exploration has led Taithe to reflect on Wilson's 'ordinary-exceptional life' and unearth the many different strands of the activism of this British humanitarian woman rooted in spirituality. Understood in this sense, the notion of intimacy (as intimate space) can contribute to the discovery of major new themes in the historiography of humanitarianism during the Second World War: for instance, the psychoanalytic and psychotherapeutic settings of Anna Freud and her colleagues working with young refugees during the Second World War;[27] or the makeshift confessional of the French military chaplain following the hospital Hadfield-Spears (mentioned at the start of this chapter).

In the English scholarship, scholars have adopted more encompassing definitions of intimacy, going beyond the lexicon of spaces and known personal connections to consider wider ties of familiarity. Michael Herzfeld has, for instance, crafted the notion of cultural intimacy. He defines cultural intimacy as 'those aspects of a cultural identity that are considered a source of external embarrassment but that nevertheless provide insiders with their assurance of common sociality'.[28] Drawing on a similar approach, Nicole Barnes uses intimacy in her study of wartime healthcare during China's war of Resistance against Japan to argue that Chinese female medical workers played a crucial role by providing the 'intimacy of healing touch' to the making of the modern Chinese nation between 1937 and 1945. According to her, through intimate acts, volunteer Chinese female medical workers played a crucial role in making the Chinese people coalesce into a national community of individuals who felt bonded to each other. In her work, she does not refer to the Chinese word for *intimacy*, but instead uses the Chinese term for compatriot '*tongbao*', meaning 'from the same womb'.[29] The notion

36    *The long Second World War, 1931–1953*

of intimacy shares meanings with a larger semantic domain that includes words like proximity, comradeship and female solidarities. To uncover intimate thoughts and acts, she adopts what she calls a 'backward reading' of the archives of provincial health administration, police reports, private and public hospitals, or foreign charitable organisations.[30] Her approach raises fascinating methodological questions, forcing us to think about whether some sources (such as letters and diaries) are more 'intimate' than others (such as censuses, police reports and hospital records), as well as the different words used by historical actors forming 'intimate communities'.

The term 'humanitarianism' is equally difficult to define. Since the beginning of the twenty-first century, scholars have debated at length about how to define humanitarianism.[31] Definitions range from considering it as a 'mode of governing',[32] a set of laws that were codified in Europe in the late nineteenth century, an impulse to assist others in dire need,[33] a sensibility,[34] a specific form of state intervention,[35] a set of practices or a logistical enterprise. Some scholars have argued that it is 'quintessentially cosmopolitan'[36] and secular,[37] while others have insisted on the importance of local charity traditions and a religious dimension instead.[38] Others have warned against the risks of 'relying on metanarratives of the globalization of Western modernity to make sense of "local" historical developments',[39] noting that humanitarianism has always been plural and fragmented.[40] Some historians have integrated military medicine and the medical care provided by voluntary aid societies to the wounded in wartime, while others have excluded it. As Pierre Fuller recently observed, the choices made in defining humanitarianism (and excluding what and who might *not* be a humanitarian) are always political and intrinsically problematic. These definitional postures can reinforce a set of liberal assumptions about charity traditions and constructed forms of culturalism.[41] Overall, there is still little scholarship that touches upon these various local conceptions and traditions of charity across spaces during the long Second World War.

This fragmentation of the scholarship on humanitarianism, combined with the many different meanings of intimacy, might partly explain why it is challenging to place the historiographies of humanitarianism and intimacy together in the same frame. However, the

## Estrangement and intimacies: new perspectives 37

rewards of doing so are compelling. Overall, the field of humanitarianism has been concerned with moving beyond biographies and hagiographic histories of self-proclaimed visionaries and has as a result tended to focus on the grand narrative of aid. But in searching for these grand narratives, historians might have contributed to the disappearance of groups whose voices are under-represented in the archives and those who did not fit in the category of humanitarian. As Bertrand Taithe and Elisabeth Piller have recently demonstrated, by adopting very clear-cut categories (humanitarianism/patriotic service/social work) and relying too heavily on humanitarians' diaries, letters and memoirs, historians of humanitarianism have helped perpetuate the idea that the noble epithet of 'humanitarian' should only be reserved for white men and reinforce narratives of heroic 'humanitarian masculinity'.[42] Thinking of humanitarianism *intimately* invites us to broaden historians' conceptions of humanitarian actors and sheds new light into the historically so-called 'humanitarian'. Reverting to biographies, Helen Dampier and Rebecca Gill have recently called for more investigation of the auto/biographical traces of humanitarian actors, in particular the subaltern biography able to 'expose the intimate and every day, the personal and the political and shifting configurations of power and authority'.[43] In this vein, Dolores Martín-Moruno has examined the various autobiographical writing and oral testimonies of Salaria Kea, an African American nurse who considered humanitarian actions during the Spanish Civil War as a manner of struggling for retributive justice. Kea's experience allows us to better understand the transnational aid networks established by the African American community in Europe and the 'emotions' which shaped them, in particular 'resentment, sympathy, love and hope'.[44] If Salaria Kea has left important written and oral traces of her experiences, other humanitarians' lives were characterised by complete anonymity. The methods of 'intimate history' offer the possibility of retrieving these anonymous lives from oblivion, providing a framework to go further in the direction of exposing the everyday and the political.[45]

From a methodological point of view, *intimating* the history of humanitarianism can in fact approximate to 'queering understanding', reflecting on the normative as well as the deviant and creating affective relations between the past and the present. To paraphrase the queer historian Carolyn Dinshaw, thinking about

38          *The long Second World War, 1931–1953*

humanitarianism *intimately* can involve a process of touching across time, an impulse towards making connections between, on the one hand, 'lives, texts, and other cultural phenomena left of [humanitarian] categories back then and, on the other, those left of current [humanitarian] categories now'.[46] Thinking about humanitarianism *intimately* offers the chance to historicise and unsettle categories (such as 'humanitarians', 'donors', 'recipients') and norms (of gender, age, class, etc.). This approach is at the heart of Saidiya Hartman's *Wayward Lives*, which offers an intimate chronicle of Black American Radicalism from 1890 to 1935. In her book, she explores the revolutionary ideals that animated the ordinary lives of young Black women in the US who rejected the socially imposed standards of respectability. Hartman is particularly attentive to what is missing from the archives, considering the structures and power relations that engender these absences. In 'notes on methods', she confesses: 'I have pressed at the limits of the case file and the document, speculated about what might have been, imagined the things whispered in dark bedrooms, and amplified moments of withholding, escape and possibility.'[47] Hartman defines her way of doing 'intimate history' in two ways: 'intimate history describes the effort to convey the revolution of black intimate life in the twentieth century' and it names the style of close narration that is utilised in the book. It reckons with the violence of history by 'crafting a love letter to all those who had been harmed'.[48] For her, intimate history, combined with 'speculative thought, radical narrative and critical fabulation' are 'ways to create other kinds of story', and to refuse a view of Black life as only 'a problem to be solved'.[49] This approach can be useful to historians of humanitarianism interested in those historical actors who rejected the terms of visibility imposed on them and fought the violence of history.

Within refugee scholarship, scholars have moved towards such approaches, showing a greater sensitivity to how refugees have manipulated and challenged the complex formal and informal hierarchies of race, class and gender that authorities attempted to impose upon them at the intimate level.[50] As many scholars have noted, refugees lived 'on the edge', in a status that makes them invisible and without the rights that come with citizenship.[51] The rich historiography on post-war refugee camps in Europe offers a good illustration of the benefit of thinking in those terms. This

*Estrangement and intimacies: new perspectives* 39

scholarship has revealed that refugee spaces were sites of humanitarian intervention where intimacy was a privileged target of control (politicisation of bodies, collective anxiety about venereal contamination, etc.) but also of resistance.[52] While not theorising intimacy, this scholarship raised important questions about the regulation of sexuality, conflicts of norms and the politicisation of intimate matters in specific micro-social and relational configurations. In this matter, the work of Esther Möller and Katharina Stornig in this volume shows promising avenues for new directions, by focusing on 'circle of intimacies' and moving beyond either top-down or bottom-up approaches.

Despite important definitional issues, thinking about humanitarianism *intimately* can thus lead to new avenues of inquiry about understudied sites (such as dreams and psychoanalytic settings), ties of solidarities (the making of an imagined national community), 'invisible' groups and radical politics. Despite important differences, approaches using intimacy have in common a keen awareness of the importance of affects and spaces, of questioning identities and of moving beyond institutional histories. For these reasons, they enable us to respond to recent calls made by historians of humanitarianism for more studies of the 'experience of humanitarian aid'.[53] They also allow us to explore the emotions behind the turning of 'compassion' into humanitarian actions,[54] and to integrate gender as a category of research in histories of humanitarianism.[55] As Ara Wilson argues, the term's 'very lack of fixity is part of its appeal'.[56] Reflecting further on how to draw together intimacy and humanitarianism, the next section considers the key promises and core difficulties in foregrounding 'intimacies' in histories of transnational medical care and aid.

## The different meanings of intimacy and the history of humanitarianism

Neither humanitarianism nor intimacy are neutral categories. These are polysemic notions, which can conceal or reveal specific social relations of inequality. If we make a brief detour into the etymology of both *intimacy* and *humanitarianism*, we see some revealing entanglements between the two concepts, at least in Europe and

40    *The long Second World War, 1931–1953*

North America. In fact, scholars have traced the development of a new humanitarian sensibility in the eighteenth century and have linked it to the development of new conceptions of the self and understandings of pain and suffering.[57] In the Enlightenment period, a new culture of intimacy emerged, when *confession* became more secular and the reading of sentimental novels became popular.[58] For Brigitte Diaz and José-Luis Diaz, the nineteenth century represented 'the century of intimacy', a period marked by the development of romantic aesthetics which promoted the self and valorised intimacy (understood by contemporaries as 'interiority') as a site of 'authenticity'.[59] In this period, the abstract 'notion of humanity' also took on new meanings, and humanitarian reform movements spread across western European and North American societies.[60] This new humanitarian consciousness and ways of feeling about 'others' did not contradict colonialism nor the global and national divisions on which Europe's liberal traditions rested. As Lisa Lowe argues in *Intimacies of Four Continents*, in the 'modern' and 'liberal' European mind of the nineteenth century, not everyone had access to these domains of 'liberal personhood' (whether it meant interiority, individual will or the possession of property and domesticity).[61] Using the concept of intimacy thus requires questioning the nature of our assumptions about agency, the nature of the individual self and the relationship between the private and the public.

### *Intimacy as a way to challenge the dichotomy between private and public, the personal and the political*

For some scholars, intimacy raises first and foremost a question of scale and enables us to move from the level of individual lives to that of the collective.[62] Lauren Berlant has crafted the notion of 'intimate public', which she has used to examine the history of public sphere femininity in the United States. In the preface of the *Female Complaint*, she defines it as 'an affective scene of identification among strangers that promises a certain experience of belonging'.[63] In other words, for her, the 'intimate public' refers to the practice of a distinct sentimental feeling culture that 'at once confirms the unity of society, regardless of its structural disparities, while also authenticating the morality and goodness of those benefitting from the disparities in question'.[64] The notion of 'intimate

*Estrangement and intimacies: new perspectives* 41

public' enables scholars of humanitarianism to question the ways in which humanitarians *feel* their way to humanitarian convictions and actions and relate to humanitarianism as a site of affective investment and emotional identification. As scholars have recently argued, historians need to engage more thoroughly with this question of how humanitarians experienced their own story as part of something social and create a collective story about the personal.[65] A particular benefit of looking at 'intimate public' is to challenge this dichotomy between private and public, the personal and the political in the history of humanitarianism.

## Regimes of intimacy

To do so, some scholars have developed the notion of 'regimes of intimacy' to explore the materialist dimension of normative constructs about intimacies.[66] Drawing on Damien Baldin's notion of regimes of sensibility,[67] they argue that historians need to enter families, homes, domestic spaces and professional organisations to apprehend the evolution of various regimes of intimacies, which are shaped by economic and social forces. For them, objects can offer insights into the emotional lives and experiences of individuals who did not leave textual traces. Scholars of wartime captivity and encampment have, for instance, highlighted how inmates relied heavily on objects to navigate the unfamiliar world of encampment and immobility. As Iris Rachamimov demonstrates, amid the uncertainties and dislocations of captivity and displacement, civilian internees and prisoners of war 'relied on artifacts to perform meaningful social scripts and deployed them to articulate a range of emotions and identities'.[68] For her, many of these scripts were aimed at sustaining pre-war notions of 'normalcy' and 'respectability'. Yet, because social scripts 'emanated from the pre-war bi-gender world, recreating them in one-gender (homosocial) settings often led to transgressions of respectable masculinity'.[69]

Despite a recent interest in material culture in the history of humanitarianism,[70] these 'regimes of intimacy' remain largely unresearched. Scholars have shown how notions of 'female nurture' were essential in legitimising women's humanitarian engagement from different national, ideological and professional backgrounds and how notions of military heroism was essential for sustaining humanitarian male engagement.[71] Yet, we still need more research into how these hegemonic norms were produced and might have co-existed and conflicted with other less hegemonic ones, as well as the role of objects in transforming these various injunctions and constraints. As Leora Auslander argues, in twentieth-century Europe, 'objects did not reflect as much as create social position (as well, some would argue, the self itself)'.[72] This also applied to humanitarian workers: vehicles, tents, uniforms (and other objects) helped them consolidate a sense of personal distinctiveness and 'position in the field' and performed socially legible scripts, even if this could also contribute to making them feel different and separate from those they work with and for.[73]

Thinking about 'regimes of intimacy' in my work on medical spaces in the French Resistance allows me to interrogate the role of objects, such as trucks, hospital tents, *guitoune* (in military slang a tent or a military shelter), personal photographs, clothing and landscapes in the formation of a care community, where new relationships were temporally formed, identities reshaped and, in the process, norms of respectability and adequate intimacy reworked. In the Hadfield-Spears unit, for example, French and British volunteers shared meals, songs and drinks in their 'trucks' and tents, but also personnel effects, such as photos from home. In the Western Desert, transforming their trucks into 'imaginary homes' could help them combat feelings of homesickness, sustain affective links with their pre-war identities and overcome the constraints of boredom and separation from home.[74] The concept of 'regimes of intimacy' also enables me to explore how, at times, spatial and bodily proximities reinforced negative feelings. In her diary, the *Directrice* (head of this hospital) Mary Spears commented on several occasions how she had to physically distance herself from others, sleeping by herself in the car – 'as [she] couldn't face being sardined'.[75] If physical proximities could lead to estrangement, it could also facilitate romantic desire and sexual fantasies. In Bir Hakeim, the Free French surgeon Vialard-Goudou related, for instance, in his diary that Irish ambulance driver Rosy Forbs often came to dine and play bridge with the French (male) doctors in their *guitoune*: 'She was an excellent girlfriend, because all of us had more or less a crush on her, because we assumed her heart was taken elsewhere, and because it had been decided once and for all – In the Desert and on

*Estrangement and intimacies: new perspectives*  43

the front line, no love stories.'[76] As this example indicates, there are many overlapping and hitherto unexplored intimacies which were squeezed into this mobile frontline community of medical care.

## Haptic and transgressive intimacies

Some scholars have argued that medical settings offer a particular valuable lens through which to study transgressive intimate bodily encounters because medical care involves asymmetrical power relations and exchanges of information perceived as deeply personal. They also entail physical touch and 'invasive' bodily practices. In the *Politics of Wounds*, Ana Carden-Coyne demonstrates how the status of 'being a patient' is bound up in dependency, and the extent to which being wounded in wartime reversed traditional gender roles.[77] In military hospitals during the First World War, the fit and virile combatant was made impotent and 'feminised', while nurses took on 'authoritative' and 'masculine' jobs. According to her, hospitals stretched the boundaries of morality and sexuality. In short, medical care made visible the complexity of gender constructs and gendered behaviours, as well as racial categorisations and sexuality.[78] In the same vein, Chris Rominger has shown that daily interactions between white nurses and Black patients in French hospitals for North African soldiers during the First World War provoked new understandings of belonging, differences and articulations of self for North African soldiers.[79]

Taken together, this scholarship has demonstrated that wartime military hospitals and dispensaries were spaces of bodily and intimate desires, where ideas about gender, race, pain and the body were negotiated and contested. Wartime hospitals were both disciplinary and transgressive spaces. These were liminal spaces, functioning as multifaceted contact zones between the civilian and military spheres, between the male and female realms, between the metropolis and the colonies, where new and transgressive intimate encounters took place.[80] While most of this research has focused on the First World War, Jane Brooks has applied this notion to her study of British wartime nursing, highlighting the ambiguities of bodily care. 'The intimacy of body care, the moment when the single young female nurse meets the young male patient, required skilful negotiations in order to alleviate the spectre of unrestrained

44 *The long Second World War, 1931–1953*

sexuality.'[81] 'The care of the male body by young single women thus placed nurses in a liminal place between the accepted face of femininity and the ambiguities of heterosexual touch.'[82]

Deploying the concept of intimacy has allowed these scholars to interrogate the role of non-verbal language and touch in shaping medical–patient encounters. But this focus on the 'intimate' has at times come at the expense of the macro-politics of care. In other words, most intimate histories of medical care tend to ignore the ways in which the intimate was shaped by the global and transnational or how colonial and transnational medical encounters shaped diplomatic and military cooperation. As Judith Surkis observes, contest over political authority and international influence took place at the level of individual bodies.[83] Moving across scales of analysis allows us to interrogate the role of intimacies in broader histories of international relations.

### Case study: intimacies, estrangement and transnational medical care in the French Resistance

Building on these various strands of scholarship, my research on medical care in the French Resistance attempts to transcend institutional and state-centred approaches that currently dominate the historiography of Allied medicine and international health cooperation to assess how intimate care relations reshaped existing colonial and inter-allied relationships. It takes as a starting point that the long Second World War elicited important new physical, cultural and bodily encounters between individuals of diverse gender, ethnic, national, class, age and religious backgrounds and that these forms of interactions have to be addressed in a transnational context and on a grassroots level. It draws on a broad definition of resistance, encompassing both official members of the Resistance as well as unofficial members who gravitated around the movement, such as members of the Free French committees scattered throughout the world and foreign volunteers who joined medical formations.

Medical workers in the Resistance had radically different wartime experiences: those who joined the Gaullist movement abroad were not confronted by the same levels of violence and repression as those in occupied France. Further, as many scholars have shown,

## Estrangement and intimacies: new perspectives    45

there was often competition between different forms of resistance, and this was also to some extent the case for medical care. Some resisters saw themselves as more legitimate than others: joining in 1940 was a badge of honour compared to those who joined in 1944 when the Allied victory was very likely.

At the diplomatic level, I have applied the concept of intimacy in my research to evaluate the role of friendships and informal networks that emerged across the world to sustain the structures for medical care and relief for Free French wounded and prisoners of war. During the war, France was in a unique position, for the Vichy regime had signed an armistice that fostered collaboration with the Third Reich and used its colonies as a bargaining chip. While most of the Empire remained faithful to Marshal Pétain until 1943, a handful of colonies, including New Hebrides, French Equatorial Africa, Cameroon, and French settlements in India and in Oceania and New Caledonia, joined the Free French camp in 1940. Yet de Gaulle's Free French organisation, in part based in London and in part Brazzaville, was never fully recognised by the Allies nor by the International Committee of the Red Cross as a government-in-exile.[84] It also lacked a fully functioning diplomatic apparatus. In this context, the Free French movement relied on a vast range of non-traditional diplomatic actors (such as philanthropists, missionaries and scientists) and committees. By August 1942, there were 412 Free French subcommittees across the world.[85] These humanitarian networks were essential to the Free French movement, serving as a vehicle of propaganda, a means of garnering Allied sympathies, accumulating resources and as a tool of social control within the Empire. Many women, including wives of important military and political figures, contributed to these committees, and their performed femininity (which reinforced traditional images of elegant French women) accounted partly for their success (in terms of fundraising and growing influence).[86]

Mobilising *intimacy* enables me to interrogate the atmospheres in which these women and informal agents of the Gaullist movement worked and the intimate spheres of connections – via the home, fundraising events and female friendships which made these networks possible. As Sun Lin Lewis recently observed, the role of hospitality that bound transnational networks together has been overlooked.[87] Retrieving these intimate spheres of connections

46    *The long Second World War, 1931–1953*

(and rivalries) from a multiplicity of archives reveals hidden aspects of the history of humanitarianism and the resistance, allowing for a more complex and less male-centric history of Free French diplomacy. It leads to a different way of understanding how the Free French gained recognition from the Allies, how they went from being considered in the international sphere as a group of dissidents to a more recognised belligerent. It also contributes to a better understanding of the complex politics of humanitarianism, with some humanitarian actors being able to be intimate with both representatives of Vichy France and the Gaullist movement, with representatives of de Gaulle and Giraud, and so on.

A second benefit of using the notion of intimacy is to better understand how French medical and military authorities politicised intimate care and drew boundaries between acceptable and unacceptable forms of corporeal intimacy.[88] The head of the Free French health service was worried about ill Free French soldiers marrying British women, as this could compromise French prestige.[89] The rate of venereal disease among Free French soldiers stationed in Great Britain was a constant preoccupation. But perhaps more importantly, Free French medical authorities were concerned about *transgressive* bodily care intimacies, white nurses touching and interacting with colonial soldiers and patients. These deepseated imperial concerns were exacerbated by the broader political context. Within the handful of colonies that followed de Gaulle, colonial authorities were confronted by the affirmation of national movements of liberation and, after 1942, the presence of American troops, which threatened French prestige on the ground. The Vichy interlude provided African critics of the Empire with new leverage against republican administrators who were keen to distance themselves from their former 'fascist' predecessor. In medical international spaces, just as French medical officers had to negotiate the bleak reality of the French Resistance's dependence on its colonies and Allies, French colonial troops could grasp and question the harsh sense of difference imposed by French colonial practice. These anxieties led to imposing strict discriminatory measures to separate Black and white medical workers, even if, in practice, care gestures could lead to their transgression.

In my research, the concept of intimacy has also enabled me to question the role of medical worker/patient relationships in the

## Estrangement and intimacies: new perspectives 47

mechanisms that hold the Free French community together and the importance of medical workers in creating collective unity among a community made up of a plurality of commitments. As Clémentine Vidal-Naquet observes, wars represent moments when intimate feelings become more visible to historians, not least because intimate thoughts are more often expressed through private correspondence and official, cultural and autobiographical representations than in peacetime.[90] I have thus paid close attention to written fragments about what it felt like to provide or receive intimate bodily care. The fragments found suggest that through touch, non-verbal language and close bodily encounters, medical workers helped the Free French to coalesce into a distinctive group who felt bonded to each other.[91] They also hint at the role of medical workers in providing a 'beautiful death', from having a hand to hold to writing a last letter. The fragments also point to the many 'small escapes' that medical workers put in place to cope with the emotional impacts of medical care on a frontline unit. For instance, the French doctor Paul Guénon wrote at length in his diary about his dreams of an imagined woman with whom he shared (imaginatively) regular drinks and romantic enchantments.[92]

In this search for written traces of the emotions expressed when attending the ill and wounded, I have also confronted important silences. The history of the self and of medical workers' intimate thoughts within occupied France requires more research. As Laurent Douzou notes, silence is an integral part of the history of the Resistance within occupied France: it is often a deliberate construction, an active choice to remain silent for a multitude of reasons.[93] The historian is confronted by different types of silences when studying the Free French movement. As far as medical care within the Free French movement is concerned, perhaps the most noticeable silences were around the issue of disgust, the impact of medical triage, the meanings of arm-to-arm blood transfusion, and the ways in which sexuality might have been at play when navigating suffering and healing. Some Free French were reluctant to write about sex as they insisted on the moral grounds of the Resistance – precisely at a moment when in occupied France, there was a widespread belief that too many French women were giving themselves to the German victors.[94] As we have seen, these silences ought to be scrutinised as a valuable signifier of the physical, psychological, sensory and emotional dimensions of medical care.

48    *The long Second World War, 1931–1953*

In some ways, I have not managed yet to write a history that is as intimate as I wished. In addition to the difficulties of fully understanding these silences, it has proven difficult if not impossible to retrieve the ways in which colonial medical auxiliaries and patients felt about the Free French community. Following Hartman's methods, I have tried to 'press at the limits' of official documentation and 'speculate about what might have been'. I have diligently collected fragments of their lived experiences in the archival records: photographs showing them carrying wounded men, surgical reports detailing the impact of their wounds on their bodies, accounts of their performance during football games, reports of the violence that they faced. But in the only biography that I have found so far written about a Cameroonian nurse, little is said about day-to-day encounters.[95] Free French 'African' views are always mediated, making it difficult to capture the complexity of their identities, perspectives and desires. While my search is not over, I am aware that I have not yet fully imagined the 'things whispered' in hospital beds, as Hartman invites us to do, and have not fully grasped how these intimate interactions imprint their marks on anti-colonial dynamics. As Clémentine Vidal-Naquet powerfully demonstrates, historians of the intimate must accept that they will not always reach what was felt nor be able to imagine it. Despite these shortcomings, focusing on the intimate life of transnational medical care suggests new ways of writing humanitarian and medical spaces in histories of French resistance, revising old historiographical questions (about the nature of Free French diplomacy, French wartime imperial anxieties, efforts at restoring France's prestige, etc.) and exploring new ones (about transnational solidarities, everyday violence, transgressions and affects in the Resistance).

## Conclusion

The chief strengths of thinking about humanitarianism as encompassing intimate acts, thoughts and relations are that it generates a keen awareness among historians of the importance of affects and spaces, of questioning identities and of moving beyond institutional histories of aid. The argument on offer here is emphatically not that all historians of humanitarianism should embrace every aspect of

*Estrangement and intimacies: new perspectives* 49

intimacy in their conceptual framework. Nor that one definition or methodological approach to the intimate past is better than another. It is instead that borrowing from the many thinking tools provided by historians of the 'intimate' can provide new insights into familiar questions of identities and self-fashioning in humanitarianism. While the concept has been stretched in many different directions, not everything is necessarily or uncritically 'intimate'. Intimacy is fundamentally about relations, from the friendly to the spiritual, the romantic to the sexual. It is about what connects past historical actors, but also, as Hartman's work suggests, what brings the past and the present together. It involves *something* shared, but not with everyone, and often reveals points of tension between various identities (e.g. political, religious, sexed, gendered, raced). As we have seen, it may be private or personal, but intimate attachments also play an important role in the formation of nation states and the shaping of international relations and vice versa.[96] In that sense, foregrounding intimacies is particularly important for the study of humanitarianism during the long Second World War because it can contribute to a better understanding of the links between giving aid and building national communities. It can also help us examine the lived experiences of medical workers and humanitarians more on the historical margins and interrogate the 'transgressive' nature of some relationships in humanitarian and medical spaces. Crucially, it allows for a more complex and nuanced assessment of how the global and transnational shaped the realm of humanitarians' everyday life and, in turn, how intimate attachments transform humanitarian organisations and international relations.

## Notes

1 The research for this article was generously funded by the Arts and Humanities Research Council (AH/T006382/1). The author would especially like to thank Craig Griffiths and Frances Houghton for their encouragement, advice and feedback at different stages of the writing up of this chapter. I would also like to thank Marie-Luce Desgrandchamps, Pierre Fuller, Eleanor Davey and Bertrand Taithe for sharing their considerable expertise on the history of humanitarianism.

50 *The long Second World War, 1931–1953*

2 Friends' Library [FL], MSS876/HIST/13, Michael Rowntree, History of the HSU [no date, 1946?], p. 10.

3 *Ibid.*, p. 11.

4 FL, FAU 1947/3/5, Ian Scott-Kilvert's obituary of Nik Alderson.

5 This is an argument that draws on the work of Harini Amarasuriya, Tobias Kelly, Sidharthan Maunaguru, Galina Oustinova-Stjepanovic and Jonathan Spencer (eds), *The Intimate Life of Dissent* (London: UCL Press, 2020). For British COs, see Tobias Kelly's chapter 'Dissenting Conscience: The Intimate Politics of Objection in Second World War Britain' in the above collection (p. 112–131); Kelly, *Battles of Conscience: British Pacifists and the Second World War* (London: Penguin, 2020).

6 Sertaç Sehlikoglu and Aslı Zengin, 'Introduction: Why Revisit Intimacy?', *The Cambridge Journal of Anthropology*, 33:2 (2015), 20–25, at p. 22.

7 Judith Surkis, 'Sex, Sovereignty and Transnational Intimacies', *The American Historical Review*, 115:4 (2010), 1089–1096; Geraldine Pratt and Victoria Rosner (eds), *The Global and the Intimate. Feminism in Our Time* (Columbia, SC: Columbia University Press, 2012).

8 Saidiya Hartman, *Wayward Lives, Beautiful Experiments: Intimate Histories of Riotous Black Girls, Troublesome Women and Queer Radicals* (New York: W. W. Norton & Company, 2019).

9 Bruno Cabanes and Guillaume Piketty (eds), Retour à l'intime au sortir de la guerre (Paris: Tallandier, 2009), pp. 11–12.

10 Laurent Douzou, 'A Perilous History: A Historiographical Essay on the French Resistance', *Contemporary European History*, 28, 1 (2019), 96–106, at p. 97.

11 *Ibid.*, p. 105. Guillaume Piketty has recently argued on the contrary in favour of an emotional history of the Resistance. *Français, libre: Pierre de Chevigné* (Paris: Tallandier, 2022); *Résister. Les archives intimes des combattants de l'ombre* (Paris: Editions Textuel, 2011).

12 Claire-Lise Gaillard, Irène Gimenez and Suzanne Rochefort, 'Introduction. Du genre des matérialités intimes aux régimes d'intimités. Définitions et mises à l'épreuve', *Genre et Histoire*, 27 (2021), online, http://journals.openedition.org/genrehistoire/6055 (accessed 20 August 2023).

13 Clémentine Vidal-Naquet, 'Intimacy: Inhabited?', *Sensibilités*, 6:1 (2019), 6–9.

14 Douzou, 'A Perilous History'.

15 Elisabeth Terrenoire, *Combattantes sans uniforme. Les femmes dans la Résistance* (Paris: Bloud et Gay, 1946). On intimacy as a 'theatre' and a 'means of violence' in another context, see Jeremie Foa, *Survivre: Une histoire des guerres de religion* (Paris: Seuil, 2024).

## Estrangement and intimacies: new perspectives 51

16 Kelly, *Battles of Conscience*, p. 15.

17 See, for example, Irène Hermann and Daniel Palmieri, 'Between Amazons and Sabines: A Historical Approach to Women and War', *International Review of the Red Cross*, 92:877 (2010), 19–30; Esther Möller, Johannes Paulmann and Katharina Stornig (eds), *Gendering Global Humanitarianism in the Twentieth Century: Practice, Politics and the Power of Representation* (London: Palgrave Macmillan, 2020); Samuel Martínez and Kathryn Libal, 'Introduction: The Gender of Humanitarian Narrative', *Humanity: An International Journal of Human Rights, Humanitarianism, and Development* 2:2 (2011), 161–170; Dolores Martín-Moruno, Brenda L. Edgar and Marie Leyder, 'Feminist Perspectives on the History of Humanitarian Relief (1870–1945)', *Medicine, Conflict and Survival*, 36:1 (2020), 2–18.

18 Didier Fassin, *Humanitarian Reason: A Moral History of the Present* (Berkeley, CA: University of California Press, 2012), p. 4.

19 George Morris, 'Historiographical Review: Intimacy in Modern British History', *The Historical Journal*, 64:3 (2021), 796–811.

20 *Oxford English Dictionary* (Oxford: Oxford University Press, 2023).

21 *Dictionnaire Larousse*, online version.

22 Vidal-Naquet, 'Intimacy: Inhabited?', pp. 6–9. Caroline Muller, *Au plus près des âmes et des corps. Une histoire intime des catholiques au XIX<sup>e</sup> siècle* (Paris: Presses Universitaires de France, 2019).

23 Françoise Simonet-Tenant, 'Pour une approche historique de l'intime', *Cliniques*, 1:19 (2020), 19–32.

24 Anne-Claire Rebreyend, *Intimités amoureuses. France, 1920–1975* (Toulouse: Presses universitaires du Mirail, 2008); Clémentine Vidal-Naquet, *Couples dans la Grande Guerre. Le tragique et l'ordinaire du lien conjugal* (Paris: Les Belles Lettres, 2014).

25 For an in-depth review of the term in French, see 'Archives et intimités', https://archivint.hypotheses.org (accessed 25 February 2025).

26 Bertrand Taithe, 'Living Humanitarian Dreams: The Oneiric and Spiritual Life and Activism of Elizabeth Wilson (1909–2000)', *Cultural Social History*, 20:3 (2023), 429–445.

27 Anna Freud and Dorothy T. Burlingham, *War and Children* (London, 1943).

28 Michael Herzfeld, *Cultural Intimacy: Social Poetics in the Nation-State*, 2nd ed. (New York:, Routledge, 2005), p. 19.

29 Barnes, *Intimate Communities*, p. 6.

30 *Ibid.*, p. 19.

31 Johannes Paulmann, 'Conjunctures in the History of International Humanitarian Aid during the Twentieth Century', *Humanity: An International Journal of Human Rights, Humanitarianism and Development*, 4:2 (2013), 215–238; Axelle Brodiez-Dolino and Bruno

52    *The long Second World War, 1931–1953*

Dumons, 'Editorial: Faire l'histoire de l'humanitaire', *Le Mouvement Social*, 2:227 (2009), 3–8.

32  Fassin, *Humanitarian Reason*.

33  Richard Wilson and Richard Brown 'Introduction' in Richard Wilson and Richard Brown (eds), *Humanitarianism and Suffering: The Mobilisation of Empathy* (Cambridge: Cambridge University Press, 2008), p. 1.

34  Thomas W. Laqueur, 'Seven Bodies, Details and the Humanitarian Narrative', in Lynn Hunt (ed.), *The New Cultural History* (Berkeley, CA: University of California Press, 1989), pp. 176–204; Karen Halttunen, 'Humanitarianism and the Pornography of Pain in Anglo-American Culture', *The American Historical Review*, 100:2 (1995), 303–334.

35  Fabian Klose, *The Emergence of Humanitarian Intervention: Ideas and Practice from the Nineteeth Century to the Present* (Cambridge: Cambridge University Press, 2015), pp. 1–28.

36  Craig Calhoun, 'The Imperative to Reduce Suffering', in Michael Barnett and Thomas G. Weiss (eds), *Humanitarianism in Question* (Ithaca, NY: Cornell University Press, 2012), pp. 73–74. For Silvia Salvatici, 'even though there is no precise definition', the 'overall deployment of the help is promoted by specific institutions and organisations, is regulated by ad hoc legislation and nowadays uses operating standards recognised at a supranational level'. *In the Name of Others: A History of Humanitarianism, 1755–1989* (Manchester: Manchester University Press, 2020), p. 6.

37  Keith D. Watenpaugh, *Bread from Stones: The Middle East and the Making of Modern Humanitarianism* (Oakland, CA: University of California Press, 2015).

38  Rebecca Gill, *Calculating Compassion: Humanity and Relief in War, Britain 1870–1914* (Manchester: Manchester University Press, 2013); Pierre Fuller, 'Decentering International and Institutional Famine Relief in Late Nineteenth-Century China: In Search of the Local', *European Review of History*, 22:6 (2015), 873–889.

39  Sho Konishi, 'The Emergence of an International Humanitarian Organisation in Japan: The Tokugawa Origins of the Japanese Red Cross', *The American Historical Review*, 119:4 (2014), 1129–1153, at p. 1133.

40  Joanne Laycock and Francesca Piana, *Aid to Armenia: Humanitarianism and Intervention from 1890s to the Present* (Manchester: Manchester University Press, 2020).

41  Pierre Fuller, 'Links and Non-links between Humanitarian Historigraphies: Setting the Scene', paper presented at Sciences Po Paris, 22 May 2023.

## Estrangement and intimacies: new perspectives 53

42 Elisabeth Piller, 'Beyond Hoover: Rewriting the History of the Commission for Relief in Belgium (CRB) through Female Involvement', *The International History Review*, 45:1 (2022), 202–224; Bertrand Taithe, 'Humanitarian Desire, Masculine Character and Heroics', in Möller, Paulmann and Stornig (eds), *Gendering Global Humanitarianism in the Twentieth Century*, pp. 35–59.

43 Helen Dampier and Rebecca Gill, 'Introduction: Humanitarianism and Biography', *Cultural and Social History*, 20:3 (2023), 317–327, at p. 321.

44 Dolores Martín-Moruno, 'The Experience of a Black Nurse in the Long Second World War: Salaria Kea', University of Manchester, 1 February 2022, https://colonialandtransnationalintimacies.com/2022/02/11/humanitarian-intimacies-gender-care-and-humanitarianism%EF%BF%BC/ (accessed 21 August 2023).

45 Hartman, *Wayward Lives, Beautiful Experiments*, p. 27.

46 Carolyn Dinshaw, *Getting Medieval: Sexualities and Communities, Pre- and Postmodern* (Durham, NC: Duke University Press, 1999), p. 1.

47 *Ibid.*, p. 9.

48 Saidiya Hartman, 'Book Forum: Intimate History, Radical Narrative', *The Journal of African American History*, 106:1 (2021), 127–135, at p. 129.

49 *Ibid.*, p. 135.

50 Jordanna Bailkin, *Unsettled: Refugee Camps and the Making of Multicultural Britain* (Oxford: Oxford University Press, 2018); Katarzyna Nowak, *Kingdom of Barracks: Polish Displaced Persons in Allied Occupied Germany and Austria* (Montreal: McGill University Press, 2023).

51 Jennifer Hyndman and Mary Giles, *Refugees in Extended Exile: Living on the Edge* (London: Routledge, 2017); for an example during the Second World War, see Jochen Lingelbach, *On the Edges of Whiteness: Polish Refugees in British Colonial Africa during and after the Second World War* (New York: Berghahn, 2020).

52 Peter Gatrell and Nick Baron (eds), *Warlands: Population Resettlement and State Reconstruction in the Soviet-East European Borderlands, 1945–1950* (Basingstoke: Palgrave Macmillan, 2009), pp. 1–22; Daniel Cohen, 'Un espace domestique d'après-guerre: les camps de personnes déplacées dans l'Allemagne occupée', in Bruno Cabanes and Guillaume Piketty (eds), *Retour à l'intime au sortir de la guerre* (Paris: Tallandier, 2009), pp. 117–131; Lisa Haushofer, 'The "Contaminating Agent": UNRRA, Displaced Persons and Venereal Disease in Germany, 1945–1947', *American Journal of Public Health*, 100:6 (2010), 993–1003; Margarete Myers Feinstein, *Holocaust Survivors in Postwar Germany, 1945–1957* (Cambridge: Cambridge

# 54    *The long Second World War, 1931–1953*

University Press, 2010); Katarzyna Nowak, 'A Gloomy Carnival of Freedom: Sex, Gender, and Emotions among Polish Displaced Person in the Aftermath of World War Two', *Aspasia*, 13:1 (2019), 113–134; Laure Humbert, *Reinventing French Aid: The Politics of Humanitarian Relief in French Occupied Germany, 1945–1952* (Cambridge: Cambridge University Press, 2021).

53 Matthew Hilton, Emily Baughan, Eleanor Davey, Bronwen Everill and Kevin O'Sullivan, 'History and Humanitarianism: A Conversation', *Past and Present*, 241:1 (2018), e1–e38.

54 Dolores Martín-Moruno and Beatriz Pichel (eds), *Emotional Bodies: The Historical Performativity of Emotions* (Champaign, IL: University of Illinois Press, 2019), p. 4.

55 Esther Möller, Johannes Paulmann and Katarina Stornig (eds), *Gendering Global Humanitarianism in the Twentieth Century: Practice, Politics and the Power of Representation* (London: Palgrave Macmillan, 2020), p. 283.

56 Ara Wilson, 'Intimacy: A Useful Category of Transnational Analysis', in Pratt and Rosner (eds), *The Global and the Intimate*, p. 32.

57 Norman S. Fiering, 'Irresistible Compassion: An Aspect of Eighteenth-Century Sympathy and Humanitarianism', *Journal of History of Ideas*, 37:2 (1976), 195–218; Lynn Hunt, *Inventing Human Rights: A History* (New York: W. W. Norton & Company, 2007).

58 Simonet-Tenant, 'Pour une approche historique de l'intime'.

59 Brigitte Diaz and José-Luis Diaz, 'Le siècle de l'intime', *Itineraires*, 2009–4 (2009), https://doi.org/10.4000/itineraires.1052

60 Fabian Klose, *In the Cause of Humanity: A History of Humanitarian Intervention in the Long Nineteenth Century* (Cambridge: Cambridge University Press, 2021), p. 39.

61 Lisa Lowe, *The Intimacies of Four Continents* (Durham, NC: Duke University Press, 2015), p. 18.

62 Lauren Berlant, 'Intimacy: A Special Issue', *Critical Inquiry*, 24, 2 (1998), 281–288, at p. 283.

63 Lauren Berlant, *The Female Complaint: The Unfinished Business of Sentimentality in American Culture* (Durham, NC: Duke University Press, 2008), p. viii.

64 Devika Sharma, 'Doing Good, Feeling Bad: Humanitarian Emotion in Crisis', *Journal of Aesthetics and Culture*, 9:1 (2017), 1–12, at p. 3.

65 Sebastien Farré, Jean-François Fayet and Bertrand Taithe (eds), *L'Humanitaire s'exhibe (1867–2016): The Humanitarian Exhibition (1867–2016)* (Geneva: Georg, 2022), p. 18.

66 Gaillard, Gimenez and Rochefort, 'Introduction'.

# Estrangement and intimacies: new perspectives    55

67 Damien Baldin, 'De l'horreur du sang à l'insoutenable souffrance animale. Élaboration sociale des régimes de sensibilité à la mise à mort des animaux (19e-20esiècles)', *Vingtième Siècle. Revue d'histoire*, 123:3 (2014), 52–68.

68 Iris Rachamimov, 'Small Escapes: Gender, Class and Material Culture in Great War Internment Camps', in Leora Auslander and Tara Zahra (eds), *Objects of War: The Material Culture of Conflict and Displacement* (Ithaca, NY: Cornell University Press, 2018), pp. 164–188, p. 169.

69 *Ibid.*, p. 169.

70 Leora Auslander and Tara Zahra (eds), *Objects of War: The Material Culture of Conflict and Displacement* (Ithaca, NY: Cornell University Press, 2018); Jennifer Way, *Deploying Craft: Crafting Wellness and Healing in Contexts of War* (New York: Routledge, forthcoming); Claire Barber, Helen Dampier, Rebecca Gill and Bertrand Taithe (eds), *Humanitarian Handicraft: History, Materiality and Trade* (Manchester: Manchester University Press, forthcoming).

71 Bertrand Taithe, 'Humanitarian Desire, Masculine Character and Heroics', in Möller, Paulmann and Stornig (eds), *Gendering Global Humanitarianism in the Twentieth Century*, pp. 35–59; Boyd van Dijk, 'Gendering the Geneva Conventions', *Human Rights Quarterly*, 44:2 (2022), 286–312.

72 Leora Auslander, 'Beyond Words', *American Historical Review*, 110:4 (2005), 1015–1045, at p. 1018.

73 Roisin Read, 'Embodying Difference: Reading Gender in Women's Memoirs of Humanitarianism', *Journal of Intervention and Statebuilding*, 12:3 (2018), 300–318.

74 Imperial War Museum [IWM], 7864, Private papers of R. N. Coates, 3 March 1942, p. 141; 7 March 1942, p. 142.

75 Spears [SPRS] 11/3/2, Manuscript diary by Mary Spears, 1 February 1942.

76 Musée de l'Ordre de la Libération, *Journal*. Chapitre VII *bis* [Diary. Chapter VII bis], pp. 110–111.

77 Ana Carden-Coyne, *The Politics of Wounds: Military Patients and Medical Power in the First World War* (Oxford: Oxford University Press, 2014).

78 Ana Carden-Coyne and Laura Doan, 'Gender and Sexuality', Susan Grayzel and Tammy Proctor (eds), *Gender and the Great War* (Oxford: Oxford University Press, 2017), pp. 91–114.

79 Chris Rominger, 'Nursing Transgressions, Exploring Difference: North Africans in French Medical Spaces during World War 1', *International Journal of Middle East Studies*, 50:4 (2018), 691–713.

## 56 *The long Second World War, 1931–1953*

80 Alina Enzensberger, 'Hospitals', in Ute Daniel, Peter Gatrell, Oliver Janz, Heather Jones, Jennifer Keene, Alan Kramer and Bill Nasson (eds), *1914-1918-Online. International Encyclopedia of the First World War*, issued by Freie Universität Berlin, Berlin, 19 May 2021, https://doi.org/10.15463/ie1418.11525 (accessed 25 February 2025); Jeffrey Reznick, *Healing the Nation: Soldiers and the Culture of Caregiving in Britain during the Great War* (Manchester: Manchester University Press, 2005); Carden-Coyne, *Politics of Wounds*; Joanna Bourke, *Dismembering the Male: Men's Bodies, Britain and the Great War* (London: Reaktion Books, 1999).

81 Jane Brooks, *Negotiating Nursing British Army Sisters and Soldiers in the Second World War* (Manchester: Manchester University Press, 2018), p. 25.

82 *Ibid.*, p. 29.

83 Surkis, 'Sex, Sovereignty and Transnational Intimacies'.

84 Marie-Luce Desgrandchamps and Laure Humbert, 'From Dissident to Recogised Belligerent? The Free French and the Red Cross Movement, 1940–43', *French History*, 37:3 (2023), 273–293.

85 Jean Baillou (ed.), *Les Affaires Etrangères et le corps diplomatique français*, II (Paris: CNRS, 1984), p. 563.

86 Charlotte Faucher, *Propaganda, Gender and Cultural Power: Projections and Perceptions of France in Britain, c. 1880–1944* (Oxford: Oxford University Press, 2022), p. 175; Laure Humbert, 'Les "rivales" Mary Spears et Marguerite Catroux. Genre, Care et "scène humanitaire", 1940–1945', *Cahiers de la Méditerranée*, 109 (2024), 63–80. For an example of it in a relief committee, see Ivy Moore, 'Le charme féminin français'. Nantes, MAE, 787PO/1/10, Mrs Moore, presidente de l'association les amis de la France, coupure de presse.

87 Su Lin Lewis, 'Women, Hospitality and the Intimate Politics of International Socialism, 1955–1965', *Past and Present*, 24 April 2023.

88 Anupama Rao and Steven Pierce, 'Discipline and the Other Body. Humanitarianism, Violence and the Colonial Exception', in Steven Pierce and Anupama Rao (eds), *Discipline and the Other Body: Correction, Corporeality, Colonialism* (Durham, NC: Duke University Press, 2006), pp. 1–35.

89 AN, 382AP/32, Le medecin General Inspecteur A Sice à MM. Les Commissaires Nationaux Militaires, 20 August 1942.

90 Nicolas Truong (ed.), *Les penseurs de l'intime* (Paris: Coédition Editions de l'Aube/Le Monde, 2021), p. 61.

*Estrangement and intimacies: new perspectives* 57

91 Laure Humbert, 'Caring Under Fire across Three Continents: the Hadfield-Spears Ambulance, 1941–1945', *Social History of Medicine*, 36:2 (2023), 284–315.
92 Musée de l'Ordre de la Libération [MOL], Paul Guénon, Diary, 25 March 1942, p. 2.
93 Douzou, 'A Perilous History'.
94 Jean-Marie Guillon and François Marcot, 'Amours et sexualité', in François Marcot (ed.), *Dictionnaire historique de la Résistance* (Paris: Robert Laffon), pp. 917–918.
95 Enoh Meyomesse, *Marcel Eyidi Bevey: Un homme politique comme il n'en existe plus* (Paris: EdkBooks, 2019).
96 Pratt and Rosner, 'Introduction: The Global and the Intimate', in Rosner and Pratt (eds), *The Global and the Intimate*, pp. 1–28.

# 2

# Colonial medicine and 'Black strength' in the French colonies of Africa during the long Second World War

*Delphine Peiretti-Courtis*

During the week of Overseas France, which took place from 15 to 22 July 1941 and was inaugurated by Marshal Pétain in Vichy, the 'greatness' of the Empire was celebrated. Colonel Gilis, a military doctor, stressed the importance of France's colonial empire after the defeat, underlining the crucial role that colonial doctors played in the survival and prosperity of the colonies:

> Without colonial doctors, both military and political efforts are ineffective, which in turn means that without the help of our Corps, colonisation is bound to fail. Is this the moment to bring French people's attention, amid a disaster, to colonisation? Yes ... [the Empire] is our country's main reason for being part of a reshaped Europe, following the aftermath of June 1940.[1]

During the Second World War, colonial medicine found new sources of legitimacy. Colonial doctors, the majority of whom were incorporated into the French military health services, tried to reassert their crucial role in the colonies. After the defeat, France needed to demonstrate its power to the world. In this context, the defeated and discredited French army sought to reaffirm its legitimacy through its medical services. More than ever, French colonies were seen as reservoirs of raw materials and labour. Since the creation of the 'Senegalese Tirailleurs' Corps in 1857, the protection of colonised populations had been perceived as essential in the 'development' and 'pacification' of the colonies. The defeat and occupation led to a renewed emphasis on the importance of colonisation in medical journals, monographs and military reports. Maintaining in good health the population of the Empire, considered as an

## Colonial medicine and 'Black strength' 59

indispensable 'human resource', became an even more pressing priority for colonial doctors in the field.[2]

In the context of war, France could rely on the resources of its Empire. This was one of the political and military strategies at the beginning of the war in September 1939. The French adopted a defensive approach to protect the territory behind the Maginot Line, hoping that German resources would soon be exhausted while counting on the colonial resources of the British and French Empires, considered to be far superior. This then became a strategy for Vichy France, which considered that the Empire could supply destitute France and provide the occupier with raw materials. Finally, it was a strategy for de Gaulle's Free France, which saw it as a territorial base and a pool of men ready to defend the occupied country. In 1940, the Empire was divided. While most of the Empire remained loyal to Pétain and the Vichy government after the armistice, a handful of colonies, including French Equatorial Africa (A.E.F.) and Cameroon, joined the Free French movement of General de Gaulle.

The organisation of health services was maintained in both parts of the Empire, whether the authorities remained loyal to Pétain or joined the dissident de Gaulle's camp.[3] French West Africa only joined the Fighting French camp after the Allied landing in North Africa in 1942. In the early days of the war, there were approximately 165 military doctors, 34 civilian doctors, some 10 pharmacists and more than 180 African doctors who had graduated from the Dakar medical school, which had been set up in 1918 in French West Africa (A.O.F.). In A.E.F., on the Free French side, around a hundred European doctors were present with African doctors and nurses.[4] The Second World War led to various shortages, a diminution of doctors and a reduction in the supply of medicines, but the colonial health services nevertheless continued. At the same time, the Second World War also contributed to the emergence of different discourses about Black bodies, linked to African soldiers' involvement in the war and the Liberation, as Anthony Guyon has clearly shown in his major work on the Senegalese infantrymen.[5] The development of anti-colonialist thinking found new support in the United States and the Soviet Union and played an important role in the evolution of the discourses about colonised people.[6]

60     *The long Second World War, 1931–1953*

After the war, the French were confronted with the establishment of new public health structures, set up by international organisations such as the World Health Organization, which challenged the place and legitimacy of French military doctors in the field. As J. L. Pearson argues, the new competition between colonial medicine, the United Nations (UN) health system and humanitarian organisations had consequences for the implementation of new public health policies in Africa.[7] Indeed, this renewed competition led to a reaffirmation of the role of French colonial doctors in the preservation of Africans. But, as Deborah Neill and Guillaume Lachenal have shown, colonial medicine was marked from the outset by the idea of competition and concerns over the assertion of its legitimacy.[8] Nevertheless, during this period, French health authorities deployed more efforts to prove that sanitary efforts to 'save' local people were numerous.[9] They wanted to demonstrate to the wider world the success of the fight against tropical diseases and progress in the protection of African mothers and children.

This chapter addresses some key questions: How did the Second World War, the defeat and the new importance of the colonial Empire for the French nation lead to a profound transformation of medical discourses, policies and health practices towards Black bodies? How far did racial stereotypes constructed by science, medicine and anthropology in France, and by colonial doctors in Africa since the previous century, continue to appear in colonial discourses and representations, even when, following the Liberation of France in 1945, racial theories had been discredited in mainstream scientific discourses? In this chapter, I examine colonial administrators' representations and discourses of 'Black bodies', meaning those of the populations of Africa and in particular those of African soldiers, famously labelled *La force noire* ('Black force') by General Mangin in 1910. Historians have shed light on the history of the 'Senegalese Tirailleurs' and their contribution to France, both in metropolitan France and in the colonies.[10] They have examined colonial administrators' constructed categories of 'warrior races' and their impacts on the recruitment of colonial troops and in the French army.[11] For instance, the works of Megan Vaughan, Anderson Warwick or Guillaume Lachenal have shed light on the close links between colonial policies and medicine in different part of European empires,[12] by applying the Foucauldian concept of biopolitics to colonial medicine. The publications by

## Colonial medicine and 'Black strength' 61

J.P. Bado, P. Chakrabarty, D. Domergue-Cloarec, M. Echengerg, D. Headrick, M. Lyons, R. MacLeod, L. Milton and R. Packard are major studies in the field of health in the colonies, showing the birth of colonial medicine and its challenges.[13]

Contributing to this fruitful historiography, this chapter sheds new light on the close links between medicine, politics and the notion of race in the colonies during the long Second World War, understood here as from the late 1920s to the 1950s. Its aim is to consider the 'political use' of bodies that had been racialised by doctors since the last century, and to assess the extent to which the war led to a rupture in both representations and treatments of Black bodies. To do so, this chapter draws on medical literature, mainly produced by health services in the colonies, reports from colonial doctors, medical and anthropological monographs and directives issued by public authorities in mainland France. It unpacks various racial stereotypes and 'uses' of Black bodies during and after the war, and critically reviews various health projects implemented to ensure the 'survival' of African populations by colonial doctors.

### The Empire and its bodies

Colonial administrators often stressed that the colonies and their inhabitants were both a political and an economic asset. Emile Perrot, a military pharmacist, member of the Academy of Colonial Sciences and university professor, claimed in 1939:

> A terrible war is unleashed ... arguments in favour of developing our colonial domain in West Africa reinforced by events, because the need for accelerated production of raw materials as well as the need for a human contribution to the battlefront is imposed more violently than ever. Our soldiers, for the second time in twenty years, will have as companions in the struggle men of colour from different parts of the world.[14]

The early days of the war exacerbated anxieties about shortcomings in medical settings in French West Africa. The annual report of the A.O.F. health services in 1940 begins with: 'The events of 1940 had repercussions on the personnel of the Health Service', the main consequences of the war being a reduction in the 'number of Health Service officers handed over to the A.M.I. [Indigenous Medical Assistance, in existence since 1905]'.[15] The war was therefore exported to the

62      *The long Second World War, 1931–1953*

colonies, with a reduction in the number of medical personnel and difficulties in obtaining medical supplies.

The bombardment of Dakar on 23 and 25 September 1940, as well as the conflict between the Gaullist forces, who were seeking to seize Dakar and establish it as a Free French base, and the colonial authorities in Senegal and Western France, who remained loyal to Vichy, thus appear in the reports as major factors in the difficulties of the health services in French West Africa. However, the pre-war organisation of the health services, based on a network of health units reproducing the administrative division of the territory into circles and subdivisions, was maintained after 1940. Most of the doctors working in the African colonies belonged to the army. The medical services in the colonies were linked to the Inspectorate General of the French Health Service and the Ministry of the Colonies. Assigned to colonial and French troops during the fighting, they were also responsible for treating the colonised population as well as colonial administrators. A director of the Colonial Health Service was responsible for coordinating medical action in the territories. Colonial doctors were assigned to the main hospitals in colonial towns but also to more isolated infirmaries, ambulances or dispensaries. They were also responsible for making medical rounds in the 'bush', according to the principle of 'mobile medicine' defined by Dr Eugène Jamot, in the 1920s, and pursued during the war, with medical staff from the Indigenous Medical Assistance. Presented as a 'civilising' and 'humanitarian' work, the mission of colonial doctors was also essentially political and economic. Because of the fear of depopulation in Africa, which had arisen during the First World War and which was accentuated in the Second World War, they were considered to be the 'guardians of the black race'.[16] Doctors were thus given important missions: to determine the state of bodies and strength, to take care of colonised people and finally to recruit the best elements: soldiers and workers useful to the Empire. Doctors were seen as the central auxiliaries of the colonial enterprise.

African soldiers were described as an essential strength for France in this period of war. This 'Black strength' was a racial stereotype popularised by General Charles Mangin in 1910 to justify the use of 'Senegalese Tirailleurs' on European soil. This imagined and fantasised 'Black strength' was valued against the supposed vulnerability of the 'civilised' peoples of Europe. In the colonial

*Colonial medicine and 'Black strength'* 63

field, doctors looked for evidence of this robustness on Black bodies. Through their studies, they contributed to the dissemination of stereotypes about the physical strength of Africans, which, until the middle of the twentieth century, was said to be an innate racial characteristic but also a character acquired through culture, environment and way of life. Physical strength was also the revealer of unfailing health.[17] The 'strong and healthy' bodies of Africans constituted real assets for the French colonial project in various ways.

Taking care of the health of the 'colonised' was considered essential for the success of colonisation by French authorities, the minister of the colonies, colonial administrators, missionaries and doctors. The colonial world was unanimous. Beyond the usefulness of 'indigenous bodies' to increase the output within the colonies and to make the French Empire prosper, 'Black strength' offered another benefit, that of defending France, in the colonies but also on European soil. In his book *La Force Noire*, Charles Mangin attempts to legitimise the recruitment of African soldiers during the European wars, using racial stereotypes about the strength and robustness of Black bodies.[18] His proposed hierarchy of 'martial races' was based on racial theories created by medicine and racial anthropology in the previous century. This hierarchy significantly evolved during the First and Second World Wars.[19] More detailed classifications were drawn up, giving pride of place to certain peoples rather than others and justifying why certain 'races' were more suited to combat than others. As Eric Jennings has demonstrated, in 1943, directives from the military command in Cameroon indicated that 'mountain people' should mainly be recruited because they would be more adaptable in 'Saharan and Mediterranean' countries. These biological and climatic considerations, which had already been applied to Senegalese infantrymen posted to Europe during the First World War, illustrated the importance attached to the deployment of these men in a region with a climate close to their own.[20] The idea was to favour certain ethnic groups over others, such as the Bambaras in West Africa, who were considered to be more suited to combat, for reasons linked to their 'race' or environment.[21] The practice of recruitment was based on voluntary service, conscription and forced enlistments.[22] As the previous war had revealed the 'weaknesses' of African soldiers and called into question the myth of Black strength, travelling draft boards

64    *The long Second World War, 1931–1953*

were set up to conduct recruitment of soldiers in French African colonies.[23] A military officer headed the board, along with a civilian group administrator, clerks in charge of administrative documents and a military doctor responsible for recruiting soldiers according to strict standards.

To rationalise and facilitate the recruitment of soldiers but also of colonial workers, military doctors created specific indices. The aim was to effectively evaluate the physical strength of men and to enable better performance. During the first half of the twentieth century, colonial physicians' knowledge of anatomy and physiology made them 'experts' in the measurement and evaluation of bodies. As such, they became essential allies of colonisation. The physical value of men, and more particularly of conscripts, was quantified in France, for all men regardless of 'race', at the end of the nineteenth century with the creation of an index established by a military doctor, M. C. J. Pignet, in 1898.[24] In the colonies, conscripts were selected according to this index until a colonial doctor, Gustave Lefrou, considered that the physical characteristics of the 'black race' were not suitable for Pignet's index. He thought that the criteria for recruiting Black men could not be the same as those for white men. Lefrou therefore created, in 1931, a 'racial' index, specific to Black populations, the 'robusticity index'.[25] Beyond the 'scientific' interest of these indices for the science of human races, they had a pragmatic purpose: they were intended to improve the selection of strong men for the colonial effort, with a 'simple, standard and considered irrefutable' means, the robusticity index.[26] Both manpower and soldiers could therefore be recruited efficiently.[27]

While the robusticity index was used to recruit labour in French East Africa but also in French West Africa, recruitment that increased during the Second World War until the abolition of forced labour in 1946,[28] this index was also used to recruit men in the colonial troops during the interwar period[29] and the Second World War. The use of this recruitment method illustrated the transition from scientific theory to colonial practice and the central role played by colonial physicians in the 'use' of the bodies of the colonised. The value of African men was thus reduced to the economic value of their bodies. The body of the 'indigenous person' became a political and economic tool that contributed to the realisation of the political aims of the colonisers. In 1949, the doctor and anthropologist

*Colonial medicine and 'Black strength'*     65

from the *École de médecine coloniale du Pharo* [the Marseille colonial school], Léon Pales, mentioned the use of the Lefrou index in the recruitment of colonial soldiers during the Second World War. While he considered the limits of this index, he also emphasised the fact that the recruitment methods and requirements could have been modified or abandoned according to the need for men during the war.[30] Various considerations, linked to the ethnicity of individuals and their strength, which recruiters were supposed to evaluate using the Lefrou index, were left aside when circumstances of war or desertions of soldiers demanded larger contingents of men. The theory existed, but the practice often varied according to the needs linked to the war, as mentioned by Eric Jennings in relation to recruitment in Chad in 1942.[31]

### Saving the 'force noire' or the awareness of 'African' vulnerability

Selecting strong and robust bodies was perceived as necessary in the context of heightened anxieties about African vulnerability stemming from the discovery of diseases such as tuberculosis, which struck the 'Senegalese tirailleurs' in the First World War, and the development of discourses around the depopulation of Africa. Beyond this awareness linked to the arrival of African soldiers in Europe, various factors played a part in the emergence of this fear: epidemics of influenza, trypanosomiasis, plague and typhus, a wave of drought and poor harvests, high infant mortality and the consequences of the First World War on the colonies, which led to several thousand deaths in West Africa. The minister of colonies Albert Sarraut declared a health emergency in the 1920s. After having long defended the idea of African invulnerability, a vision inherited from slavery and reinforced by racial anthropology and medicine in the nineteenth century, 'Black strength' now had to be restored. Colonial doctors were given a health mission of the utmost importance: the African population had to be preserved to ensure the prosperity of the colonies.

From the First World War onwards, French medical elites considered that the 'Senegalese tirailleurs', weakened in Europe during the fighting or their confinement in camps, were illustrative of

66        *The long Second World War, 1931–1953*

a broader phenomenon. Discourses around 'African vulnerability' challenged the myth of the exceptional and innate strength of Africans. In a book entitled *Les Noirs*, published in 1919, Alphonse Séché, a writer and journalist, reflected on the gap between idealised representations of 'Black strength' and the perceived reality of colonial troops, which were sometimes made up of sickly individuals who had been too hastily recruited on the African continent. He referred to the notion of 'warrior races',[32] and seemed to regret the fact that these soldiers were not recruited according to racial characteristics and were not sufficiently prepared for combat. He also mentioned the 'resenegalisation' cures undergone by African soldiers in a hospital in Menton, after their mobilisation, before their return to Africa to allow for their gradual re-acclimatisation.[33] According to him, '[t]he cold [had] decimated them and the cannon deprived them of their means. In short, the Senegalese had gone bankrupt'.[34] This experience of 're-acclimatisation' and these considerations about 'Senegalese tirailleurs' in the First World War was central to the evolution of the conception and recruitment practices of soldiers during the Second World War. Selection became essential. Anthony Guyon examined the figure of the 'Senegalese infantrymen', who, in the discourse of officers, colonial administrators and doctors, were seen as valiant and courageous on the one hand and, on the other, as weakened by the fighting, illnesses, the context and the European climate.[35] As Claire Miot has demonstrated, military officials justified in 1944 the withdrawal of colonial soldiers, called 'blanchiement (whitening) campaigns', using climatic and biological arguments mentioned in medical texts dating from the nineteenth and early twentieth centuries, as well as the example of infantrymen weakened in the First World War. Indeed, the many warnings issued by doctors at the beginning of the century about the use of Black troops in Europe were later used as a pretext for the military's 'whitening campaigns' and the withdrawal of Black troops from battalions at the Liberation. When political interests prevailed, soldiers from the African continent were massively recruited to fight in Europe, regardless of doctors' recommendations;[36] on the other hand, when African soldiers had to be gradually removed from the battalions that liberated France in 1944, they were replaced by the Forces françaises de l'intérieur (FFI), with the argument of climate resistance. In order to 'whiten' the troops, the soldiers mentioned in

## Colonial medicine and 'Black strength' 67

the sources were most often 'white soldiers' who had to embody the French Resistance. In this context, the considerations expressed by doctors several decades earlier reappear in the writings of military leaders such as Marshal De Lattre de Tassigny or General de Gaulle in his *Memoirs*.[37] So, in their discourse, the deadly effects of the climate on African soldiers required their immediate repatriation. While military officials continued to refer to climatic arguments, doctors no longer seemed particularly concerned about the question of the acclimatisation of Black bodies in the 1940s. There are very few references to this subject in their writings. This is a question that had been widely addressed more than a century earlier at the Société d'Anthropologie de Paris by many scientists such as Boudin, Perrier and Lagneau. The debates had lasted several years, and the conclusions had been formalised before the end of the nineteenth century. It was recognised by the scientific community that populations of different races could acclimatise in other countries. They took the example of Black populations in the United States. Although the difficulties encountered by different 'races' could be numerous, linked to diseases or different climates, acclimatisation was nevertheless possible. At that time, it was less the climate that was questioned than other influences such as the psychological effects of 'uprooting', tuberculosis or nutrition.[38] Moreover, doctors did not seem to have been asked to justify the need for repatriation and therefore the 'whitening' of troops in 1944, but their arguments, which had already been used, were once again employed.

### Health and medicine in African colonies: issues for colonisation and war

In 1943, in *Le Noir d'Afrique* (The Black of Africa), the colonial doctor Gustave Lefrou wrote that '[t]he colonisation of this immense territory is subordinated above all to the human factor … Africa is unfortunately a continent that is being depopulated, the Black race, a race that is dying.' He then raised the question of '[h]ow [one should] make Blacks if we do not know who they are?'.[39] His book demonstrates how the preservation of the 'Black force', which was now considered vulnerable, became an urgent concern for the prosperity of France.

68    *The long Second World War, 1931–1953*

During the first half of the twentieth century, 'making Blacks' meant above all ensuring the protection of mothers and the survival of children, but also effectively combating deadly epidemics in order to preserve the men and women who constituted an indispensable 'human resource pool' for colonisation. This colonial health policy was implemented through different poles, organisations and structures from the beginning of the twentieth century. Treatments against sleeping sickness were administered to the populations with the help of 'bush tours' organised in the 1920s in Cameroon by Dr Jamot and his mobile hygiene teams, a fight that was continued by Dr Gaston Muraz in the 1930s to 1940s and during the Second World War. A vaccine against yellow fever was developed in 1932 at the Pasteur Institute in Dakar by several 'pastorians' such as Jean Laigret. The pastorians considered that in order to overcome the disease and reduce mortality in Africa, it was necessary to act on individuals through prophylactic treatments to protect them from various viruses and parasitic diseases. This sanitary struggle was therefore actively pursued during the long Second World War and the results were set out in annual reports sent to the health services in metropolitan France to show the effectiveness and above all the usefulness of medicine in the colonies. The annual reports of the direction of health services to the colonies, for both the A.O.F. and the A.E.F., whose head was Adolphe Sicé from 1940, general physician of the Colonial Health Service and eminent member of the Gaullist movement during the war, give us an indication of the main health challenges facing the French Empire during the Second World War. The issues were not specifically linked to the war, the health emergencies remaining the same as those which existed before the war. Across the empire, colonial authorities nevertheless needed to compensate for the inadequacies and difficulties linked to the war context, such as the reduction in medical staff, organisational problems within services and supply difficulties. The fight against major endemics such as sleeping sickness remained the priority, addressed by Muraz, in A.E.F., A.O.F., Togo and Cameroon,[40] but also the fight against infant mortality throughout the colonies, a fight led in France a few decades earlier and by the World Health Organization after the war.

African motherhood became a real colonial issue in the interwar period. The Black woman, who had been elevated to the rank of

## Colonial medicine and 'Black strength' 69

model mother during the nineteenth century, notably for her supposed closeness to nature, was now denigrated and held responsible for infant mortality. Colonial physicians considered that women's work, supposed ignorance of the rules of hygiene and nutritional deficiencies were responsible for the high mortality rate among young children. According to them, mothers needed to be educated and civilised. Moreover, this colonial mission continued the civilising logic stated by Jules Ferry in 1885 and supported by many physicians such as Dr Perrot in 1939. The French colonial project was conceived as a humanitarian project with an assumed economic benefit: 'for the greater glory of France, effective protector from now on of black childhood ... this is a humanitarian work including a benefit for the tutelary nation which, indeed, is eager, for various imperious reasons, to see the populating of its vast African domain increase'.[41] Humanitarian mission and civilising mission thus become closely linked and indistinctly employed. In many reports entitled 'Protection de la maternité et de l'enfance indigène dans les colonies françaises' (Protection of Indigenous Maternity and Childhood in the French Colonies) since the 1940s, the regular monitoring, protection and consultation of mothers and newborns were presented as one of the main missions of physicians in the French colonies.[42] The infantilisation of African mothers was permanent and this paternalism justified surveillance and coercion. In the 1960s, pamphlets on the 'Education of African Women' written by 'bush doctors' testified to the persistence of the 'civilising' and paternalistic spirit of the colonialists at the dawn of independence.[43]

The conferences on obstetrics organised in Brazzaville in 1944 discussed the issue of 'maternal and child health; in Africa and claimed to take stock of progress made. The successes of colonial medicine in the field of indigenous maternity were highlighted in these conferences. The aim was to legitimise the actions and request additional resources to open dispensaries and maternity hospitals. The doctors boasted that they had succeeded in preserving health in the colonies during the war in France, for women: 'The year 1940 saw the continuation, despite difficulties of all kinds due to the state of war and armistice and to the blockade, of the work of protecting indigenous mothers and children in the various territories of the Empire.'[44] Maternal and child protection was one of the most important components of medical action in the colonies during this

# 70    *The long Second World War, 1931–1953*

period and, for medical and colonial authorities, it embodied an aspect of France's civilising mission. It also reflected the alleged success of the colonial enterprise. For the missionary doctor Louis-Paul Aujoulat and the colonial troops doctor-lieutenant Georges Olivier in 1946: 'The future of the black race is linked, in part, to its numerical development. This will be achieved, on the one hand, by protection against the various endemic diseases (purely medical work) and, on the other hand, by the development of the birth rate; this shows the importance of obstetrics for blacks.'[45]

In the middle of the twentieth century, colonial doctors presented themselves as the heirs of those who had worked since the nineteenth century to protect the health of the colonised people. Moreover, the civilising mission that justified the colonial conquest presented colonial medicine as social and humanitarian. In 1941, Dr Gilis described the A.M.I. during the Overseas France Week as follows: 'the social and profoundly humanitarian work that the Assistance Médicale Indigène represents'.[46] Created in 1905, it was promoted and presented as one of the most concrete achievements of the civilising work accomplished by military doctors, as demonstrated by Alice Concklin in her book *A Mission to Civilize: The Republican Idea of Empire in France and West Africa 1895–1930*.[47] Colonial doctors presented themselves as the only ones who could protect the populations. Their goal was to highlight the long past of their health action in the colonies in the face of new humanitarian organisations.

Colonial medicine gradually took on the characteristics of humanitarian medicine. For the World Health Organization, humanitarian medicine is, among other things, humanitarian assistance to victims of natural disasters and emergency situations. For the humanitarian doctor, this involves treating populations in a crisis context, setting up prevention and care development programmes, and training on-site medical teams. The end of the Second World War saw the birth of numerous humanitarian associations. While colonial medicine became 'cooperation medicine' after independence, the 'humanitarian' tone was given to these military doctors from the nineteenth century with the formulation of civilising ideology as an argument justifying colonisation. However, after the war, the presence of the World Health Organization, along with other humanitarian organisations, threatened the medical ambitions of French colonial power.

## Colonial medicine and 'Black strength' 71

The provision of medical care now needed to be shared. Colonial medicine defended the pursuit of its mission and the protection of its 'protégés'. The rhetoric of development replaced that of civilisation. Guillaume Lachenal and Bertrand Taithe studied the case of the famous missionary doctor Louis-Paul Aujoulat and the interdependence between religion, medicine and politics in the colonial field at the time of the development of humanitarianism in continuity with the colonial period.[48] Several major studies have shown that humanitarianism, which was born in a colonial context, had difficulty in freeing itself, at least in its first decades, from the paternalistic prism of colonial medicine.[49] The notion of development aid was linked to the 'civilising mission'. Jessica Lynn Pearson demonstrates that, in the face of this new competition, one of the key objectives of French health policies was to reassert France's power and to prevent international organisations from 'interfering' in the French colonies. In particular, she explains that UN experts wanted to use international health programmes to free colonised peoples from the control of and dependence towards their colonisers, which were also imposed by means of a health trusteeship. The French, for their part, hoped to deepen their control over the territories and their populations by taking over the healthcare of the inhabitants.[50]

The ideological anti-colonialism of the United States, the USSR and the UN, which proclaimed the right of peoples to self-determination in 1945, was a threat to colonising countries like France. The legitimacy of colonisation had to be reaffirmed.

Colonial authorities, and in particular doctors, who were the key agents of the colonial enterprise, thus attempted to demonstrate the necessity of their mission in the face of the upheavals that shook the Empire, both inside and out. After the war, Dr Marcel Vaucel, inspector of the Pasteur Institutes and director of the health service at the Ministry of Overseas France created in 1946, defended the central role of colonial doctors in the protection of the colonised people while recognising their new aspirations. This modest recognition of the claims of the colonised was also seen as an essential guarantee of the maintenance of colonial power, as the creation of the French Union in 1946 shows.[51] While France tried to adapt itself to the post-war international context and to the demands of the colonised, the challenge was above all to adapt in order to maintain its hold on its colonies. The central political role played

72      *The long Second World War, 1931–1953*

by Vaucel at the time of the war embodies the different missions – medical, political and military – that some doctors carried out in the colonies during this period. In Cameroon in the summer of 1940, he joined the Free French as director of the territorial health service in Cameroon. Together with Adolphe Sicé and other dissident doctors, he helped created a military health service for Free French troops. As Guillaume Lachenal has shown, he also supported the experiment conducted by Dr David in the Haut-Nyong region.[52] Director of the health service for Free French Africa from 1942, he then became director of the health service for the colonies after the reunification of the Empire under the banner of Free France in 1943. He played a central role in the Brazzaville conference, highlighting the health challenges facing the Empire and seeking to continue and expand the fight against various tropical endemics that had begun before the war.

Public health programmes have continued to focus on the issue of maternal and child protection, through the fight against infant mortality but also through new studies and actions in the field of food, a central pillar of humanitarian aid.

### Food, health and race

The international directives issued by the UN after its creation to combat malnutrition and undernourishment in the so-called 'under-developed countries' had an impact on the thinking of French scientists and the health policies implemented in the French colonies. The question of food and the preservation of a nutritional balance became a global concern in the post-war period. Many UN experts were convinced that political stability depended on the health of the population. The Food and Agriculture Organization of the United Nations (FAO) was founded in October 1945, drawing on an earlier international venture dating from 1904 as the International Institute of Agriculture. In this context, French experts wanted to keep their status of expert in their 'own' territories and actively intervened to avoid external interference.

Since the 1920s to 1930s, the question of nutrition had been of particular interest to race scientists, physicians and anthropologists. In parallel with the continuing interest in racial, biological and innate characteristics, studies on cultural, dietary and climatic factors emerged to explain and determine the share of innate and acquired factors in the physical and moral differences between peoples. Sociology, cultural anthropology, ethnography and psychology, which emerged at the turn of the twentieth century, contributed to changing the way we look at bodies and otherness. In this context, the question of the environment and external factors, such as diet, became central to qualifying the role played by the innate factor in the human constitution, in the intellectual, physical and moral capacities of beings. In January 1937, national surveys on diet were launched in France, in a context of strong development of research in the field of nutrition.[53] The objective was to evaluate the nutritional characteristics of foods and eating habits with a view to health and education, but also with the aim of advancing scientific and medical research. It was at this time that a doctor proposed a project for the physical and moral transformation of races, in particular Black African populations, through food from a eugenic perspective. In his article in the *Bulletin of the Society of Exotic Pathology*, Dr Alexandre Gauducheau, a renowned colonial doctor, proposed a 'project ... of exotic experimentation', summarised by the question 'Is it possible to transform human races through "food and hygiene?"'[54]

The aim of scientific studies was to understand the effects of food on human constitution and physiology, but investigations on the food issue also had a pragmatic interest, that of taking charge of African health in the face of the malnutrition and undernourishment experienced by certain colonised populations. As Vincent Bonnecase explains,[55] that attention and particular focus on the colonies and the colonising countries became even more important in the post-war context, with the creation of international institutions, because the colonising powers had to justify to the world that they were concerned about the living conditions of the peoples they had placed under their control. The new international organisations requested information on the nutritional status of the populations, and periodic reports had to be submitted on the food situation in the colonised territories. In this context, the 'Investigation organization for the anthropological study of the indigenous populations of A.O.F. (food and nutrition)' (Organisme d'enquête pour l'étude anthropologique des populations indigènes de l'AOF) was created

74    *The long Second World War, 1931–1953*

in 1946. The ambivalence of this undertaking is well illustrated by Vincent Bonnecase. This 'anthropological mission' quantified food intake in the African colonies but continued to use racial anthropology in its study procedures, explaining food behaviour through the racial prism. Léon Pales, a famous military physician and anthropologist, was the head of this Mission. Numerous publications of the results of this Mission showed the interweaving of ancient anthropometric and raciological methods with more recent research on nutrition and the effects of acquired cultural and environmental traits on bodies.[56] For example, the doctor and anthropologist Léon Pales talked about the fact that the 'tirailleur' (African soldier) has evolved with the war, contact with Europeans and a different diet:

> The tirailleur improves his physical condition during service, much more than if he had stayed at home. In his unit, he finds a regular and relatively well-balanced life, which is in any case superior, in quality and quantity, to that of his fellow soldiers who stayed in the village. The tirailleur thus becomes, physically, a test of what could be.[57]

He was thus responding to the hypotheses formulated a decade earlier by his predecessor, Dr Gauducheau. According to Léon Pales, African soldiers reflected what 'the material improvement of life, essentially food and nutrition, is likely to bring to African populations'. While the notion of race took a back seat to culture in shaping bodies, the idea of a beneficial civilisation remained omnipresent at the end of the war and on the eve of independence.

In the first half of the twentieth century, food, individual psychology and environment were the main cultural factors for understanding human diversity. At the same time, the pseudo-racial science of the late nineteenth century continued to exist, and new focus on hereditary and blood characteristic breathed fresh life into raciology. Following the discovery of blood groups at the beginning of the twentieth century, interest in blood and its racial characteristics was revived. More than a thousand articles on sero-anthropology were published in scientific journals in the 1930s and 1940s, based on the cooperation of colonial physicians and laboratory researchers. A wave of blood sampling was carried out in the colonies during this period. The presence of groups of soldiers in the colonies, but also in France, with the war context, was an opportunity for anthropological research. They were supposed to represent their 'race'. A few

## Colonial medicine and 'Black strength' 75

drops of blood on a slide was enough to detect the blood group of people. Léon Pales continued his research on the racial, anthropometric and serological characteristics of peoples, even after the concept of biological race had been invalidated. In 1945, he provided the conclusions of a study carried out by a colleague using the blood of several Sudanese tirailleurs from West Africa who had been displaced to an environment very different from their original one: France. This study was conducted at the École du Pharo at the end of the 1930s.[58] The results of the blood tests of the 140 'Senegalese tirailleurs' analysed forced Dr Pales to question the racial character of the blood components because the climate, food and lifestyle modified the innate characteristics. It was impossible to determine race through the study of blood. However, other criteria were brought to light, such as diet and its influences. These doctors' conclusions highlighted the importance of acquired characteristics in human diversity in the middle of the twentieth century. Despite the discourse that developed in Europe against the concept of race after 1945, this did not prevent scientific research on race from continuing in the African colonies. Thus, there was no clear break in race science after the Second World War and the condemnation of race by scientists meeting under the aegis of UNESCO after 1945.[59]

Studies on the racial properties of blood were carried out by the Pasteur Institutes in A.O.F., A.E.F. and Indochina until the midtwentieth century. The physician-captain Robert Koerber continued to examine the distribution of blood groups according to race in A.O.F. in 1948, in parallel with Pales' research, by observing nearly four hundred men, Ouolofs, Malinkés, Bambaras and Peuls, also concluding, after a great deal of research, that it was difficult to establish a precise correlation between ethnic groups and blood groups due to the numerous crossbreedings.[60] The diversity that existed within African territories was thus demonstrated, as were the limits of this technique – sero-anthropology – in a classificatory sense. In the 1950s, this unwavering desire to determine the racial markers of individuals faded and research on food was directed towards investigations solely related to the health of populations and the fight against malnutrition. In 1953, the former 'Mission anthropologique' became the 'Office for Research on African Food and Nutrition (Organisme de Recherches sur l'Alimentation et la Nutrition africaines)' (ORANA).

76 *The long Second World War, 1931–1953*

Despite the scientific changes and the changing political context in the years 1945–1950, the quest for the pure biological identity of human groups continued in the minds of many doctors, some of whom participated in the UNESCO conferences on race. Dr Claude Chippaux still stated in 1948 that 'blood is the reflection of all individual or racial variations'.[61] The war had repercussions for the organisation of colonial health services. Although it contributed to the establishment of new health organisations, such as the World Health Organization, it did not mean that colonial doctors disappeared. The war helped to change the conception and representation of the colonised body. But it did not eliminate racial stereotypes. Research into 'human races' is continuing, with new interpretations focusing more on cultural but also genetic factors. War and science sometimes met, but sometimes evolved in parallel ways. Although interest in studies on race diminished in the medical literature after independence, racial prejudices concerning the bodies and minds of 'Africans', which were still essentialised, persisted. In the book *Afrique noire, terre inconnue. La croisière noire de la santé* (1951), with a preface by Léopold Sédar Senghor and written by André. Gautier-Walter, there were several references to the arrival of a new period; ethnocentrism and racism were explicitly condemned and racial equality was proclaimed. However, in what was presented as a 'health' and 'humanitarian' expedition, with the distribution of several 'tons of medicine', the paternalism that was characteristic of colonial medicine persisted:

> Socially speaking, the blacks must recognise that the West is playing, for a long time to come, the role of 'father' to a young boy who needs to be awakened to certain forms of modern life … It is a sort of 'puberty crisis' that Africa is going through. The child can be in no way inferior to his parents.[62]

This paternalistic and inferiorising view, apparently unconscious on the part of its author, reveals that if the moral, ideological, scientific and political context was certainly accompanied by important ruptures in the perception of African populations, humanitarianism and 'cooperation' sometimes replaced colonial medicine without any profound change in the mentalities of the doctors present in the field. The military doctors who belonged to the École du Pharo at the time of colonial medicine were often the same ones who later belonged to the medicine attached to 'international cooperation' perceived as humanitarian medicine, such as Claude Chippaux, a

## Colonial medicine and 'Black strength'

famous military doctor, surgeon and professor of anthropology. The mission of caring for the Other, already present at the time of colonisation, persisted, and if the category of race disappeared little by little, the hierarchical relationship that was present at the time of colonisation melted into a new climate but did not disappear. This scientific, medical and anthropological research also had a political and economic purpose a few years after the war. In 1954, André Mayer, a professor at the College of France and member of the Academy of Medicine, who was behind the 1937 national food survey, reaffirmed French responsibility in Africa in a book by the physician Léon Pales, in the international context of the United Nations.[63] He also reaffirmed the importance of preserving, caring for and feeding African populations for the prosperity of colonisation, while acting as a spokesperson for the colonial thinking of the time:

> We don't want to leave these lands unproductive. We want to 'enhance' them and use the methods we have invented to do so. But who will implement these methods? We cannot do it alone. And how could sick, malnourished and ignorant populations do it without us? One cannot 'enhance' a part of the world without 'enhancing' the people who occupy it.[64]

This 'Black strength', and its study by doctors, therefore remained essential in the 1950s, at the end of the long Second World War, in order to continue to 'develop' the colonies and thus participate in France's 'greatness'. The humanitarian, sanitary and civilising mission of colonisation remained an ideal supported by many actors in the colonial system after the war and the economic and political objective of medical action in the colonies remained strongly present. For Marshal De Lattre de Tassigny or Adolphe Sicé, it was French physicians who enabled the 'black race' to survive and it was for this reason, and as a way of thanking the 'Fatherland' (French homeland), that the 'tirailleurs' defended France during the two world wars.[65] The medical, civilising and humanitarian work therefore had an economic and military counterpart. While racial anthropology continued to influence the way bodies were conceived after 1945, racism was condemned in medical writings, but this did not prevent paternalistic reflexes and the idea of 'European superiority' from continuing to spread insidiously in the minds, discourses and practices of so-called cooperative medicine or humanitarian medicine, which succeeded colonial medicine.

78     *The long Second World War, 1931–1953*

## Notes

1 Louis Gilis, 'La participation du Corps de Santé colonial à la semaine de la France d'Outre-mer', in *Médecine tropicale: Revue du corps de santé colonial* (Marseille: Ecole d'application du service de santé des troupes coloniales, 1941), p. 175.

2 Jacques Cantier and Éric T. Jennings (eds), *L'Empire colonial sous Vichy* (Paris: Odile Jacob, 2004); Éric T. Jennings, *La France libre fut africaine* (Paris: Perrin, 2014).

3 Guillaume Lachenal, *Le Médecin qui voulut être roi. Sur les traces d'une utopie coloniale* (Paris: Seuil, 2017).

4 Mody Kanté, *L'école de médecine de Dakar. Creuset de la formation d'une élite médicale africaine (1918–années 1950)* (Paris: L'Harmattan, 2023); Pascale Barthélémy, *Africaines et diplômées à l'époque coloniale (1918–1957)* (Rennes: Presses universitaires de Rennes, 2010).

5 Anthony Guyon, *Les tirailleurs sénégalais, de l'indigène au soldat de 1857 à nos jours* (Paris: Perrin, 2022).

6 Robert Gildea, *L'Esprit impérial. Passé colonial et politiques du présent* (Paris: Passés Composés, 2020).
   J. P. Daughton, 'Behind the Imperial Curtain: International Humantiarian Efforts and the Critique of French Colonialism in the Interwar Years', *French Historical Studies*, 34:3 (2011).

7 Jessica L. Pearson, *The Colonial Politics of Global Health: France and the United Nations in Postwar Africa* (Cambridge, MA: Harvard University Press, 2018).

8 Deborah Neill, *Networks in Tropical Medicine: Internationalism, Colonialism, and the Rise of a Medical Specialty, 1890–1930* (Stanford, CA: Stanford University Press, 2012); Lachenal, *Le Médecin qui voulut être roi*.

9 Delphine Peiretti-Courtis, *Corps noirs et médecins blancs: la fabrique du préjugé racial XIXe-XXe siècles* (Paris: La Découverte, 2021).

10 Guyon, *Les tirailleurs sénégalais*.
   Eric T. Jennings, *Free French Africa in World War II: The African Resistance* (Cambridge: Cambridge University Press, 2015); Cantier and Jennings, *L'Empire colonial sous Vichy*; Myron Echenberg, *Les tirailleurs sénégalais en Afrique Occidentale Française (1857–1960)* (Paris: Karthala, 2009).
   Jean-François Mouragues, *Soldats de la république. Les tirailleurs sénégalais dans la tourmente. France mai-juin 1940* (Paris: L'Harmattan, 2010).
   Martin Mourre, *Thiaroye 1944. Histoire et mémoire d'un massacre colonial* (Rennes: Presses universitaires; Baltimore, MD: de Rennes, 2017).

## Colonial medicine and 'Black strength'    79

11 Richard S. Fogarty, *Race and War in France: Colonial Subjects in the French Army, 1914–1918* (Baltimore, MD: Johns Hopkins University Press, 2008); Antoine Champeaux, Éric Deroo and János Riesz, *Forces noires des puissances coloniales européennes* (Paris: Lavauzelle, 2009); Claire Miot, 'Le retrait des tirailleurs sénégalais de la Première Armée française en 1944. Hérésie stratégique, bricolage politique ou conservatisme colonial?' *Vingtième Siècle: Revue d'histoire*, 125:1 (2015), 77–89; Stéphanie Soubrier, *Races guerrières. Enquête sur une catégorie impériale. 1850–1918* (Paris: CNRS, 2023).

12 Warwick Anderson, *Colonial Pathologies, American Tropical Medicine, Race and Hygiene in the Philippines* (Durham: Duke University Press, 2006); Guillaume Lachenal, *Le Médecin qui voulut être roi. Sur les traces d'une utopie colonial* (Paris: Seuil, 2017); Megan Vaughan, *Curing Their Ills: Colonial Power and African Illness* (Cambridge: Polity Press, 1991).

13 Jean-Paul Bado, *Médecine coloniale et grandes épidémies en Afrique* (Paris: Karthala, 1996); Pratik Chakrabarti, *Medicine and Empire, 1600–1960* (New York: Palgrave Macmillan, 2014); Danielle Domergue-Cloarec, *La santé en Côte d'Ivoire, 1905–1958* (Toulouse: Publications de l'Université de Toulouse le Mirail, 1986); Myron Echenberg, *Black Death, White Medicine: Bubonic Plague and the Politics of Public Health in Colonial Senegal, 1914–1945* (Portsmouth: Heinemann, 2002), Daniel R. Headrick, *The Tools of Empire: Technology and European Imperialism in the Nineteenth Century* (New York: Oxford University Press, 1981); Maryinez Lyons, *The Colonial Disease: A Social History of Sleeping Sickness in Northern Zaïre 1900–1940* (Cambridge: Cambridge University Press, 1992); Roy Macleod and Lewis Milton (eds), *Disease, Medicine and Empire: Perspectives on Western Medicine and the Experience of European Expansion* (London: Routledge, 1988); Randall Packard, *The Making of a Tropical Disease: A Short History of Malaria* (Baltimore: Johns Hopkins University Press, 2007).

14 Émile Perrot, *Où en est l'Afrique Occidentale Française? Mission en Côte d'Ivoire, Haute-Guinée, Soudan, Sénégal* (Paris: Larose éditeurs, 1939).

15 Archives nationales du Sénégal, fonds A.O.F., Rapport annuel du Service de Santé, 1940.

16 Gustave Lefrou, *Le Noir d'Afrique. Antropo-biologie et raciologie* (Paris: Payot, 1943).

17 Léon Pales, 'Physiologie comparative des races humaines. Les constituants biochimiques du sang des Noirs soudanais occidentaux transplantés en France', *Bulletins de la Société d'Anthropologie de Paris*, 6:9 (1945), 114–121.

# 80    *The long Second World War, 1931–1953*

18  Charles Mangin, *La force noire* (Paris: Hachette, 1910); Fogarty, *Race and War in France*; Soubrier, *Races guerrières*; Vincent Joly, 'Races guerrières' et masculinité en contexte colonial. Approche historiographique, *Clio*, 33 (2011), 139–156.

19  Julie Le Gac and Nicolas Patin, *Guerres mondiales. Le désastre et le deuil. 1914–1945* (Paris: Armand Colin, 2022), pp. 103–131; Julie Le Gac, 'Races guerrières', *Encyclopédie d'histoire numérique de l'Europe* [en ligne], https://ehne.fr/fr/node/21460 (accessed 11 December 2020); Frédéric Garan and Jean-François Klein, 'Le "soldat indigène": un auxiliaire indispensable aux empires, XIXe-XXe siècles', *Revue Historique des Armées*, 306:3 (2022), 3–8.

20  Eric T. Jennings, *La France libre fut africaine* (Paris: Perrin, 2014), pp. 147–178.

21  Soubrier, *Races guerrières*.

22  Danielle Domergue-Cloarec, 'Une histoire en partage: les tirailleurs sénégalais dans la Première Guerre mondiale', *Humanisme*, 305: 4 (2014), 95–99; Guyon, *Les tirailleurs sénégalais*; Cantier and Jennings, *L'Empire colonial sous Vichy*; Jennings, *La France libre fut africaine*.

23  Alphonse Séché, *Les Noirs (d'après les documents officiels)* (Paris: Payot et Cie, 1919), pp. 17–21.

24  M. C. J Pignet, 'Valeur numérique de l'homme', *Bulletin médical* (s.l., 1898).

25  Gustave Lefrou, 'Un nouvel indice de robusticité chez les Noirs', *Bulletins de la Société de Pathologie exotique*, vol. 24 (Paris: Masson, 1931).

26  Henri Sergent, 'Contribution à l'étude d'un nouvel indice de robusticité chez les Noirs (indice de Lefrou)', *Annales de médecine et de pharmacie coloniales*, no. 30 (Paris: Imprimerie nationale, 1932), p. 493; Pierre Millous, 'Le coefficient de robustesse ou indice Pignet chez les Noirs de la côte occidentale d'Afrique', *Journal de la Société des africanistes*, 3 (1933), 57–72.

27  Séverin Abbatucci, *Médecins coloniaux* (Paris: Editions Larose, 1928), p. 82; Jules Guiart, Charles Garin and Marcel Léger, *Précis de médecine coloniale. Maladies des pays chauds* (Paris: Librairie J.B. Baillière et Fils, 1929), p. 391; Loiselet Thilliez, *Bréviaire médical à l'usage des missionnaires et des coloniaux* (Paris: Vigot frères éditeurs, 1930); Brau Paul, *Trois siècles de médecine coloniale française* (Paris: Vigot frères éditeurs, 1931), p. 194.

28  Babacar Fall, *Le travail forcé en Afrique Occidentale Française, 1900–1945* (Paris: Karthala, 1993).

29  Dr Chaigneau, 'Application dans un bataillon de Sénégalais du nouvel indice de robusticité pour Noirs', *Annales de médecine et de pharmacie coloniales*, no. 29 (Paris: Imprimerie nationale, 1931), pp. 652–661.

# Colonial medicine and 'Black strength'  81

30 Léon Pales and Marie Tassinde deSaint-Péreuse, 'Raciologie comparative des populations de l'A.O.F. [I. Parallèle anthropométrique succinct (stature) des militaires et des civils]', *Bulletins et Mémoires de la Société d'anthropologie de Paris*, 9th Series, Volume 10, fascicule 4–6 (1949), p. 193.

31 Jennings, *La France libre fut africaine*, pp. 147–178.

32 Fogarty, *Race and War in France*; Soubrier, *Races guerrières*; Joly, ' "Races guerrières" et masculinité en contexte colonial'.

33 Alphonse Séché, 'Les Noirs sur la Côte d'Azur: deux hôpitaux de Sénégalais', *La Revue hebdomadaire*, 29 (1916), 370–383; Elizabeth Rechniewski, 'Resénégalisation and the Representation of Black African Troops during World War One', in Ben Wellings and Shanti Sumartojo (eds), *Commemorating Race and Empire in The First World War Centenary* (Aix-en-Provence: Presses universitaires de Provence, 2018), pp. 79–91.

34 Séché, *Les Noirs (d'après les documents officiels)*, pp. 20–21.

35 Guyon, *Les tirailleurs sénégalais*.

36 Charles-Victor Berger, 'Considérations hygiéniques sur les tirailleurs sénégalais', *Archives de médecine navale*, no. 14 (Paris: J.-B. Baillière, 1870), p. 450; Gustave Reynaud, 'L'armée coloniale au point de vue de l'hygiène pratique', *Archives de médecine navale et coloniale*, no. 58 (Paris: Octave Doin, 1892).
Jean-Marie Gravot, 'Hygiène générale. Morbidité et mortalité des troupes originaires des colonies (tirailleurs sénégalais, malgaches, indochinois),' *Annales de médecine et de pharmacie coloniales*, no. 24 (Paris: Imprimerie nationale, 1926), p. 207.

37 Quoted in Guyon, *Les tirailleurs sénégalais*, pp. 260–262.

38 François Toullec, 'La tuberculose des Sénégalais', *Annales de médecine et de pharmacie coloniales*, no. 29 (Paris: Imprimerie nationale, 1931), pp. 635–652; Laurence, 'L'invasion primitive tuberculeuse chez le tirailleur sénégalais', *Annales de médecine et de pharmacie coloniales*, no. 30 (Paris: Imprimerie nationale, 1932), pp. 516–531.
René Martial, 'Contribution à l'étude de l'alimentation du tirailleur sénégalais en Afrique occidentale française', *Annales de médecine et de pharmacie coloniales*, no. 29 (Paris: Imprimerie nationale, 1931), p. 532.

39 Lefrou, *Le Noir d'Afrique*, p. 16.

40 Gaston Muraz, 'Lutte contre la maladie du sommeil en AOF et au Togo', *Académie des Sciences Coloniales* (1943).

41 Perrot, *Où en est l'Afrique Occidentale Française?* pp. 394–444, at p. 444.

42 Anne Hugon, 'L'historiographie de la maternité en Afrique subsaharienne', *Clio. Histoire, femmes et sociétés*, 21 (2005), 212–229;

# 82

*The long Second World War, 1931–1953*

Anne Hugon, *Être mère en situation coloniale* (Paris: Éditions de la Sorbonne, 2020).

43 L. Aubry, 'L'éducation de la femme africaine,' *Journées africaines de pédiatrie*, Dakar, 1960.

44 Médecin-colonel Giordani, 'Protection de la maternité et de l'enfance indigènes pendant l'année 1940', in Médecin-colonel Le Gall (ed.), *La Situation sanitaire de l'Empire français pendant l'année 1940* (Paris: Charles Lavauzelle et Cie, 1943), p. 519.

45 Louis Aujoulat and Georges Olivier, 'L'obstétrique chez les Yaoundé', in *Médecine Tropicale*, no. 3 (Marseille: Ecole d'Application du Service de Santé des Troupes Coloniales, 1946), p. 159.

46 Gilis, 'La participation du Corps de Santé colonial à la semaine de la France d'Outre-mer', p. 175.

47 Alice Concklin, *A Mission to Civilize: The Republican Idea of Empire in France and West Africa, 1895–1939* (Stanford, CA: Stanford University, 1997).

48 Guillaume Lachenal and Bertrand Taithe, 'Une généalogie missionnaire et coloniale de l'humanitaire: le cas Aujoulat au Cameroun, 1935–1973', *Le Mouvement Social*, 227:2 (2009), 45–63.

49 Michael Barnett, *Empire of Humanity: A History of Humanitarianism* (Ithaca, NY: Cornell University Press, 2011); Marie-Luce Desgrandchamps, 'En quête de légitimité. Le Comité international de la Croix-Rouge et l'Afrique durant les années 1960', *Monde(s)*, 19:1 (2021), 221–239; Bronwen Everill and Josiah Kaplan, *The History and Practice of Humanitarian Intervention and Aid in Africa* (Basingstoke: Palgrave Macmillan, 2013); Didier Fassin, *La raison humanitaire. Une histoire morale du temps présent* (Paris: Le Seuil, 2010); Irène Herrmann, *L'humanitaire en question* (Paris: Éditions du Cerf, 2018); Bernard Hours, 'Les ONG: outils et contestation de la globalisation', *Journal des anthropologues* (2003), 94–95, https://shs.cairn.info/revue-journal-des-anthropologues-2003-3-page-13?lang=fr(accessed 15 May 2023); Philippe. Ryfman, *Une Histoire de l'humanitaire* (Paris: La Découverte, 2008).

50 Pearson, *The Colonial Politics of Global Health*.

51 Médecin-général Vaucel, 'Médecine aux colonies et médecins des troupes coloniales', *Revue des troupes coloniales* (1946), p. 52.

52 Lachenal, *Le Médecin qui voulut être roi*.

53 Thomas Depecker, Anne Lhuissier and Aurélie Maurice (eds), *La juste mesure. Une sociologie historique des normes alimentaires* (Rennes: Presses universitaires de Rennes, 2013).

54 Alexandre. Gauducheau, 'Dans quelle mesure est-il possible de transformer les races humaines par l'alimentation et l'hygiène? Projet

*Colonial medicine and 'Black strength'* 83

d'expérience exotique', *Bulletin de la Société de pathologie exotique*, vol. 30 (Paris: Masson, 1937), pp. 496–500.

55 Vincent Bonnecase, 'Avoir faim en Afrique occidentale française: investigations et représentations coloniales (1920–1960)', *Revue d'Histoire des Sciences Humaines*, 21 (2009), 151–174.
Vincent Bonnecase, *La pauvreté au Sahel: du savoir colonial à la mesure internationale* (Paris: Karthala, 2011).

56 Léon Pales, *Organisme d'enquête pour l'étude anthropologique des populations indigènes de l'A.O.F. Alimentation-Nutrition. Rapport N°1 (Sénégal)* (Dakar: Direction générale de la santé publique, 1946); Léon Pales, *Organisme d'enquête pour l'étude anthropologique des populations indigènes de l'A.O.F., Alimentation-Nutrition, Rapport N°3: Guinée occidentale, Dakar, Sénégal et Soudan, A.O.F.* (Dakar: Gouvernement général de l'Afrique Occidentale Française, 1947).

57 Pales and TassindeSaint-Péreuse, 'Raciologie comparative des populations de l'A.O.F., p. 209.

58 Pales, 'Physiologie comparative des races humaines'.

59 In the middle of the twentieth century, a group of scientists, doctors, geneticists and anthropologists brought together by UNESCO after the Second World War played a major role in the deconstruction of the concept of race. UNESCO, created in 1945, has the mission of fighting racism. This organisation is setting up a series of conferences on race during which many scientists speak.

60 R. Koerber, 'Contribution à l'étude de la répartition des groupes sanguins chez quelques races de l'Afrique occidentale française', *Bulletins et Mémoires de la Société d'anthropologie de Paris*, 9 (1948), p. 170.

61 Claude Chippaux, *Eléments d'anthropologie* (Marseille: Bibliothèque Paul Rivet, 1948).

62 André Gautier-Walter, *Afrique noire terre inconnue. La croisière noire de la santé* (Paris: Frédéric Chambriand, 1951), p. 125.

63 André Mayer, in Léon Pales, *L'alimentation en A.O.F., Milieux-Enquêtes-Techniques-Rations* (Dakar: ORANA, 1954), p. 5.

64 *Ibid.*, p. 8.

65 Adolphe Sicé, *L'Afrique équatoriale française et le Cameroun au service de la France (26–27–28 août 1940)* (Paris: PUF, 1946), p. 35. Médecin and inspecteur général of colonies, he contributed to Congo joining the Free French in 1940; he took part in the Conseil de Défense de l'Empire and directed the Service de Santé of Free French Africa.

# 3

# Africa, the Africans and the Red Cross: assessing the impact of the long Second World War

*Marie-Luce Desgrandchamps*

In the 1960s, sub-Saharan African countries and people, which had been almost entirely excluded from Red Cross activities and structures, became not only one of the main targets of the Red Cross Movement's activities but also active members.[1] They created national Red Cross societies, became members of the League of Red Cross Societies – the international body gathering all Red Cross societies – and worked actively toward the 'decolonisation' of the Geneva Conventions. In this chapter, I argue that the long Second World War constituted an important first step in this evolution. By situating the Italo-Ethiopian War and the Second World War in the same analytical framework, I suggest that the Red Cross Movement, which sat somewhere between the colonial order (as exemplified by the colonial sections of national Red Cross societies) and the international order with its international actors, the League and the International Committee of the Red Cross (ICRC) was significantly transformed by the upheavals of this period on the continent. Crucially, I revisit the old question of the links between Red Cross activism and colonialism, shedding new light on race relations in the Movement during this period.

As some recent studies have demonstrated, not only was the theatre of hostilities in East (1940–1941) and the North Africa (1940–1943) crucial to the war's military outcomes, but the African continent provided crucial human and economic resources for the belligerents.[2] For the French, in particular, Eric Jennings has shown that Free French Africa (Cameroon and French Equatorial Africa) played a key role in the French external resistance, which did not hesitate to exploit these territories fully.[3] In the French and British

Empires, the specific conditions of the war, the proximity the conflict established between Black and white soldiers, the condition of captivity of French colonial soldiers in Europe and the strategic role the African continent played in terms of resources profoundly transformed the relationship between the metropolis and its colonial spaces and population.[4] It also significantly shaped the relationship between European Red Cross activists and the African continent. More generally, as Timothy L. Schroer has demonstrated, between 1929 and 1949 the category of race emerged and then disappeared from the Geneva Conventions on prisoners of war.[5] Drawing on ICRC archives (Central Agency and general archives), in this chapter, I investigate two key questions: How and why did the long Second World War foster the inclusion of sub-Saharan Africa actors and territories within the scope of the Movement? Did this in turn lead to a change in the dominant perception among European Red Cross actors from seeing African people as essentially 'people to civilise' to considering them as more 'equal human beings'?

I have divided this chapter into four sections. First, I present the historiographical landscape on the relationship between the Red Cross Movement and colonial Africa. Second, I argue that the Italo-Ethiopian War was a key moment that led to the inclusion of the first 'Black' African national Red Cross Society in the Movement. Third, I show that the long Second World War led to the first contacts between African soldiers and their families through the Red Cross apparatus, the Central Agency of the ICRC for prisoners of war (PoWs), which set up a tracing service dedicated to the prisoners from French colonies. This Central Agency offered these prisoners the same kind of services as it did their European counterparts. Fourth, the division of the French Empire, particularly the rupture created by the split between the Vichy regime and the Gaullist movement, as well as the presence of European PoWs on the continent, fostered the creation of an embryonic Red Cross network in sub-Saharan Africa comprising ICRC delegates and Red Cross colonial branches. This evolution carried the seeds for a new, although limited, interest in the situation and the inclusion of Black African people in the Movement. By exploring the ambiguities and sometimes contradictions of these early Red Cross initiatives and various dimensions of Red Cross developments in sub-Saharan Africa during the long Second World War, this chapter contributes to a

86    *The long Second World War, 1931–1953*

better understanding of the tensions that emerged in the Movement in the following decades, when new African actors started to call more loudly for independence, the decolonisation of the Red Cross Movement and full inclusion in it.

### The historiographical landscape: tracing the Red Cross's colonial origins

Historical studies of humanitarianism's 'colonial origins' fall into several categories: analysis of the impact of 'civilising mission' discourses and hierarchies on humanitarian ideas, the legacies of colonial practices on humanitarian actions and the ways Red Cross conventions deprived the colonised population of legal subjectivity. As numerous scholars have demonstrated, humanitarian discourses, practices and actors maintained close ties with Western imperialism during the nineteenth and twentieth centuries.[6] Studied through the lens of the civilising mission, or through the activities of missionaries and anti-slavery movements, these links have been particularly scrutinised for the British Empire.[7] More generally, the legacies of colonial knowledge and practices in humanitarian actions are also well documented in very different contexts,[8] whereas non-occidental traditions of humanitarianism have been neglected.[9]

The history of the Red Cross Movement is no exception. Historians have begun to examine the role of national Red Cross societies as 'agents of empire' and to scrutinise the ICRC's/League's lack of involvement on the continent until the Ethiopian war. As Albert Wirz and Andreas Eckert have shown, in the nineteenth century, Red Cross humanitarianism shared ideological roots with colonialism through notions of modernity, civilisation and racial hierarchy. Gustave Moynier, the 'batisseur' of the International Committee of the Red Cross during its first decades, was actively involved in Léopold II's colonial venture in the Congo at the end of the nineteenth century.[10] In addition, national Red Cross societies, thought of as auxiliaries of the armies' health services, often accompanied occidental armies in colonial wars without paying much attention to the African population. This was particularly clear during the Boer Wars and the Rif War and during the Italian

# Africa, the Africans, and the Red Cross 87

campaigns in Libya.[11] The empires also used the creation of Red Cross colonial sections in the colonies to increase their medical presence in these areas. Dispensaries or clinics were established by the Red Cross colonial sections but often were run by missionaries who were dedicated to providing care first and foremost for the settlers and to a lesser extent for the colonised population.[12] They also became places of social activities for the settler communities, which organised charity dinners or fundraising in schools, for example.

In sub-Saharan Africa, the activities of these overseas branches of the Red Cross often remained quite marginal before the Second World War. When they occurred, they were embedded in the imperial health apparatus/policy, which extended the impact of colonialism into one of the most intimate parts of the colonised people's lives, such as birthing, child rearing and sexuality.[13] The South African Red Cross was a notable exception. It had started to develop at the end of the previous century during the Boer Wars.[14] After the conflict, as South Africa evolved from a British colony to an independent country (1910), the South African Red Cross developed into an independent Red Cross society, which was admitted into the League in 1919 and recognised by the ICRC in 1928. The society remained in white hands and practised segregation.[15]

The Movement's two international bodies, the ICRC and the League, remained relatively uninvolved in sub-Saharan Africa before the Italo-Ethiopian War (1935–1936). Although the ICRC had visited some internment camps in North Africa during the First World War, it did not consider the continent part of its scope of activities. Likewise, the League paid little attention to the continent. Created in 1919 by the representatives of the Western Red Cross, the League was a relatively young organisation in the inter-war period, which had other priorities than the development of Red Cross activities in sub-Saharan Africa.

Although the historiography has shown that the Red Cross Movement's primary interests did not include sub-Saharan Africa until the middle of the 1930s, some of its members also acted as reactionary forces during the decolonisation process and did not count among the most progressive and emancipatory humanitarian

88          *The long Second World War, 1931–1953*

bodies.[16] As Andrew Thompson has argued, the decolonisation period put the Red Cross's fundamental principles to the test. Some Red Cross societies were heavily involved in counterinsurgency policies and activities.[17] For instance, focusing on the Mau Mau Crisis in the 1950s, Emily Baughan has highlighted that the British Red Cross and Save the Children, far from being emancipatory movements, participated in the rehabilitation of the British Colonial Empire.[18]

The period of the long Second World War remains the notable absentee in this historiography. The Italo-Ethiopian War has been well studied in itself,[19] but other activities of the Red Cross Movement in Africa or for the Africans during the war remain understudied. The historiography has mainly focused on other issues, such as the European national Red Cross societies and the ICRC's attitudes towards concentration and extermination camps in Europe, displaced persons, the treatment and protection of the prisoners of war and food aid.[20] Recently, historians have started to decentre the narrative by showing that the war opened up new spaces, such as Latin America, for the League of Red Cross Societies and local branches of national societies.[21] Speaking more broadly about the Movement, this was also the case for sub-Saharan Africa. The three following examples illustrate that the long Second World War was indeed a fundamental period when sub-Saharan African people began to be seen as more than just 'people to civilise' even though paternalism did not disappear.

### The Italo-Ethiopian War and the inclusion of the first Black African Red Cross

Although it claimed to be universal, before the Italo-Ethiopian War, the ICRC considered 'Black African people' not civilised enough to join the Movement. Although some of their prejudices toward them – often understood as a whole – remained even after the war,[22] the aggression by a European power against an independent and recognised African state changed the game: it led to the inclusion of the first Black African national Red Cross society in the Movement. In this section, I analyse the conditions under which this development was possible and reveal this process's limits.

Africa, the Africans, and the Red Cross 89

The Italo-Ethiopian War (1935–1936) was part of the Italian construction of a colonial empire in Africa but implied the conquest of an independent and recognised state, which was a member of the League of Nations.[23] This specific configuration as well as the methods of warfare the Italians employed attracted international attention. The atrocities Italian troops committed as well as the use of poison gas and the deliberate bombings of ambulances and hospitals by the Italian Air Force have been thoroughly discussed.[24] As the historians Nicola Perugini and Neve Gordon have argued, Ethiopian sovereignty was considered less inviolable than that of other nations because of a colonial trope. Because Ethiopia was considered 'uncivilised' and therefore unable to apply the basic principles of international law, European powers felt justified to apply them partially.[25] During the interwar period, the idea of European powers having a right and even a duty to colonise less civilised nations remained widespread among European conservative elites. In the case of Ethiopia, as Amalia Ribi has demonstrated, before the war, anti-slavery groups played an important part in depicting Ethiopia as a backward country and society because of the persistence of slavery.[26]

The Red Cross Movement's involvement in the conflict took place in this context. In his book *Between Bombs and Good Intentions*, Rainer Baudendistel explores the range of humanitarian activities the ICRC coordinated and their shortcomings. Above all, he shows that some ICRC members' ambiguity towards the fascist regime influenced the ICRC's perceptions and attitude in the conflict: the ICRC became caught up in Italian propaganda and failed to take a stand on the use of poison gas or on the bombing of the Red Cross hospitals.[27] Despite these failures, the conflict still represented the Red Cross Movement's first involvement with an African belligerent in a colonial conflict and led to the recognition of the first African Red Cross society, the Ethiopian Red Cross. In comparison, the Rif War, which occurred a few years earlier, did not raise the same amount of concern and mobilisation among the Movement.[28] During the Italo-Ethiopian War, several other Red Cross national societies sent mobile hospitals into the field, close to the front (Dutch, Egyptian, Finnish, British (2), Norwegian and Swedish).[29] To coordinate the deployment of this aid in Ethiopia,

90 *The long Second World War, 1931–1953*

the ICRC sent two delegates, Marcel Junod and Sydney Brown. Caught by the events and the difficult situation of the Ethiopian Red Cross, its presence in the field lasted longer that the ICRC initially envisaged but resulted in two trajectories. Marcel Junod's first mission for the ICRC marked the beginning of a long and spotlighted involvement with the ICRC whereas Sydney Brown's career in the organisation came to an end because he was too quick to denounce the ICRC's shortcomings during the conflict and was accused of having adopted anti-fascist opinions during the war.[30]

The hybrid nature of the conflict – between an interstate conflict and a war of colonial conquest – and the specific situation and perception of Ethiopia in the 1930s explained the Red Cross Movement's ambivalence towards this conflict. For example, the international Red Cross Movement's recognition of the Ethiopian Red Cross was not without tensions. Unsurprisingly, the Italian Red Cross decried the acceptance of a Red Cross that was insufficiently civilised. Privately, ICRC leaders also questioned the relevance and validity of such recognition, as Baudendistel points out.[31] They constantly suspected that it was only a facade to encourage Red Cross solidarity, but at the same time, a movement claiming to be universal could not simply dismiss this organisation.

Comprising high-ranking Ethiopian dignitaries, Westerners working for the government and doctors from missionary societies, the Ethiopian Red Cross reflected Ethiopia's particular situation in an Africa surrounded by empires.[32] The Ethiopian Foreign Minister asked a US missionary, Thomas Lambie, who had acquired Ethiopian nationality in 1934, to become the executive secretary. Despite difficulties in setting up and organising mobile units, the Ethiopian Red Cross deployed seven of them in a context in which the Ethiopian army health service was non-existent. To do so, it relied on the commitment of missionary doctors present in Ethiopia and on the wave of solidarity generated by the conflict in Europe and the United States, especially in anti-fascist and Afro-American circles. Multiple Red Cross and Red Crescent national societies also responded by sending money, material or teams.

The hybrid nature of this independent African country, which also had a strong missionary presence and in which Westerners were well represented, probably played an important role in the solidarity shown with the Ethiopian Red Cross. On the one hand,

# Africa, the Africans, and the Red Cross 91

racial solidarity was important in gathering the support of Afro-American associations and churches in the United States.[33] On the other hand, the specific image of Ethiopia that European travellers had constructed since the nineteenth century established a form of proximity with this country. It was depicted as an essentially Christian nation inhabited by a population of 'white negros' to recall the title of a wildly spread publication of the time.[34] This conception arose due to the legacies of the myth of the kingdom of Priest John and the Hamitic theory developed during the nineteenth century but still very en vogue in the 1930s.[35] According to these conceptions, if the Ethiopian people were not yet considered civilised enough to be treated on an equal footing with the Westerners, their features suggested a potential for a civilisation conducive to the development of the Red Cross.

The Red Cross Movement's first involvement in an African state in a colonial conflict resulted from this specific conjuncture. The conflict sets a precedent for the Red Cross Movement and shows that it was possible for the ICRC to develop activities and send representatives to 'Black' Africa; it also showed that 'Black' Africans could be integrated into it. More generally, the conflict and its consequences changed the way African people were perceived in humanitarian networks.[36] Although the Ethiopian Red Cross formally ceased to exist during the Italian occupation, it was unofficially re-formed in 1946 and then officially in 1947 and became one of the first Red Cross societies to be recognised in an African country, with the exception of South Africa.[37] In the 1960s, it managed a nursing school and a hospital in Addis Ababa with the support of the League, the Swedish Red Cross and the Soviet Red Cross Alliance. At the time, other Red Cross societies in sub-Saharan countries were only beginning to be set up.

## The colonial section of the ICRC's Central Agency for the prisoners of war

The Second World War led to other important transformations, including the development of relief activities for colonial PoWs and the creation of a specific section in the ICRC for French colonial PoWs. This led to the first contacts among many African soldiers,

92    *The long Second World War, 1931–1953*

their families and the Red Cross, inscribing the Movement in their everyday lives. In the case of the soldiers from the French Empire, these encounters took place through the French Red Cross, which distributed relief in prisoners' camps or through visits by ICRC delegates.[38] They were also the result of a specific policy of the ICRC's Central Agency for the PoWs.[39] For the first time, the ICRC's Central Agency for the PoWs set up a tracing service dedicated to the prisoners from the French colonies. Focusing on this move, in this section, I analyse why it became important for the Swiss institution to care specifically for these prisoners and this move's effects on the extension of the Red Cross network on the continent.

In 1939, unlike Britain, which favoured the use of colonised soldiers above all in its colonies, France did not hesitate to deploy its colonial soldiers in the European theatres of war. Around 520,000 African soldiers (from North Africa, French West Africa and French Equatorial Africa) fought in the French campaign in 1940.[40] A recent and growing historiography has examined these PoWs' experiences and the conditions,[41] but very little has been written about the way the Central Agency of the Red Cross dealt with this specific category of PoWs.[42]

The Central Agency's aim was to gather information on the PoWs and help restore the connections between them and their families. In the Agency, the work was organised by sections that collected information on PoWs according to their nationality: there was a French section, a British section, a German section, and so on. During the First World War, information about colonial soldiers had followed an imperial logic, which means that their situation was treated by the section of the empire from which they came, such as French or British. But in 1940, things changed when the Central Agency decided to create a specific section for the numerous French colonial prisoners resulting from the Battle of France. According to an ICRC report, the main reason for this decision was technical: many of the soldiers coming from the Empire were illiterate and the complexity of African and Asian onomastic systems made their identification and registration almost impossible. Because of these problems, the risk was that the cards referring to native soldiers would be 'lost forever in the French card-index'.[43] To overcome these difficulties, three interrelated files had to be established: a nominative file and two numerical files (one

*Africa, the Africans, and the Red Cross* 93

by prisoner number and one by military number). Many efforts were deployed: about fifty experts of African and Asian cultures and geography (essentially repatriated Swiss nationals and former legionnaires in the French colonial army) were hired to correct name errors and trace or verify family addresses in places of origin.[44]

Even if this transformation occurred above all for technical reasons, it set an important precedent and led the Central Agency to take people from the empires into account to an extent that had not been reached previously. From the moment the Central Agency started to do so, it became difficult to go back, as the discussions in the first months of the colonial section's existence showed. In December 1940, as the colonial section was struggling to trace these soldiers, the directorate started to wonder whether it was worth keeping the section in the Agency. Some people thought that it would be better to give the information about these prisoners to French organisations, which were better equipped than the Agency to make connections with colonial territories. This option was nonetheless soon abandoned because it seemed impossible for the Agency to disregard the fate of a category of prisoners without contradicting its humanitarian mission.[45]

The sequence of events and the gradual disconnection between Vichy France and the growing part of the colonial empire under Free French control vindicated this decision: if the Agency had given up in 1941, the connections between the colonial PoWs and their families would have been even more jeopardised. The colonial section was the only organisation to have a full overview of the captured soldiers from the colonial empire who had fought in the campaign of 1940 and later with the Free French or during the liberation of Europe from 1943 onwards. According to French authorities, this made the files the section gathered invaluable.[46] About 4,000 to 5,000 letters or messages passed through Geneva each month in 1941, increasing by 190 per cent to just under 15,000 letters per month in subsequent years. During the whole war, the colonial section dealt with about 80,000 cases of PoWs as well as deceased or missing persons from the Empire.

For many African soldiers and their families, the colonial section and its relays in the field represented the first contacts with the Red Cross. As early as December 1940, the head of the section emphasised that 'the numerous communications and requests for

94        *The long Second World War, 1931–1953*

information that we send out every day strengthen the link between the Agency and Africa'.[47] Four years later, in a note to an ICRC committee member, the section's director made similar comments, stressing the 'confidence shown by the natives' in the Agency and 'the ever-increasing number of calls addressed to it and the expressions of gratitude it received'.[48] It remains difficult to assess to what extent this section contributed to the creation of a positive memory of the Red Cross among the colonial soldiers in the long term. Nonetheless, it is quite clear that during their captivity, they were in contact with the Red Cross emblem or idea, whether through parcels, messages or volunteers. For example, Eugène Mallot, a Cameroonian member of the YMCA, visited the ICRC in 1953. In a conversation he had with Pierre Gaillard of the ICRC headquarters, he expressed the great gratitude of the Cameroonian veterans for the Red Cross and their wish to see the Red Cross firmly established on the African continent.[49] Although this person might have wished to flatter his Swiss interlocutor with kind words, this example shows that African veterans of the Second World War had a memory of their interaction with the Red Cross. According to one of the former presidents of the Senegalese Red Cross, Rito Alcantara, when Léopold Sedar Senghor asked him to become the president of this institution in 1964, he mentioned his first encounter with the Red Cross – he did not specify which one exactly – during his captivity in France during the war.[50]

By deciding to set up a specific colonial section, the Agency's directorate made it clear that the colonial soldiers' fate was not only a matter for the imperial metropolis but also deserved to be considered by the Central Agency for the PoWs, just as the fate of other PoWs was. Marguerite Gautier-van Berchem, who had worked for the Agency during the First World War and who became the director of the colonial section when it was officially created in 1941, shared this concern. She was well aware of the stakes involved in what she considered a first move toward a more 'humanitarian treatment' of the colonial question, as she explained to her colleagues in 1944:

> I would also add that the action undertaken in Geneva in favour of the indigenous populations is of a scope which exceeds that of the agency's other national sections because it is aimed at peoples towards whom the white races have been guilty of many abuses. In post-war Europe, if the colonial question is not dealt with on another level, a

# Africa, the Africans, and the Red Cross

more humanitarian level, it is to be presumed that these races of colour which today have judged us will no longer accept foreign interference in the running of their country. The work the ICRC, faithful to its principle of considering all men as brothers, has undertaken in favor of the colored races should then serve as an example.[51]

Like many European people at the time, she was well aware of the need to reform the colonial system but did not plead for its abolition, as her close work with the colonial administration in France demonstrates at the end of the war.[52] Her sensibility regarding these questions was probably linked with her specific background. A daughter of Max van Berchem, a scholar specialist of Islamic culture in Egypt, she was an archaeologist and had participated in various archaeological excavation campaigns in the South of Algeria before working for the Central Agency's colonial section.[53]

## An embryonic Red Cross network in sub-Saharan Africa

Beyond the establishment of a colonial section in Geneva, the war also paved the way for the future development of Red Cross structures and networks in Africa. The division of the French Empire as well as the presence of European PoWs and civilian internees on the continent fostered the creation of an embryonic Red Cross network in sub-Saharan Africa, comprising ICRC temporary delegates and Red Cross colonial branches. As this section demonstrates, this embryonic network laid the foundation for the Movement's development on the African continent more broadly even though it remained in white hands.

As mentioned earlier, the territories south of the Sahara occupied a more than marginal place in the Red Cross before the Second World War. Apart from the recognition in 1921 of the white-led South African Red Cross in the Movement, the ephemeral existence of the Ethiopian Red Cross in 1935–1936 and the creation of local branches in the Belgian and British Empires, such as in Congo or in Gold Coast before the 1930s, the Red Cross's development in these regions was almost non-existent and the ICRC had no delegate on the continent. Because of the upheavals it caused in the empires, the war led to the burgeoning of Red Cross activities in sub-Saharan Africa even though they remained essentially in white hands.

96    *The long Second World War, 1931–1953*

First, the necessities of the war fostered the development of colonial sections in territories under French, Belgian and British jurisdictions, where the metropolitan Red Cross and the states made appeals of solidarity. Activities such as collecting funding for the war-torn metropolis, preparing parcels for soldiers and restoring connections between the settlers' communities and their relatives engaged as soldiers or impacted by the war became these sections' raison d'être. This was particularly the case in the territories that were cut off from their metropolis. For example, the Belgian Red Cross in the Congo experienced considerable growth during the conflict because it had to deal with the severing of connections between the colony and the metropolis in addition to its usual activities (maintaining dispensaries etc.). In the French Empire, the war encouraged the development of colonial Red Cross sections, particularly in French Equatorial Africa and Cameroon, which rallied to Free France in 1940, unlike the rest of French Africa, which remained loyal to Vichy France. Setting up a colonial section in Brazzaville was a way for the Free French to benefit from American solidarity through the American Red Cross, for example.[54]

However, these dynamics were not limited to the dissident regions in the French Empire. Therefore, the French Red Cross network grew not only in Free French Africa (Mgr Biéchy in Brazzaville, Mgr Le Mailloux in Cameroon) but also in the other parts of the French Empire: in Dakar and Saint-Louis (Mr Felix Martine, Mr Mathis and Ms Pichon) and also in Bamako, Madagascar (Dr Fontoynont) and Ouagadougou (Mr Jean Blay). At first specifically dedicated to the re-establishment of connections between the settlers and their relatives in Europe, these representatives of the French Red Cross in the field also became crucial relays in the field for the Central Agency's colonial section. As its work grew, they played an increasingly important role in transmitting messages between detained colonial soldiers and their families living in their regions of activity.[55]

Second, the ICRC's involvement in sub-Saharan Africa grew because of the presence of a large number of civilian internees and PoWs on the continent. For example, at the end of 1940, the German Red Cross contacted the ICRC to enquire about the treatment of German civilians living in French Equatorial Africa who had been interned after this region had rallied to de Gaulle.[56]

## Africa, the Africans, and the Red Cross

On the Allied side, in 1940, the South African Red Cross, which had already asked the ICRC to designate a representative in the country,[57] emphasised the need to send someone to visit their prisoners on the East African front, where South African troops were fighting against the Italians alongside the British.[58] The ICRC relied on Swiss citizens established on the African continent to represent the organisation and report on the internment conditions of the various prisoners or internees. The profile of these Swiss citizens varied (consulate agents, employees of Swiss firms, missionaries), but they all belonged to the circle of Swiss elites living in colonial or ex-colonial empires.[59] For example, in South Africa, the ICRC called on Edmond Grasset, who was working at the South African Institute for Medical Research at the time and who later became a professor of hygiene and bacteriology in Geneva and headed the Institut d'Hygiène. In the Belgian Congo, it was Robert Maurice, a geologist working in Elizabethville, who started to visit the German internees for the ICRC before leaving the country in 1941. He later started a diplomatic career and became the Swiss ambassador to Spain in the 1960s. Although many of these collaborations faded after the end of the war, two of them became central to the ICRC's work during the following years: those with Henri-Philippe Junod and Geoffrey Senn. Remaining the only representatives of the ICRC in sub-Saharan Africa after the war, they played a central role in ICRC African policy during the decolonisation period in operational terms and in terms of information.

The Allied fighting in East Africa, which involved many South African troops, led to the recruitment of Henri Philip Junod. The cousin of Marcel Junod, Henri-Philippe Junod began his collaboration with the ICRC in this context. At the time he was a member of the Swiss Mission in Pretoria and was involved in various South African institutions.[60] In November 1941, the South African Red Cross suggested Henri-Philippe Junod be nominated as a delegate in East Africa to take care of South African prisoners.[61] The ICRC accepted,[62] but the Allied victory in the region led to a change of attribution in Junod's work. He finally had to take care of the Italian prisoners and civilian internees detained by the British. After having visited the prisoners in Ethiopia, Somalia and Eritrea, he went back to South Africa, where many Italian prisoners

98     *The long Second World War, 1931–1953*

were interned during the war. Junod then became the deputy delegate of the ICRC's representative, Edmond Grasset, who was trying to control and improve the internment conditions of these 175,000 detainees.[63] The small ICRC delegation (Grasset, Junod and a secretary) also cultivated positive relationships with the South African Red Cross. This was very important for the headquarters in Geneva, which tried to strengthen its relationships with Red Cross actors in this region. In 1943, two members of the ICRC's committee, Lucie Odier and Suzanne Ferrière, undertook the first ICRC official mission in Southern Africa. They saw what was done for the European prisoners and refugees and met with South African and British authorities and Red Cross local committees to improve the collaboration with the ICRC,[64] especially in terms of relief provision and communication delays. One of this mission's results was an increase in the South African Red Cross's financial contribution to the ICRC.[65]

At the end the war, when Edmond Grasset was appointed a professor at the University of Geneva, the question arose regarding replacing him because many European PoWs and civilian internees were still detained in South Africa. Junod, who had been his deputy delegate since 1941, was naturally solicited to take over the delegation to continue to visit the camps until all prisoners had been liberated.[66] In 1950, Junod paid a visit to the ICRC headquarters in Geneva because he was planning to travel to Switzerland for other purposes. After congratulating him for his work in a region where they admitted they had not been able to follow closely what had happened during the war, ICRC members took advantage of Junod's presence to enquire about the situation in South Africa. They asked him to reflect on a 'possible role of the ICRC in the event of a delicate situation in South Africa',[67] where tensions between the communities had been growing since the National Party's victory in 1948 and the promulgation of apartheid laws. For the first time, their interest shifted from the prisoners' fate to the overall situation of a country in the grip of major racial tensions. Junod's answers emphasised the complexity of a situation he did not clearly condemn. He did not favour any initiatives from the ICRC, especially in a context in which Switzerland had started to develop investments in the country.[68] Junod acknowledged that the first aid

Africa, the Africans, and the Red Cross    99

network and relief networks for non-white people should be better prepared for conflicts. However, he advised above all not mingling too much and working as closely as possible with the South African Red Cross. Other suggestions ranged from encouraging the miners to attend safety-first courses to preparing communication material to make ICRC history and activities more widely recognised.[69] As a result, the ICRC decided only to intensify its contact with the South African Red Cross and to plan a communication campaign to showcase ICRC activities and history.[70] If such decisions did not lead to a radical shift in ICRC policy in this country, the preceding discussion shows that the ICRC was starting to wonder how to take care of the African population.

The establishment of another delegate, Geoffrey Senn, during the Second World War also encouraged the ICRC in this direction.[71] The need to visit prisoners and civilian internees in South Africa and in the British Empire, especially its Eastern part, was behind the recruitment of Geoffrey Senn. He began working as Grasset's deputy delegate for Rhodesia but became quickly identified as an excellent delegate. He was responsible for Southern Rhodesia. He then asked the ICRC for an extension of its mandate to Nyassaland and Northern Rhodesia.[72] His work consisted of visiting many Italians (civilians) who had settled in Ethiopia but had been interned in Rhodesia after the country's liberation by the Allies. He also visited thousands of Italian and German civilian internees and PoWs interned in the British Empire and witnessed the plight of thousands of Polish refugees who were placed in camps once they arrived in the British Empire.[73] When the delegation in Salisbury was closed in 1947, the ICRC headquarters in Geneva asked him to remain an ICRC correspondent.[74] However, one year later, in 1948, Senn asked for his title of delegate again and was then considered a voluntary delegate.[75] The headquarters understood Senn's move as a sign of him wanting recognition from the ICRC for his work during the war. However, Senn's project was rather different. In 1948, he wrote to the ICRC complaining about the British Red Cross's poor work in the Federation of Rhodesia and Nyassaland and then started to create a new section of the Red Cross in Rhodesia.[76] He said that the British Red Cross branch had accomplished great things during the war but had since then ceased

100    *The long Second World War, 1931–1953*

its activities. Put in an uncomfortable position vis-à-vis the British Red Cross, the ICRC curbed Senn's enthusiasm. This episode shows quite well how the ICRC's involvement in the case of European civilian internees planted a seed for other activities. Even if this was not a linear process, the war resulted in a growing network of white Red Cross structures on the continent. Their permanence after the war, once their primary tasks for white soldiers and detainees had been accomplished, opened a space for new developments in territories that had not been fully considered until then.

## Conclusion

Although long ignored by historiography, the long Second World War in Africa marked an important moment for the development of the Red Cross Movement on the continent. The multiple dimensions of the Red Cross Movement's commitment to Africa enrich a historiography that has focused primarily on the development of humanitarian practices in the British Empire. They show how non-imperial actors, such as the ICRC, took advantage of the gaps the war created to penetrate empires and engage with Black Africans, whom some in the Red Cross Movement had essentially perceived as not civilised enough to be subjected to the norms of the Geneva Conventions.[77] From the Second Italo-Ethiopian War onwards, there was an inflection in the conception of the African populations and their possible inclusion in the Movement as well as in the possibility of developing local sections in these areas, even if they remained essentially in white hands.

The fact that this development began with the Italo-Ethiopian War is significant. The particular situation of this independent African country, fighting against the Italian colonial project on the one hand, and the particular conception of the Ethiopian population, on the other hand, allowed for the inclusion for the first time of an African Red Cross society dedicated to the Ethiopians. More generally, as Bronwen Everill has emphasised, the Italo-Ethiopian War also marked a rupture in the way African victims were viewed in British humanitarian circles. It shifted from anti-slavery rhetoric to more universal language regarding refugees.[78] Therefore, this

# Africa, the Africans, and the Red Cross     101

moment marked a new step towards the inclusion of Black Africans in the mental map of some humanitarians not only as people to civilise and rescue from slavery through the 'benevolent' presence or trusteeship of empires but as victims of war and refugees, among others.

A couple of years later, the attention the Central Agency of the ICRC paid to the fate of colonial soldiers from the French Empire also confirmed this evolution. According to its supporters, especially Marguerite Gautier-van Berchem and her deputy, Marguerite Divorne, their initiative for a greater consideration of the needs of the colonised soldiers during the war should have been part of a wider movement to reform empires, based on a more humane and inclusive conception of the colonised people. Rather than an anticolonial stance, this way of seeing can be linked to the developmentalist turn the empires took during the war.

Finally, because of the upheaval of empires it provoked, the war encouraged the development of a Red Cross network on the continent, comprising the South African Red Cross as well as French, British and Belgian Red Cross committees and delegates in the colonies. They played a crucial role in the transmission of news between the soldiers engaged in other continents and their families living in Africa (whether they were settlers or autochthonous families). The deployment of ICRC delegates in the field also helped put the African continent on the Movement's agenda. Because their primary mission was to check the detention conditions of the European soldiers or civilian internees on the African continent, some of them remained delegates once they accomplished this mission, and became the main relay of the ICRC in the field during the decolonisation conflicts.

## Notes

1 The research for this chapter was carried out during the project 'Colonial and Transnational Intimacies: Medical Humanitarianism in the French External Resistance' funded by the Arts and Humanities Research Council (AH/T006382/1). The author would like to thank Laure Humbert, Bertrand Taithe and the anonymous reviewers for their advice and feedback on this chapter.

102    *The long Second World War, 1931–1953*

2 Nicola Labanca, David Reynolds and Olivier Wieviorka, *La guerre du désert. 1940–1943* (Paris: Perrin, 2019); Judith A. Byfield, Carolyn A. Brown, Timothy Parsons and Ahmad Alawad Sikainga, *Africa and World War II* (Cambridge: Cambridge University Press, 2015); Catherine Akpo-Vache, *L'AOF et la seconde guerre mondiale* (Paris: Karthala, 1996); LéonModeste Nnang Ndong, *L'effort de guerre de l'Afrique: Le Gabon dans la Deuxième Guerre mondiale (1939–1947)* (Paris: L'Harmattan, 2011); Michel Ostenc, 'Les Italiens en Afrique du nord pendant la Seconde Guerre mondiale', *Guerres mondiales et conflits contemporains*, 275:3 (2019), 143–146; Camille Lefebvre, 'Combattants, travailleurs, prisonniers, les africains dans la guerre', in Alya Aglan and Robert Frank (eds), *1937–1947: La guerre-monde* (Paris: Gallimard, 2015), pp. 527–564; David Killingray and Martin Plaut, *Fighting for Britain: African Soldiers in the Second World War* (Woodbridge: James Currey, 2012).

3 Eric Jennings, *Free French in Africa in World War II* (Cambridge: Cambridge University Press, 2015); Géraud Létang, 'Mirage d'une rebellion. Être français libre au Tchad (1940–1943)' (PhD dissertation, Institut d'études politiques de Paris, 2019).

4 Jean-François Muracciole, 'La conférence de Brazzaville et la décolonisation: Le mythe et la réalité', *Espoir*, 152 (2007) ; Martin Thomas, *The French Empire at War, 1940–1945* (Manchester: Manchester University Press, 1998). On the impact on the Commonwealth, see Jonathan Fennell, *Fighting the People's War: British Army and the Second World War* (Cambridge: Cambridge University Press, 2019). On war captivity: Armelle Mabon, 'Solidarité Nationale et Captivité Coloniale', *French Colonial History*, 12:1 (2011), 193–207; Armelle Mabon, *Prisonniers de guerre Indigènes: Visages oubliés de la France occupée* (Paris: La Découverte, 2010); Raffael Scheck, *French Colonial Soldiers in German Captivity during World War II* (New York: Cambridge University Press, 2014); Sarah Frank, *Hostages of Empire: Colonial Prisoners of War in Vichy France* (Lincoln, NE: University of Nebraska Press, 2021); Raffael Scheck, 'Les prémices de Thiaroye: L'influence de la captivité allemande sur les soldats noirs français à la fin de la Seconde Guerre Mondiale', *French Colonial History*, 13:1 (2012), 73–90; Martin Mourre, *Thiaroye 1944. Histoire et mémoire d'un massacre* colonial (Rennes: Presses Universitaires de Rennes, 2017).

5 Timothy L. Schroer, 'The Emergence and Early Demise of Codified Racial Segregation of Prisoners of War under the Geneva Conventions of 1929 and 1949', *Journal of the History of International Law*, 15 (2013), 53–75.

# Africa, the Africans, and the Red Cross     103

6 Marie-Luce Desgrandchamps and Damiano Matasci (eds), 'De la 'mission civilisatrice' à l'aide internationale dans les pays du Sud: Acteurs, pratiques et reconfigurations au XXe siècle', *Histoire@Politique*, 41 (2020).

7 Fae Dussart and Alan Lester, *Colonization and the Origins of Humanitarian Governance: Protecting Aborigines across the Nineteenth-Century British Empire* (Cambridge: Cambridge University Press, 2014); Emily Baughan, *Saving the Children: Humanitarianism, Internationalism and Empire* (Berkeley, CA: University of California Press, 2021); Emily Baughan, Alan Lester, Rob Skinner and Bronwen Everill (eds), 'Empire and Humanitarianism', *Journal of Imperial and Commonwealth Studies*, 40:5 (2012).

8 Tahila Sasson, 'From Empire to Humanity: The Russian Famine and the Imperial: Origins of International Humanitarianism', *Journal of British Studies*, 55 (2016), 519–537.

9 Pierre Fuller, 'Links and Non-links between Humanitarian Historiographies: Setting the Scene' (workshop 'Researching the History of Medical Care, Humanitarianism and Violence in Asia during the "long" Second World War: New Approaches, Challenges and Limits', Institut d'études politiques de Paris, 22 May 2023); Ester Moeller and Maria Framke, 'From Local Philanthropy to Political Humanitarianism: South Asian and Egyptian Humanitarian Aid during the Period of Decolonisation', *Zentrum Moderner Orient (ZMO) Working Papers*, 22 (2019).

10 Albert Wirtz and Andreas Eckert, 'The Scramble for Africa: Icon and Idiom of Modernity', in Olivier Petré-Grenouilleau (ed.), *From Slave Trade to Empire: Europe and the Colonisation of Black Africa* (London: Routledge, 2004), pp. 133–153; Fabio Rossinelli, *Géographie et impérialisme. De la Suisse au Congo entre exploration géographique et conquête coloniale* (Neuchâtel: Alphil, 2022).

11 Martínez-Antonio and Francisco Javier, 'Resilient Modernisation: Morocco's Agency in Red Cross Projects from Hassan I to the Rif Republic, 1886–1926', *Asclepio*, 66:1 (2014); Elizabeth Van Heyningen, 'The South African War as Humanitarian Crisis', *International Review of Red Cross*, 97:900 (2015), 999–1028; André Durand, *De Sarajevo à Hiroshima* (Geneva: Institut Henry Dunant, 1978), p. 10.

12 The first of these overseas branches was the Croix-Rouge congolaise et africaine, which Leopold II established in Belgium to accompany the 'civilizing mission' in the Congo.

13 Holly Ashford, 'The Red Cross and the Establishment of Maternal and Infant Welfare in the 1930s Gold Coast', *The Journal of Imperial and Commonwealth History*, 47:3 (2019), 514–541. Nancy Rose Hunt,

104    *The long Second World War, 1931–1953*

'"Le bébé en brousse": European Women, African Birth Spacing, and Colonial Intervention in Breast Feeding in the Belgian Congo', in Frederick Cooper and Ann Stoler (eds), *Tensions of Empire: Colonial Cultures in a Bourgeois World* (Berkeley, CA: University of California Press, 1997), pp. 287–321); Anne Hugon, *Être mère en situation coloniale Gold Coast, années 1910–1950* (Paris: Editions de la Sorbonne, 2020).

14 Heyningen, 'The South African War'; Rebeca Gill, 'Network of Concerns, Boundaries of Compassion: British Relief in the South African War', *The Journal of Imperial and Commonwealth History*, 40:5 (2012), 827–844.

15 Candice Rey, 'Entre prétentions universelles et pratiques ségrégationnistes: Histoire de la Croix-Rouge sud-africaine (1896–1966) (Master's thesis, University of Fribourg, 2023).

16 Marie-Luce Desgrandchamps, 'En quête de légitimité. Le Comité international de la Croix-Rouge et l'Afrique durant les années 1960', *Monde(s)*, 19:1 (2021), 221–239; Ana Guardião, 'A Matter of Control: Colonial and Humanitarian Population Management Strategies, Angolan Refugees' Resistance, and the Politics of Difference (1961–1964)', *e-Journal of Portuguese History*, 19:2 (2021), 51–75.

17 Andrew Thompson, 'Humanitarian Principles Put to Test: Challenges to Humanitarian Action during Decolonization', *International Review of the Red Cross*, 97:897/898 (2016), 45–76; Jennifer Johnson, 'The Limits of Humanitarianism: Decolonization, the French Red Cross and the Algerian War', in A. Dirk Moses, Marco Duranti and Roland Burke (eds), *Decolonization, Self-determination and the Rise of Global Human Rights Politics* (Cambridge: Cambridge University Press, 2021), pp. 79–108.

18 Emily Baughan, 'Rehabilitating an Empire: Humanitarian Collusion with the Colonial State during the Kenyan Emergency, ca. 1954–1960', *Journal of British Studies*, 59 (2020), 57–79.

19 Rainer Baudendistel, *Between Bombs and Good Intentions: The ICRC and Italo-Ethiopian War, 1935–1936* (New York: Berghahn, 2006).

20 Jean-Claude Favez, *Une mission impossible? Le CICR, les déportés et les camps de concentration nazis* (Lausanne: Editions Payot, 1988); Isabelle Vonèche Cardia, *Neutralité et engagement. Les relations entre le Comité international de la Croix-Rouge et le gouvernement suisse (1938–1945)* (Lausanne: SHSR, 2012); Delphine Debons, *L'assistance spirituelle aux prisonniers de guerre. Un aspect de l'action humanitaire durant la Seconde Guerre mondiale* (Paris: Editions du Cerf, 2012); Sébastien Farré, 'The ICRC and the Detainees in Nazi Concentration Camps (1942–1945)', *International Review of the Red Cross*, 88 (2012),

## Africa, the Africans, and the Red Cross    105

1381–1408; Gerald Steinacher, *Humanitarians at War: The Red Cross in the Shadow of the Holocaust* (Oxford: Oxford University Press, 2017); Irène Herrmann, *L'humanitaire en question* (Paris: Editions du Cerf, 2018); James Crossland, *Britain and the International Committee of the Red Cross, 1939–1945* (London: Palgrave Macmillan, 2014); Daniel Palmieri, 'Le Comité International de la Croix-Rouge et les organisations pour les réfugiés, 1943–1948', *Relations internationales*, 152:4 (2012), 17–28; Jean-Pierre LeCrom, *Au secours Maréchal! L'instrumentalisation de l'humanitaire (1940–1944)* (Paris: Presses universitaires de France, 2013).

21 Neville Wylie and Melanie Oppenheimer, 'Irrelevant Backwater? Latin America as a Field of Activity for the League of Red Cross Societies, 1938–1945', unpublished paper, online seminar series: 'New Approaches to Medical Care, Humanitarianism and Violence during the "long" Second World War, c. 1931–1953', 4 April 2023; Leo van Bergen, 'A Humanitarian and National Obligation: A Comparison between the Dutch Red Cross, 1940–5, and the Dutch East-Indies Red Cross, 1942–50', in Neville Wylie, Melanie Oppenheimer and James Crossland (eds), *The Red Cross Movement: Myths, Practices and Turning Points* (Manchester: Manchester University Press, 2020), pp. 282–295; Marie-Luce Desgrandchamps and Laure Humbert, 'From Dissident to Recognized Belligerent? The Free French and the Red Cross Movement, 1940–1943', *French History*, 20 (2023), 1–21.

22 On prejudices towards Kenya and Central Africa, see Pringle Yolana, 'Humanitarianism, Race and Denial: The International Committee of the Red Cross and Kenya's Mau Mau Rebellion, 1952–60', *History Workshop Journal*, 84 (2017), 89–107; Marie-Luce Desgrandchamps, 'Entre ambitions universalistes et préjugés raciaux', *Histoire@ Politique*, 41 (2020), 1–11.

23 Bahru Zewde, *A History of Modern Ethiopia, 1855–1974* (Oxford: James Currey, 1991); Ruth Ben-Ghiat and Mia Fuller (eds), *Italian Colonialism* (Basingstoke: Palgrave Macmillan, 2005). Nicola Labanca, *Oltremare: Storia dell'espansione coloniale italiana* (Bologna: Il Mulin, 2007); Angelo Del Boca, *Italiani, brava gente? Un mito duro a morire* (Vicenza: Neri Pozza, 2005); Nicolas Labanca, *Una guerra per l'Impero, Memorie della campagna d'Etiopia 1935–36* (Bologna: Il Mulino, 2015).

24 Georgio Rocha, 'The Italian Air Force in the Ethiopian War (1935–1936)', in Ben-Ghiat and Fuller (eds), *Italian Colonialism*, pp. 37–46; Alberto Sbacchi, 'Poison Gas and Atrocities in the Italo-Ethiopian War (1935–1936)', in Ben-Ghiat and Fuller (eds), *Italian Colonialism*, pp. 47–56.

# 106    *The long Second World War, 1931–1953*

25 Nicola Perugini and Neve Gordon, 'Between Sovereignty and Race: The Bombardment of Hospitals in the Italo-Ethiopian War and the Colonial Imprint of International Law', *State Crime Journal*, 8:1 (2019), 104–125, at p. 3.

26 Amalia Ribi, *Humanitarian Imperialism: The Politics of Anti-Slavery Activism, 1880–1940*, Oxford Historical Monographs (Oxford: Oxford University Press, 2015).

27 Baudendistel, *Between Bombs and Good Intentions*.

28 Pascal Daudin, 'The Rif War: A Forgotten War?', *International Review of the Red Cross*, 105:923 (2023), 914–946; Francisco Javier Martínez-Antonio, 'Weak Nation-states and the Limits of Humanitarian Aid: The Case of Morocco's Rif War, 1921–1927', in Johannes Paulmann (ed.), *Dilemmas of Humanitarian Aid in the Twentieth Century* (Oxford: Oxford University Press, 2016) pp. 91–114.

29 Baudendistel, *Between Bombs and Good Intentions*, pp. 322–324.

30 Baudendistel, *Between Bombs and Good Intentions*; Marcel Junod, *Warrior without Weapons* (London: Jonathan Cape, 1951); Sydney Brown, *Für das Rote Kreuz in Aethiopien* (Zurich: Europa Verlag, 1939).

31 Baudendistel, *Between Bombs and Good Intentions*, pp. 36–44.

32 Zewde, *A History of Modern Ethiopia*.

33 William R. Scott, *The Sons of Sheba's Race: Africa Americans and the Italo Ethiopian War, 1935–1941* (Bloomington, IN: Indiana University Press, 1993); W. E. B. DuBois, 'Inter-racial Implications of the Ethiopian Crisis: A Negro View', *Foreign Affairs*, 14:1 (1935), 82–92.

34 Alejandro Liano, *Ethiopie: Empire des nègres blancs* (Paris: Pierre Roger, 1931). On these debates among the Afro-American supporters of Ethiopia, see Scott, *The Sons of Sheba's Race*, pp. 192–207.

35 Charles Seligman, *Races of Africa* (London: Thornton Butterworth, 1930).

36 Bronwen Everill, 'The Italo-Abyssinian Crisis and the Shift from Slave to Refugee', *A Journal of Slave and Post-Slave Studies*, 35:2 (2014), 349–365.

37 On the specific case of the South African Red Cross, see Rey, 'Entre prétentions universelles'.

38 Mabon, 'Solidarité Nationale et Captivité Coloniale'; Daniel Palmieri, 'D'hommes à hommes. Le Comité international de la Croix-Rouge et les Frontstalags', in Fabien Theofilakis (ed.), *Les prisonniers de guerre français en 1940* (Paris: Fayard, 2022), pp. 177–186.

39 On the agency, see https://blogs.icrc.org/cross-files/fr/guide-recherche-agence/#_Toc41125056 (accessed 25 September 2023).

40 Lefebvre, 'Combattants, travailleurs, prisonniers'.

## Africa, the Africans, and the Red Cross    107

41 Johann Chapoutot and Jean Vigreux (eds), *Des soldats noirs face au Reich: Les massacres racistes de 1940* (Paris: Presses Universitaires de France, 2015); Julien Fargettas, 'Sind Schwarze da? La chasse aux tirailleurs sénégalais. Aspects cynégétiques de violences de guerre et de violences raciales durant la campagne de France, mai 1940–août 1940', *Revue Historique des Armées*, 271 (2013), 42–50; Raffael Scheck, *Hitler's African Victims: The German Army Massacres of Black French Soldiers in 1940* (Cambridge: Cambridge University Press, 2006); Scheck, *French Colonial Soldiers*; Frank, *Hostages of Empire*; Mabon, *Prisonniers de guerre Indigènes*; Martin C. Thomas, 'The Vichy Government and French Colonial Prisoners of War, 1940–1944', *French Historical Studies*, 25:4 (2002), 657–692.

42 Palmieri, 'D'hommes à hommes'; Marie Allemann, 'Marguerite Gautier-Van Berchem, une figure emblématique', https://blogs.icrc.org/cross-files/fr/marguerite-gautier-van-berchem/ (accessed 17 July 2023).

43 ICRC, *Report of the International Committee of the Red Cross on its Activities during the Second World War, 1 September 1939 – 30 June 1947*, vol. 2 (Geneva: ICRC, 1948), p. 209.

44 *Ibid.*, p. 210.

45 Archives of the International Committee of the Red Cross (AICRC), PV, Sous-commission de l'Agence B, 3 January 1941.

46 AICRC, C G2 FR C-015, Mission de Marguerite van Berchem à Paris, du 12 novembre 1944 au 5 février 1945.

47 AICRC, Agence, C G2 FR C 001, Report from C. Gautier, 26 December 1940.

48 Marie Allemann, 'Marguerite Gautier-Van Berchem, une figure emblématique'.

49 AICRC, BAG 209 003, Pierre Gaillard, PV d'entretien, 23 October 1953.

50 Rito Alcantara, *Rito, Une vie* (Paris: La Banque des femmes, 2008), p. 262; Raffael Scheck, 'Léopold Sédar Senghor prisonnier de guerre allemand: Une nouvelle approche fondée sur un texte inédit', *French Politics, Culture & Society*, 32:2 (2014), 76–98.

51 AICRC, C G2 FR C-015, note à Monsieur Lombard de Marguerite van Berchem, 23 October 1944.

52 AICRC, C G2 FR C-015.

53 Diego Fiscalini, 'Des élites au service d'une cause humanitaire: Le Comité international de la Croix-Rouge' (Master's thesis, University of Geneva, 1985), p. 119.

54 Desgrandchamps and Humbert, 'From Dissident to Recognized Belligerent?', p. 13.

108 *The long Second World War, 1931–1953*

55 AICRC, C G2 FR C-021, C G2 FR C-022, C G2 FR C-023, C G2 FR C-024, C G2 FR C-025, C G2 FR C-026, C G2 FR C-027.

56 Desgrandchamps and Humbert, 'From Dissident to Recognized Belligerent?', p. 13.

57 AICRC, PV, Commission centrale, 5 February 1940.

58 Ian van der Waag (ed.), *Sights, Sounds, Memories: South African Soldier Experiences of the Second World War*, 1st ed. (Stellenbosch: African Sun Media, 2020); Fennell, *Fighting the People's War*.

59 Beatrice Veyrassat, *Histoire de la Suisse et des Suisses dans la marche du monde* (Neuchatel: Alphil, 2018); Patricia Purtschert and Harald Fischer-Tiné (eds), *Colonial Switzerland: Rethinking Colonialism from the Margins* (Basingstoke: Palgrave Macmillan, 2015).

60 Eric Morier-Genoud, 'Missions and Institutions: Henri-Philippe Junod, Anthropology, Human Rights and Academia between Africa and Switzerland, 1921–1966', *SZRKG*, 105 (2011), 193–219.

61 AICRC, PV, Journal, 25 November 1940.

62 AICRC, PV, 29 November 1940.

63 AICRC, PV, Commission des activités extérieures, 30 August 1950.

64 Lucie Odier, 'Mission en Afrique', *Revue internationale de la Croix-Rouge*, 297 (1943), 730–747.

65 AICRC, PV, 8 July 1943.

66 AICRC, PV, Commission des délégations, 17 July 1945.

67 AICRC, PV, Commission des activités extérieures, 30 August 1950.

68 Sandra Bott, *La Suisse et l'Afrique du Sud, 1945–1990, Marché de l'or, finance et commerce durant l'apartheid* (Zurich: Chronos, 2013).

69 AICRC, PV, Conseil de présidence, 30 November 1950.

70 AICRC, PV, Commission des activités extérieures, 29 November 1950.

71 On Senn's work in South Africa in the 1960s, see Andrew Thompson, ' "Restoring Hope Where All Hope Was Lost": Nelson Mandela, the ICRC and the Protection of Political Detainees in Apartheid South Africa', *International Review of the Red Cross*, 98:3 (2016), 799–829.

72 AICRC, PV, Journal, 30 September 1941.

73 AICRC, PV, séance des délégations, 24 December 1942. On these refugees, see Jochen Lingelbach, *On the Edges of Whiteness: Polish Refugees in British Colonial Africa during and after the Second World War* (New York: Berghahn, 2020).

74 AICRC, PV, Commission des délégations, 5 February 1947.

75 AICRC, PV, Commission des délégations, 23 July 1948.

76 AICRC, PV, Conseil de présidence, 23 July 1949.

77 Palmieri, 'D'hommes à hommes'.

78 Everill, 'The Italo-Abyssinian Crisis and the Shift from Slave to Refugee'.

# 4

# (Un)Settling intimacies: boundaries of aid in a North African refugee camp, 1944–1946

*Esther Möller and Katharina Stornig*

This chapter deals with the boundaries of aid in El Shatt, a refugee camp established in the Sinai Peninsula, mainly for Europeans, by the Allied powers in 1944 and maintained until 1947, when the last of its inhabitants left the site. In particular, we analyze the various social and political groups and institutions that were not only present in the camp but also interacted closely and on day-to-day level, and thus actively participated in both care work and the organization of camp life. Introducing the notion of intimacy to the study of the social, political, and cultural relations in the camp as well as in the extended and transnational humanitarian structures and social surroundings in which it existed, we argue that El Shatt's main protagonists constituted several "circles of intimacy," which were central to the organization of both camp life and humanitarian aid. Among these protagonists were not only the humanitarian organizations, the British military, and the Egyptian and international staff working in El Shatt, but also the refugees themselves, Egyptian political and juridical authorities, and international donors and supporters of humanitarian aid in Great Britain and the United States. We use the notion of "circles of intimacy" in order to highlight the ways in which the engineers and organizers of the refugee camp drew on certain visions of social bonding during the parallel experiences of un- and resettlement on the one hand,[1] and the workings of "cultural intimacy," understood as "the recognition of those aspects of a cultural identity … that … provide insiders with their assurance of common sociality" on the other.[2] As we will show, these "circles of intimacy" were partly separated from each other and partly overlapped, but all contributed to the

110    *The long Second World War, 1931–1953*

construction of social and cultural relations in the camp, which housed peoples of different age, gender, nationality, professional background, social or professional status, and religion.

El Shatt was the largest of five refugee camps established by the Allied powers during the Second World War in the Middle East. Located in the Egyptian desert east of the Suez Canal, it accommodated up to thirty thousand men, women and children, mostly from the Dalmatian coast, who had fled from Nazi occupation or were evacuated by partisans and the British navy after the Italian capitulation in September 1943.[3] Most of the refugees left the camp in 1946 and either returned to Yugoslavia or departed for other destinations, especially the United States. The camp was first run by MERRA, the Middle East Relief and Rehabilitation Administration of the Allied Forces, and then taken over by the United Nations Relief and Rehabilitation Administration (UNRRA), an international agency founded by forty-four states in 1943 in order to provide and administer relief to the millions of war victims and refugees in their territories categorized and administrated as "displaced persons."[4] Even though UNRRA was designed as an international organization with member countries from all continents, it was dominated by the United States, which also provided the largest amount of funding. In addition to MERRA and UNRRA, several other humanitarian organizations sent staff to El Shatt until its closure in 1947.

Even though historical research has dedicated considerable attention to the study of humanitarian work and assistance in post-war European refugee camps,[5] El Shatt, along with other camps for European refugees in the Arab world from Morocco to Lebanon, has only recently been rediscovered by historians.[6] On the one hand, historians of Yugoslavia have studied El Shatt as an important step in the history of nation building, in particular with regard to Yugoslavia.[7] Scholars such as Kornelija Ajlec have drawn not only on the memories of former camp inhabitants but also on UN and Croatian state archives in order to retrace this piece of entangled Yugoslavian and especially Croatian history.[8] On the other hand, historians as well as political scientists, sociologists, and anthropologists have started to investigate refugee camps in the Middle East more generally as important spaces of political and social interaction.[9] Taking their cue from the case study of camps for Palestinian refugees, scholars have realized that

## (Un)Settling intimacies in a refugee camp          111

these camps – though somewhat exceptional, as Michel Agier and Francoise Saulnier-Boucher have remarked[10] – often turned into permanent habitations with their own structures of governance and exchange with other institutions. These studies complement those of historians who emphasize the need to analyze refugee camps in a global perspective, as "forgotten portals of globalization."[11] While aspects of social relations among refugees and between refugees and staff of the humanitarian organizations have already been touched upon in the studies on El Shatt, they examine neither the sphere of the intimate nor social constructions of gender and age as analytical categories by which to understand the social and cultural dimensions of day-to-day life in the camp.

Finally but importantly, recent scholarship on refugee camps in the Middle East has emphasized the agency of the refugees themselves. For a long time, refugees – and once again the Palestinian refugees offer an instructive example – have been considered passive recipients of aid whose main preoccupation consisted in waiting for the next steps taken by other actors. Yet both Ilana Feldman (with regard to Palestinian refugees) and Peter Gatrell (with regard to refugees in general) have stressed the refugees' own involvement in the definition of their status as refugees and in shaping the conditions of their lives and political possibilities.[12] Gatrell's suggestion that we should speak of "refugeedom" in order to emphasize the value of refugees as political and social beings seems very helpful in order to shed light on the multiple interactions with governments and state institutions, but also with the populations living in proximity with refugees, either in camps or in individual dwellings. These latter interactions have often been absent from studies on refugee camps that focused exclusively on the camp sites and failed to consider potential interactions with neighboring populations.[13] Yet, especially in the context of refugee camps for Europeans in colonial and postcolonial settings, it seems crucial to look at these interactions in order to understand the different relations the refugees had with the Western humanitarian organizations on the one hand, and with people from (formerly) colonized societies on the other.

This chapter aims to contribute to this scholarship by studying the social and cultural relations in El Shatt through the lens of intimacy. More particularly, it suggests analyzing the (re)making and blurring of social, personal, and cultural boundaries between the

112    *The long Second World War, 1931–1953*

diverse people present in El Shatt – including men, women, and children of different origins and status (e.g., as refugees, civilian workers, or military or humanitarian personnel) – through humanitarian aid. While at first sight, refugee camps – as sites resettling and thus containing, housing, and administrating large numbers of displaced persons – seem the incarnation of (enforced) intimacy, this study also shows that close or even personal relationships and interactions were reinforced or enhanced by the different actors involved. Camp life in El Shatt was shaped by different groups of actors (Allied authorities, international aid workers, Egyptian people, and the refugees themselves) and their relationships to the "outside" world.[14] El Shatt saw multiple and complex – voluntary and involuntary – encounters, intimacies, constellations, and social relationships. It thus invites us to engage critically with a strand in research on humanitarianism that conceives of refugee camps primarily as "exceptional" and "humanitarian" spaces cut off from the surrounding environment, where particular social relations sometimes developed even in conflict with the social norms of the environment.[15] Indeed, as Jordanna Bailkin has shown with regard to refugee camps in Britain in the twentieth century, camps both clearly distinguished and blurred boundaries between refugees and the surrounding population. As the Egyptian population also experienced the war's privations, and some were themselves displaced, they and the refugees "moved in and out of moments of closeness and distance, structured by timelines of war and poverty."[16] Consequently, their relations alternated between a clear hierarchy and moments of more equal encounters.[17]

El Shatt constitutes an interesting case in point to study the intimacies created, used, or recreated through humanitarian relief because it was administered not only by Western military and humanitarian bodies but also by some of the refugees themselves. This means that some refugees in the camp were at the same time donors and recipients of aid. As administrators, they could speak on behalf of other refugees, but they could also gain power through access to material and knowledge. What is more, it was a very large camp and its organizers produced copious documentation, much of which is preserved and accessible to researchers, for instance in the historical archives of the United Nations or in the form of published and personal accounts by humanitarian workers. This chapter uses these sources and supplements them with research on both the perspectives of

*(Un)Settling intimacies in a refugee camp*        113

Croatian refugees and Egyptian perspectives on the Second World War. Indeed, we particularly seek to highlight the roles of Egyptians in the camp, which outlived the war years and thus underlines the idea of a "long" Second World War in a global perspective.[18] Finally, the case of El Shatt forcefully reminds us that migration and flight occurred not only from the Middle East to Europe but also vice versa, thus challenging the humanitarian organizations' perceptions of and forms of cooperation with host societies.

In the following, we introduce what we call different "circles of intimacies" – that is, circles of (presumed, attempted, or prevented) human bonding and emotional or intuitive closeness despite the disruptive experiences of un- and resettlement due to the war. We use the notion in order to highlight both (cultural, emotional, ideological, etc.) proximity and social hierarchies as they worked out in day-to-day camp organization and life. We thus suggest that these circles related both to the specific organizational logics of El Shatt as a largely closed humanitarian enclave in the Egyptian desert and to the transnational relations in which it was embedded.

## Family and community

The accommodation of refugees in El Shatt was structured according to – real or imagined – social and cultural bonds as well as status. Members of biological families were accommodated together in the same tent, thus presuming good relations between different generations. Yet living together could also provoke conflicts, and it therefore sometimes occurred that "camps prompted uneasy ties between refugees of different … generations."[19] When space became scarce, tents were to be shared either with relatives or with refugees from similar geographical and cultural backgrounds. The idea was that, by accommodating refugees from the same Dalmatian communities together, social ties would be strengthened, and entire villages ideally be recreated within the space of the camp.[20] Thus, while the camp's administration not only enabled but even encouraged intimacy to family and kin, it strove to limit enforced proximity to strangers considering the overall situation of a crowded refugee camp, ensuring that refugees of a similar cultural and national background and origin were grouped together.

114     *The long Second World War, 1931–1953*

Furthermore, refugees in El Shatt were grouped according to social status and the humanitarian infrastructure available: for instance, orphans were gathered in an on-site orphanage, forming part of an imagined community of displaced children that the UNRRA official Martha Branscombe, in an article published in 1945, called "The Children of the United Nations."[21] In turn, partisan fighters were accommodated in British military tents, which created another spatial and social unit in El Shatt. UNRRA officials generally administrated people according to gender and age, distinguishing in their reports between "men and boys," "women and girls," and "children under 14," at least for the Greek and Yugoslav refugees.[22] That means that at fourteen years or over, young people were gendered male or female and no longer considered "children." Finally yet importantly, ethnicity and national belonging were deeply inscribed in the camp's social order. Yugoslavs were housed together and in separation from other refugee groups present, such as Greeks or European Jews.

This categorization and organization of the camp inhabitants by the administrators can also be seen on the lists set up by the latter, in which the number of refugees was recorded "by nationality."[23] However, this category was not used in a consistent manner, as next to "Yugoslavs" or "Greeks," the list of late 1946 also included a number of "Dodecanese" or "Armenians" and thus linguistic groups that at the time did not correspond to a sovereign nation state. This may point to the fact that the camp administrators took the refugees' own (ethnic, national, or linguistic) self-identification as a starting point. The list is also interesting for listing fifty "Ethiopians," thirteen "Somalis," and sixteen "Eritreans" as housed in El Shatt. The presence of refugees from African countries has been little observed in research. While this aspect cannot be developed further in this chapter, it would be highly interesting to analyze how colonial or racial divides worked out within the camp structure and social relations, thereby substantiating the claim that camps were also spaces of encounters between people from very different ethnic backgrounds.[24] In this vein, it would be valuable to study potential contacts and interactions between European and African refugees, as well as to ask if their treatment by humanitarian organizations and the camp administration differed.

Altogether, the accommodation of refugees in El Shatt points to – existing or presumed – bonds between families as well as

# (Un)Settling intimacies in a refugee camp                115

within social, cultural, or national communities. According to the administrative logic, these bonds served as the structuring principles of social order and thus also of regulating intimacy. The camp's organizers tried to rebuild social structures and human bonds as they presumed them to have existed in the refugees' lives before evacuation or as they expected them to work out once the war was over. Indeed, some sources suggest that (presumed) intimacy and solidarity within these groups were seen as sources of prosocial behavior and a strategy not only of dealing with the confinement of camp life but also of building a post-war society. As the British newspaper *The Sphere* put it in an article on "the Partisans of Yugoslavia" in May 1944: "Living in Army huts and tents, they are rebuilding their individual and family lives. The camp is valuable experience in preparation for the bigger job of helping the liberated peoples of Europe along the road to reconstruction."[25]

At the same time, however, it is important to note that the closeness and intimacies in El Shatt were enforced politically, since its inmates were not allowed to leave the site and to visit (for instance) the nearby city of Suez.[26] Here, the Egyptian government comes into play as an important stakeholder not yet considered sufficiently by research: in 1946, it further restricted the movements and mobility of refugees, with the result that, according to an UNRRA official, "El Shatt has become more of a concentration camp."[27] The sources suggest that the Egyptian government was very suspicious of any influence that the refugees, many of them communists, might have on the Egyptian population. Therefore, it had permitted the camp to be set up only on condition of its being located in the desert, far from areas inhabited by Egyptians,[28] and tried to limit the refugees' external contacts as much as possible. This policy only proved partially successful, as we will see below.

## Gender- and age-based institutions and sociability

Day-to-day life in El Shatt was to a large extent structured around constructions of gender and age.[29] This was also the case for separate spheres of humanitarian work as well as for refugee sociability: workspaces, but also sports and leisure clubs for men and women as well as schools, kindergartens, and playgrounds in the

116     *The long Second World War, 1931–1953*

camp offered opportunities for refugee men, women, and children. The primary sources suggest that more of these spaces were established for men and children than for women. Some Yugoslav camp administrators even argued that men, although fewer in number, were the pillars of social and political structures in the camp.[30]

Furthermore, work opportunities were created especially for men. Most women seem to have worked as nurses, cooks, and teachers.[31] Other workshops, not designated for any particular sex, repaired shoes or produced handcrafts. The latter were even presented and sold at exhibitions, including embroidery, knitwear, paintings, and lace. The fact that there were more work opportunities for men was partly due to the prominent role played by Yugoslav partisans in organizing camp activities, though there had also been female partisans, if fewer in number.[32] The partisan movement was officially known as the "People's Liberation Movement" and was dominated by the Communist Party, though it also included people with other political backgrounds.[33] Its members present in Egypt had fought against the Axis powers, which had destroyed their state in 1941, and they now sought to rebuild Yugoslav society in Egypt.[34] The partisans conceived of working as an important aspect of this endeavor and saw it, moreover, as a way to prove the refugees' high motivation.[35] As most of the partisans who feature in the historical records on work in El Shatt were men, workplace sociability relied on an all-male community. However, an administrative report also mentioned the avoidance of boredom, existing skills, interest in being part of a group, and the desire to get away from wives and children as other motivations for men to engage in – unpaid, owing to partisan rules – labor.[36] This brings us to the next circle of intimacy, that made up of the partisans who were camp organizers but also increasingly claimed roles as political and decidedly masculine leaders.


## Camp administrations and aid workers

Although established, managed, and supplied by the British and American allies as well as by UNRRA, camp life was to a considerable extent organized by the Yugoslav refugees. In particular, former partisan fighters who formed the so-called Refugee Central Committee emerged as leaders in El Shatt. Aiming to turn the

## (Un)Settling intimacies in a refugee camp 117

refugees into citizens of a future Yugoslavia and to display their aptitude at successfully managing the complicated situation to the Allies, the committee established what the historian Florian Bieber has called the "de facto self-government of the refugees."[37] While another camp in Egypt, Al-Arish, housed the royalist or supposedly royalist refugees from Dalmatia, the majority of those gathered at El Shatt shared the partisans' political convictions. Thus, political identification also served as a basis for intimacy, trust, and close collaboration in the organization of camp life.[38] Moreover, the partisans sought to maintain good relations with the British army in order to win support for the partisans' work in both the camp and the future state of Yugoslavia.[39] Yet, as Bieber observes, "their relations were marked by both mutual admiration and suspicion",[40] as both groups sought to gain as much control over the camp as possible.

In terms of gender, refugee leadership in El Shatt was built on exclusively male representation. Women were not addressed as potential fighters themselves but only as partisans' wives. When asked to hold free elections for the camp's administration board by UNRRA and some critics, the Refugee Central Committee replied that the camp mainly consisted of women and children who were not representative of the future society they sought to build, as many husbands and fathers were still fighting in the war.[41] This clearly shows that the all-male committee in the camp was not willing to accept either elections or women voters.

Apart from the partisans, El Shatt was administered by international military and humanitarian institutions. At the beginning, the camp was organized by the British army who had evacuated the refugees from Dalmatia and brought them to Egypt. In 1942, the British army had created the Middle East and Refugee Administration (MERRA), which was responsible for the various refugee camps in the region. In May 1944, MERRA was replaced by UNRRA, which sent administrators and medical staff to Egypt. Other humanitarian organizations working at El Shatt included the American and British Red Cross societies and the Quakers, as well as the Greek Red Cross and the British Save the Children Fund. As a British nurse recalled in 1945, "the staff has been a truly international group."[42] While she mentions positive moments of understanding, she also encountered difficulties

118        *The long Second World War, 1931–1953*

in cooperating in humanitarian relief, for instance due to "varying ideas on medical care."[43]

With regard to relations between aid workers and refugees in El Shatt, a complex configuration of intimacy and distance can be observed, as "the camps offered opportunities for both selfishness and service."[44] On the one hand, aid workers were taught to keep professional distance in order to perform their activities according to their organizations' and not the refugees' priorities. On the other hand, however, the crowdedness and lack of physical separation in terms of walls and houses brought aid workers and refugees into close contact. This was reinforced by the isolated location of the camp in the desert and the attempt to organize all forms of sociability within it. In addition, the sources suggest that a certain intimacy, especially between health workers and children, was helpful to ensure the refugees' cooperation.[45] These contacts can be traced in personal diaries such as that of the British nurse Dorothy Hamilton Des Quartiers, who worked for the British Red Cross in the Middle East between 1943 and 1945, at El Shatt as well as in the camps of Nuseirat and Al-Khatabta. For instance, she writes of "undernourished babies" who had died as "pathetic little bodies" of "distracted parents".[46] Her pity for the babies speaks of a sense of closeness, while she maintains a critical distance from the refugee parents.

Other examples are photographs depicting aid workers in the camp. Certain photos show physical closeness between aid workers and refugee children, revealing the workers' acceptance of bodily contact. Besides, due to a constant lack of medical staff, aid workers had to rely on the assistance of refugees. A central factor was language. As most aid workers did not speak the refugees' language – most of whom, in turn, did not speak English – physical contact was important in order to instruct refugee women, who assisted in care work. As a nurse recalled: "If we want an aide [as the women assistants were called] to do something and can't tell her, we may have to lead her by the hand the length of a long ward and then use the gestures necessary."[47] While most of the international aid workers and especially the nurses were women, the international camp administrators in charge were men. Thus, care work was mostly performed by women, while men dealt with juridical and political questions. Yet, female aid workers were also aware of

## (Un)Settling intimacies in a refugee camp    119

a political dimension of their activities when describing their work with refugee staff as having "the objective of preparing them for life and work in their country when they return."[48] Other sources represented female humanitarian work as an experience that was also socially and personally rewarding. For instance, a newspaper article about Mary W. Lumb, a staff officer with the British Cross who had worked at El Shatt as well as Volos (Greece) between 1944 and 1945, not only referred to the woman's humanitarian contributions as a "backbreaking job" but added that it was "a great satisfaction to Mrs Lumb to be able to help in the distribution of food and medical supplies to people who had been without these vital necessities for so long."[49]

Finally, it should be added that the social and cultural relations in El Shatt at least in one case permitted the blurring of boundaries between the international staff and the refugees in the camp. While we have not come across complaints or reports of gender-based violence or abuse in the sources, the *West London Observer* reported on an "UNRRA Refugee Camp Romance" in June 1946. The article reproduced the generally positive representation of the Yugoslav refugees in the British press as brave and cheerful people and reported that a "pretty young Dalmatian ... – one of the 20,000 Yugoslav Partisans who fled from Nazi persecution to the sanctuary of an UNRRA Displaced Persons camp on the fringe of the Sinai" had fallen in love with a British sergeant. Furthermore, the article mentioned a wedding dress made "with exquisite taste and care, by refugee seamstresses" and stated that the couple was married in a church in Suez before relocating to Britain in the summer of 1946.[50] El Shatt was thus depicted in highly positive terms as a site of romantic love that facilitated intimacy even between male military personnel and female refugees rather than as a site of enforced resettlement due to the war.

### Local population, staff and the Egyptian authorities

While there was a certain degree of intimacy between aid workers and refugees, another group of people is almost wholly absent from many Western primary sources and even the secondary literature in spite of being very much present in the camp: the local population

120    *The long Second World War, 1931–1953*

and staff as well as the Egyptian authorities. Indeed, there were more points in common and moments of encounter between them than is often presumed. In the case of El Shatt, there were three groups of Egyptians concerned by the refugee camp: Egyptian state authorities and their representatives, Egyptian civilians working for or in the camp, and Egyptians living near the camp. The Egyptian authorities certainly did intervene in the organization and running of the camp but often in an indirect manner.[51] The Egyptian government gave permission to open and maintain the camp in Egypt, yet its freedom of action at that time was limited because during the Second World War the British army had established its headquarters in Egypt and exploited the country and its resources with scant regard for the interests of the population.[52] Historical research has long overlooked the active participation of Egyptian institutions and individuals in the war,[53] and this seems also to apply to the running of refugee camps in Egypt. In Western sources, Egyptians are either completely absent or represented in very negative terms. Moreover, only men appear in these sources, although Egyptian women most probably were also in contact with El Shatt. In her diary, the Red Cross nurse Dorothy Hamilton Des Quartiers, who worked in different refugee camps in the Middle East during the Second World War, mentions the local population, when she does so at all, only in very negative terms. For example, she notes "great troubles with Arab thieves"[54] who "were dressed naked and oiled their bodies, so that if they were caught they were impossible to be held."[55] As for Bedouins, it is worth recalling that in Great Britain at the time there was much concern about "unsettled" people, be they refugees or others without a stable home, and with seeing such people settled,[56] and this cultural background may have reinforced Hamilton Des Quartier's orientalist view of parts of the population in Egypt.

A close reading of the UNRRA reports reveals that the population near the camp also provided refugees and staff with food and groceries, either by running the canteens or by bringing fresh food to the camp. As many Egyptians were also in precarious economic conditions due to the war and thus in similar need of food themselves, boundaries between the population and the refugees became blurred. This may have been one reason why the presence

## (Un)Settling intimacies in a refugee camp 121

of the Egyptians in the camp, for example, as kitchen staff, is described in UN reports as a source of infection, "as they had no conception of proper sanitation," according to UNRRA sanitary engineer Frederick F. Alderidge.[57] He reported that as a consequence "it was found necessary to discharge them and substitute refugee women."[58] Another function of the local population was to provide guards for the camp. Interestingly, the UNRRA reports refer to these guards as "ghaffirs," using the Arabic word for guard.[59] This reveals a certain appropriation of the local language and customs, but probably also the necessity of using certain Arabic terms for communication. Yet Egyptian staff members are mentioned when problems occur, such as conflicts over finances, disagreements between Arab staff, or the escape of refugees from the camp. For example, in July 1946, the camp director reported to the security officer that an Egyptian *ghaffir* had been found in a tent that was out of bounds to him but that nothing had been stolen. The *ghaffir* was dismissed.[60] Moreover, Britain's semi-colonial rule meant that Egyptian authorities had only limited jurisdiction over the camp. In summer 1946, when acid had been thrown within the camp, the Egyptian police wanted the accused to be tried in Suez, but the case was instead taken to the Mixed Court in Cairo.[61] These Mixed Courts were a legacy of the historically strong influence of the European powers in Egypt: established in the nineteenth century by the Khedive to deal with the affairs of the many Europeans involved in Egypt, it was a legal system which exempted Europeans from being judged by Egyptian courts and as such part of an imperial legal infrastructure that consolidated unequal relations.[62]

Yet the Egyptian population encountered the refugees and their administrators not only in professional or commercial contexts but also during leisure activities. For instance, there was a camp choir that performed in various Egyptian cities and also a football team that appears to have played matches against Egyptian sides.[63] However, it is doubtful whether the local population also interacted as consumers of goods produced by refugees in the camp, as was the case in other camps for European refugees in Syria and Lebanon,[64] since El Shatt was much more remote from the nearest villages than other camps in the Middle East.

122     *The long Second World War, 1931–1953*

All Western sources completely ignore that at the same time, Egyptians were themselves running charitable and medical associations that took care of refugees.[65] While their main focus was on Arab refugees, either from within Egypt or from neighboring countries such as Libya, these organizations also sent money, food, clothes, and blankets to people who had to leave their homes in, for instance, Poland, Hungary, or Yugoslavia.[66] The next step for research will be to find out about these organizations' contacts with Europeans finding refuge in Egypt.

### Transnational humanitarian community

A last important circle of intimacy that we traced in the sources relates to what humanitarians imagined as a transnational community of aid givers. Some texts indeed suggest that El Shatt was interpreted not in isolation from but in relation with transnational humanitarian efforts during the Second World War. This transnational humanitarian community provided an important frame of reference. It was cited by humanitarian actors and institutions in El Shatt, who strove to bridge distance and to make the camp an object of humanitarian emotions, assistance, and donations in Britain and the United States.

In this context, professional photography played a crucial role, as the camp's administrators created specific and staged views of the refugees' lives, producing a certain sense of intimate insight into refugees' lives as well as their joys and sorrows. Thereby, the work of the American photographer Otto Gilmore deserves mention. Gilmore was a renowned photographer who also experimented with new techniques,[67] and visited the camp in 1944. He did so in the service of the US Office of War Information and with the explicit aim of bearing witness to UNRRA's work.[68] His photographs aimed at representing a distant "reality" from the Egyptian desert to spectators in other parts of the world. This effort of producing and distributing photographic images of El Shatt certainly related not only to humanitarian or informative concerns but also to established strategies in humanitarian campaigning and fundraising.[69] Gilmore's photographs were and still are widely seen and offer good examples of what scholars have studied as humanitarian

(Un)Settling intimacies in a refugee camp 123

photography. What is more, they testify to the ideal visions of camp life as developed by UNRRA in line with its guiding principle, "help the people to help themselves."[70]

Gilmore's photographs provide insights into the ways in which Yugoslav refugees were constructed as civilian victims and survivors of the war, and as somewhat exotic yet nonetheless allied Europeans. The images include individual and group portraits of men, women, and children going about their day-to-day camp life in the Egyptian desert. Gilmore pictured the Yugoslav refugees as active in organizing camp life collectively, thereby representing a kind of social order with gender and age-based arrangements to which viewers in Britain and the US could easily relate. In his photographs, we see girls and women cooking, children playing, and the elderly waiting for the war to end. All seem eager to return to Dalmatia but also able to cope with their complicated situation. Gilmore's photographs certainly also provided tools that could be used in humanitarian communication and fundraising.

Seen from this angle, it comes as no surprise that children were central to these images as well as to promotional articles in newspapers.[71] In 1944, the Coventry branch of Save the Children published a fundraising article which told the emotional story of seven-year-old Lepa Marinkovic, a Yugoslav girl who had ended up in El Shatt after escaping from the Nazis while her father had joined Tito's forces.[72] The narrative invited a compassionate response from readers by representing the war as a disruptive experience of a young girl's childhood in "rugged, widely lovely Dalmatia." Accordingly, Lepa "saw men and women shot, and houses looted and burned," suffered from hunger and missed her partisan father, until her mother took the opportunity to escape and she found herself in a "city of tents in the Sinai desert."[73] There, the girl, together with thousands of other refugee children, was provided with food, water, and other material supplies by an international group of welfare workers, among them "administrators and welfare specialists" sent by the Save the Children Fund. Finally, the article turned to local contributions for the rescue of young war victims by reporting on "Coventry-built ambulances" in the three camps housing refugees from Dalmatia, as well as by reporting on a new healthcare project that included the training of refugee girls in hygiene, providing medical care for convalescents, and advising mothers in childcare.

124     *The long Second World War, 1931–1953*

What is more, it mentioned a teacher-training course launched in order to give six thousand children like Lepa the opportunity to return to school after two years of absence. In conclusion, the article pointed to the great reconstructive task ahead once the war had ended and invited donations to send a Coventry mobile unit "to help the destitute children of the devastated lands of Europe."[74] Hence, it used the individual story of a young girl from Dalmatia and her existence in a far-off refugee camp located in a northern African desert in order to prepare and promote humanitarian relief and reconstruction in the wake of the Second World War.

## Conclusion

This chapter has focused on the refugee camp of El Shatt in Egypt and its many internal and external connections. As most of the refugees only returned to their countries of origin or moved on to other destinations in 1947, it underlines that enlarging the geographical focus in which we consider the Second World War also changes its chronological boundaries. In addition, the chapter's interest in questioning gender and age as organizing categories for life in the camp has revealed that there were many factors predating the war that shaped social relations, but that these relations were also transformed by the war and the conditions of life in the camp. First, by choosing intimacy as a lens to analyze relations between all actors involved in humanitarian and medical care, this chapter has pointed to both the reconstruction and transformation of social relations in El Shatt. On the one hand, tents were assigned families and people from the same regions and grouped accordingly, and work spaces were organized according to gender. On the other hand, photos taken or commissioned by the camp administrators also privileged nuclear families over particular age groups – such as children or the elderly – and thus suggested other forms of intimacy. Second, the focus on intimacy has shown that, although social, national, and economic differences existed between the recipients and donors of humanitarian aid in the camp, living together in close quarters as well as the need for medical and other staff at times also blurred the boundaries between these groups: refugee women were trained

*(Un)Settling intimacies in a refugee camp* 125

as nurses and a humanitarian worker married a refugee. Third, the lens of intimacy has allowed us to highlight actors that are often invisible in Western sources, notably the Egyptian staff working in the camp, but also the Egyptian political and juridical authorities concerned with the regulation of the camp as part of a specific region and country.

## Notes

1 With respect to refugee camps in post-war Britain, Jordanna Bailkin has argued that "being 'resettled' was deeply unsettling." Jordanna Bailkin, *Unsettled: Refugee Camps and the Making of Multicultural Britain* (Oxford and New York: Oxford University Press, 2018), p. 8.

2 Michael Herzfeld, *Cultural Intimacy: Social Poetics and the Nation State* (New York and London: Routledge, 1997), p. 3.

3 Florian Bieber, "Building Yugoslavia in the Sand? Dalmatian Refugees in Egypt, 1944–1946," *Slavic Review*, 79:2 (2020), 298–322, at p. 298.

4 Silvia Salvatici, *A History of Humanitarianism, 1755–1989: In the Name of Others* (Manchester: Manchester University Press, 2019), 116–132.

5 See, for example, Daniel G. Cohen, *In War's Wake: Europe's Displaced Persons in Postwar Order* (New York: Oxford University Press, 2012); Silvia Salvatici, "Professionals of Humanitarianism: UNRRA Relief Officers in Post-War Europe," in Johannes Paulmann (ed.), *The Dilemmas of Humanitarian Aid in the Twentieth Century* (Oxford: Oxford University Press, 2016), pp. 235–262; Silvia Salvatici, "'Fighters without Guns': Humanitarianism and Military Action in the Aftermath of the Second World War," *European Review of History: Revue européenne d'histoire* (2017), 1–19; Laure Humbert, *Reinventing French Aid: The Politics of Humanitarian Relief in French-Occupied Germany, 1945–1952* (Cambridge: Cambridge University Press, 2021).

6 Katherine Mackinnon and Benjamin Thomas White, "What Becomes a Refugee Camp? Making Camps for European Refugees in North Africa and the Middle East, 1943–1946," *Journal of Refugee Studies*. https://doi.org/10.1093/jrs/fead042; Laura Robson, "UNRRA in North Africa: A Late Colonial History of Refugee Encampment," *Past & Present*, 261:1 (2023), 193–222.

7 Bieber, "Building Yugoslavia in the Sand?"

126 *The long Second World War, 1931–1953*

8 While Ajlec's PhD thesis was in Croatian, she has also published in English on the topic: "Yugoslav Refugees and British Relief Workers in Italian and Egyptian Refugee Camps, 1944–6," in David Brydan and Jessica Reinisch (eds), *Internationalists of Europe: Rethinking the Twentieth Century* (London: Bloomsbury Academic, 2021), pp. 105–123.

9 See Baher Ibrahim, "Refugee Settlement and Encampment in the Middle East and North Africa, 1860s–1940s," https://static1.squaresp ace.com/static/5748678dcf80a1ffcaf26975/t/614ca66b9294e2269 debb27a/1632413293154/Baher+Ibrahim%2C+Research+guide+ to+refugee+settlement+and+encampment+in+the+Middle+East+ and+North+Africa%2C+1860s-1940s.pdf (accessed 24 November 2022); Benjamin T. White, "Humans and Animals in a Refugee Camp: Baquba, Iraq, 1918–20," *Journal of Refugee Studies*, 32:2 (2018), 216–236. https://doi.org/10.1093/jrs/fey024; Kjersti Berg, "Mu'askar and Shu'fat: Retracing the Histories of Two Palestinian Refugee Camps in Jerusalem," *Jerusalem Quarterly*, 88:4 (2021), 30–52.

10 Michel Agier and Françoise Bouchet-Saulnier, "Espaces Humanitaires, Espaces d'exception," in Fabrice Weissman (ed.), *Á l'ombre Des Guerres Justes: L'ordre International Cannibale et l'action Humanitaire* (Paris: Flammarion, 2003), 297–313.

11 Jochen Lingelbach, "Refugee Camps as Forgotten Portals of Globalization: Polish World War II Refugees in British Colonial East Africa," *Comparativ. Zeitschrift für Globalgeschichte und vergleichende Gesellschaftsforschung*, 27:3 –4 (2017), 78–93.

12 Ilana Feldman, "The Challenge of Categories: UNRWA and the Definition of a 'Palestine Refugee,'" *Journal of Refugee Studies*, 25:3 (2012), 387–406; Peter Gatrell, "Refugees—What's Wrong with History?" *Journal of Refugee Studies*, 30:2 (2017), 170–189.

13 Lingelbach, "Refugee Camps," p. 79.

14 According to the retrospective report of a doctor who had worked in El Shatt, the refugees there acted on "orders from home," refusing, for instance, to accept money for their labor. Henry R. O'Brien, "Other Nurses," *The American Journal of Nursing*, 47:10 (1947), 676–679, at p. 676.

15 See Agier and Bouchet-Saulnier, "Espaces Humanitaires, Espaces d'exception," pp. 297–313.

16 Bailkin, *Refugee Camps*, p. 5.

17 See Bailkin, *Refugee Camps*, p. 10.

18 For this "long" Second World War, see, for example, Andrew N. Buchanan, *World War II in Global Perspective, 1931–1953: A Short History* (London: Wiley, 2019).

## (Un)Settling intimacies in a refugee camp     127

19 Bailkin, *Refugee Camps*, p. 11.
20 Ajlec, "Yugoslav Refugees," p. 114.
21 Martha Branscombe, "The Children of the United Nations: UNRRA's Responsibility for Social Welfare," *Social Service Review*, 19:3 (1945), 310–323. Recent studies have focused especially on the situation and humanitarian treatment of unaccompanied children in post-war Europe, whose national and social identities were anything but clearly defined. See, for instance, Tara Zahra, *The Lost Children: Reconstructing Europe's Families After World War II* (Cambridge, MA: Harvard University Press, 2011); Lynne Taylor, *In the Children's Best Interests: Unaccompanied Children in American-Occupied Germany, 1945–1952* (Toronto: University of Toronto Press, 2017).
22 See United Nations Archives, New York (hereafter UN Archives), S 1450 0000 0068 00001, "U.N.N.R.R.A. Middle East Office. Twentieth Native Report of the Chief of the Middle East Office, October 1st–31, 1946," p. 10.
23 See UN Archives, S 1450 0000 0068 00001, "U.N.N.R.R.A. Middle East Office. Twentieth Native Report of the Chief of the Middle East Office, December 1st–31, 1946," p. 7.
24 See Bailkin, *Refugee Camps*, p. 10.
25 "The Partisans of Yugoslavia and their Continued Offensive Against the German Forces of Occupation," *The Sphere* (27 May 1944), p. 276.
26 See UN Archives, S 1450 0000 0068 00001, "U.N.N.R.R.A. Middle East Office. Twentieth Native Report of the Chief of the Middle East Office, December 1st–31, 1946," p. 1.
27 *Ibid.*
28 Ajlec, "Yugoslav Refugees."
29 For the roles of specific ideas of gender and family in post-war humanitarian contexts and understanding of rehabilitation, see Tara Zahra, "'The Psychological Marshall Plan': Displacement, Gender, and Human Rights after World War II," *Central European History*, 44 (2011), 37–62.
30 For example, the partisan camp leaders refused to hold elections because of the high number of women and children in the camp and the resulting "incomplete" population. See Bieber, "Building Yugoslavia in the Sand?" p. 311.
31 *Ibid.*, p. 306.
32 Ajlec, "Yugoslav Refugees," p. 110; Bieber, "Building Yugoslavia in the Sand?" p. 303.
33 See Bieber, "Building Yugoslavia in the Sand?" p. 298.
34 Bieber, "Building Yugoslavia in the Sand?"
35 *Ibid.*, p. 306.

128    *The long Second World War, 1931–1953*

36  Report by Henry G. Russel, cited in Bieber, "Building Yugoslavia in the Sand?" p. 306.
37  Bieber, "Building Yugoslavia in the Sand?" p. 303.
38  This can also be seen in photographic representations of the committee, which showed men in uniform working or consulting together and – as in a British newspaper feature from 1944 – sitting in front of "a portrait of their leader, Marshall Tito." "The Partisans of Yugoslavia and their Continued Offensive Against the German Forces of Occupation," *The Sphere* (27 May 1944), p. 276. See also Bieber, "Building Yugoslavia in the Sand?" p. 310.
39  See Bieber, "Building Yugoslavia in the Sand?" pp. 301–302.
40  *Ibid.*, p. 302.
41  *Ibid.*, p. 311.
42  Margaret G. Arnstein, "Nursing in UNRRA Middle East Refugee Camps," *The American Journal of Nursing*, 45:5 (1945), 378–381, p. 379.
43  *Ibid.*
44  Bailkin, *Refugee Camps*, p. 10.
45  *Ibid.*, p. 381.
46  Archives of the British Red Cross, London (hereafter ABRC), 1629, Diary of Dorothy Hamilton Des Quartiers, 1939–1945, p. 16.
47  Arnstein, "Nursing," p. 379.
48  *Ibid.*, p. 380.
49  "Did Red Cross Work in Greece," *Halifax Evening Courier* (3 October 1945), p. 2.
50  "UNRRA Refugee Camp Romance," *West London Observer* (14 June 1946), p. 2.
51  This phenomenon was not specific to El Shatt but common in other refugee camps for Europeans in the Middle East as well, such as the camp for Greek refugees at Moses Wells, not far from El Shatt. See Alex Lamprou, "From Displaced Memory to the Memory of Displacement: Refugees from Greece to the Middle East during World War Two," *Migration Erinnern, Hypotheses Academic Blogs* (2021), https://migrer.hypotheses.org/283 (accessed April 24, 2025).
52  See Helmut Mejcher, *Der Nahe Osten im Zweiten Weltkrieg* (Paderborn: Ferdinand Schöningh, 2017), pp. 87–114.
53  See Emad Ahmed Helal, "Egypt's Overlooked Contribution to World War II," in Heike Liebau (ed.), *The World in World Wars: Experiences, Perceptions and Perspectives from Africa and Asia* (Leiden: Brill, 2010), pp. 217–247.
54  ABRC, 1629, Diary of Dorothy Hamilton Des Quartiers, 1939–1945, p. 16.

## (Un)Settling intimacies in a refugee camp        129

55 *Ibid.*

56 See Bailkin, *Refugee Camps*, pp. 4–5.

57 Frederick F. Aldridge, "Contributions of the Sanitary Engineering Program of UNRRA to International Health," *Public Health Reports (1896–1970)*, 62:50 (1947), 1729–1739, p. 1731.

58 *Ibid.*

59 See UN Archives, S 1450 0000 0068 00001, "U.N.N.R.R.A. Middle East Office. Twentieth Native Report of the Chief of the Middle East Office, October 1st–31, 1946," p. 4.

60 UN Archives, 671, Camp El Shatt, Letter from Camp director to Security Officer, 25 July 1946.

61 *Ibid.*

62 Mai Taha, "Drinking Water by the Sea: Real and Unreal Property in the Mixed Courts of Egypt," in Daniel S. Margolies, Umut Özsu, Maïa Pal and Ntina Tzouvala (eds), *The Extraterritoriality of Law: History, Theory, Politics* (London: Routledge, 2019), pp. 119–133.

63 Bieber, "Building Yugoslavia in the Sand?" p. 304.

64 See Alex Lamprou, "Negotiating Sexuality: Greek Refugees in the Middle East and Africa (1942–45)." Presentation at the International Organizations and Body Politics in MENA History conference, 27–29 June 2022, Institute of European History, Mainz.

65 Esther Möller and Shaimaa Esmail El-Neklawy, "Between Local Philanthropic Traditions and State Politics: Endowments and Charitable Associations in 19th- and 20th- Century Egypt," *Endowment Studies*, 6 (2022), 192–220.

66 For the case of the Egyptian Red Crescent, see the newspaper articles in *Rūz alYūssif*, 11 February 1941, p. 7: "Jamʿiyyat al-salīb al-aḥmar al-dawlī tashīd bi-māʾthir jamʿiyyat al-hilāl al-aḥmar" (The International Red Cross Society Praises the Achievements of the Egyptian Red Crescent Society) or in *Al-Balāgh*, 29 June 1944, p. 2: "Li-muʿāwanat muslimī yūghuslāfiyya" (For the Help of the Muslims of Yugoslavia).

67 He invented the "Gilmore Colors": https://filmcolors.org/timeline-entry/1254/ (accessed April 11, 2023).

68 The photo taken by American photographer Otto Gilmore at the El Shatt camp in September 1944 has the caption: "Refugees come to refugees elected by themselves with their day to day problems. The Central Committee composed of officers selected by the refugees takes care of all the many daily problems at El Shatt, UNRRA's largest camp in the Middle East." www.loc.gov/item/2005675128/ (accessed April 11, 2023).

69 The history of humanitarian photography is traced in Heide Fehrenbach and Davide Rodogno (eds), *Humanitarian*

130    *The long Second World War, 1931–1953*

*Photography: A History* (Cambridge, MA and New York: Cambridge University Press, 2015), with a focus on UNRRA: Silvia Salvatici, "Sights of Benevolence: UNRRA's Recipients Portrayed," in Fehrenbach and Rodogno (eds), *Humanitarian Photography*, pp. 200–222.

70 On the motto and its ultimate vagueness, see: Silvia Salvatici, "'Help the People to Help Themselves': UNRRA Relief Workers and European Displaced Persons," *Journal of Refugee Studies*, 25:3 (2012), 428–451.

71 For the centrality of children to the modern humanitarian imagination, see Heide Fehrenbach, "Children and Other Civilians: Photography and the Politics of Humanitarian Image-Making," in Fehrenbach and Rodogno (eds), *Humanitarian Photography*, pp. 165–199; Katharina Stornig, "Promoting Distant Children in Need: Christian Imagery in the Late Nineteenth and Early Twentieth Centuries," in Johannes Paulmann (ed.), *Humanitarianism and Media. 1900 to the Present* (Oxford and New York: Berghahn, 2018), pp. 41–66.

72 "Little Lepa! Her Story is the Story of a Great Need," *The Coventry Evening Telegraph* (1 November 1944), p. 4.

73 *Ibid.*

74 *Ibid.*

# 5

# "National Defense Medicine": Chinese-style physicians and medical relief during the war against Japan

*Jean Corbi*

In 1938, one year after the Japanese invasion of China, a daily newspaper based in Chongqing, *Xinan ribao*, published a weekly column entitled "National Defense Medicine" (*Guofang yiyao*). The meaning of this term was clear: Chinese medicine was a key element in defending the nation against Japan. This column was sponsored by the Central Institute of National Medicine (CINM) and its director, Jiao Yitang, whose name was written below the title. The CINM and its director played a crucial role in enhancing the status of Chinese-style physicians when they were increasingly marginalized by the Ministry of Health (founded in 1928), which sought to promote Western, scientific medicine.[1] Jiao himself was a prominent figure in the Guomindang (GMD), the nationalist party led by Chiang Kai-shek that seized power in 1927 and established a new capital in Nanjing. He became a member of the legislative Yuan (equivalent to a parliament) in 1928, before he became the head of the CINM when it was founded in 1930.[2]

The CINM's creation closed a major episode of heightened tensions between the government and the world of Chinese medicine. In 1929, an advisory board in the Ministry of Health had passed a proposition to abolish Chinese medicine. However, the proposition was eventually withdrawn in the face of a massive mobilization of Chinese-style physicians and drug sellers. Their mobilization, in turn, led to the CINM's creation.[3] In other words, the Ministry of Health considered Chinese medicine a major obstacle to improving the population's health, and even a danger to public health. Yet less than ten years later, Chinese medicine was framed as a force to defend the nation from the Japanese threat.

132      *The long Second World War, 1931–1953*

Although Chinese-style physicians were overshadowed by the practitioners of Western medicine who were the main actors in state medicine before and during the war, they also played a role in trying to alleviate the suffering of the Chinese people during the conflict. But since Western medicine was the official medicine under the GMD, Chinese medicine was almost excluded from medical institutions affiliated with the state.[4] Chinese-style physicians thus had to participate in wartime medical efforts through non-state organizations, including the CINM and their local professional organization associations. Wartime relief efforts took many different forms: directly healing the wounded soldiers and civilians; helping the refugees and those whose homes had been destroyed, facing cholera outbreaks that regularly struck the cities; and educating the population and popularizing methods to recognize and treat common ailments.

This chapter discusses how Chinese-style physicians, at various levels and through different means, contributed to humanitarian work during the war, with a focus on the province of Sichuan. After 1938, when the Chinese government retreated to Chongqing, the province's first commercial city, Sichuan became the center of free China until 1945, breaking almost two decades of instability and isolationism.[5] Indeed, since the fall of the Qing dynasty in 1911, Sichuan was torn between rival warlords (*junfa*); one warlord never managed to dominate the entire province. Of course, the situation of wartime Sichuan was no better – if not much worse: Chongqing was targeted by at least two hundred air raids, and other cities were also heavily bombed.[6] The national government's location in Chongqing led to the province's reunification, the reaffirmation of the civil administration previously overshadowed by military apparatus, and, more specifically, a renewed attention to health and medical questions.[7] For example, the Sichuan Provincial Health Administration was formed in 1939. The documents produced and gathered by the provincial bureaucracy shed some light on the attitude of Chinese-style physicians during the war.

Since the 1980s, Chinese medicine has been the subject of a great deal of historical research, both in China and abroad. This literature has explored many facets of the history of Chinese medicine, including the physicians themselves and their position within Chinese society.[8] However, most historiography has focused on a portion of the Chinese territory, namely the Jiangnan region

*Chinese-style physicians and medical relief* 133

(including the provinces of Jiangsu, Zhejiang, and Anhui) for the late imperial period and major cities such as Shanghai (the most foreign-influenced city) or Nanjing (China's capital from 1927 to 1937 and 1945 to 1949) for the twentieth century.[9] But this focus is not a purely geographical problem. These works have paid special attention to governmental policies toward Chinese medicine and to the discourse and work of major intuitions or prominent figures— what we will call the spokespersons of Chinese medicine. Authors such as Bridie Andrews and Sean Lei Hsiang-lin have clearly shown that "Chinese" medicine was produced by interactions with Western medical knowledge via the mediation of a modernizing Chinese state.[10] Chinese-style physicians thus emerged as a group, unified by their opposition to, or difference from, Western medicine. But to what extent was the competition with Western medicine actually a concern for anonymous practitioners? And what other meaning could gain their collective engagement for a common cause? The present chapter provides some answers to these questions through a local approach encompassing the work of branches of national institutions as well as grassroots organizations.

This chapter also aims to integrate the Second World War into the history of Chinese medicine. As Nicole Barnes has explained, the war has been portrayed "as a period of stagnation, a figurative black hole of medical development" in China, with most research ending around 1937 or starting from 1949.[11] Barnes, along with other scholars, has shown that public authorities continued to promote public health during the conflict.[12] But their works have focused mostly on state medicine; that is, Western medicine. As a result, Chinese-style physicians are quite absent from this history.[13] In China as elsewhere, the war changed the configuration of medical services or fostered medical innovations in biomedicine. The war also affected Chinese medicine and, as this chapter will show, the way Chinese-style physicians organized themselves as a profession and engaged collectively in medical relief activities.

We usually have only a few sources on work done outside of state-controlled institutions; they left scant traces in governmental archives. Moreover, smaller organizations' actions were seldom reported in newspapers or official publications. In contrast with the easy access to materials on the CINM, for example, the column "National Defense Medicine," it is harder to find sources tracing

134    *The long Second World War, 1931–1953*

the activities of local associations of physicians. To consider the different types of institutions and the most prominent one, this chapter uses a combination of materials published in the newspaper *Xinan ribao* and archives kept in the province of Sichuan, especially in the Sichuan Provincial Archives (SPA).[14] The materials include applications filed by physicians to obtain a license, records of associations established in the province, and different documents about their operations. In the SPA, we collected a total of 1,963 application files, including an applicant's resume. Most were filed between 1939 and 1946. We conducted in depth quantitative and qualitative analysis on a random sample of three hundred resumes produced by Chinese-style physicians. They include, along with other information, a succinct presentation of their professional experience. For many reasons, these sources are most often scarce or fragmentary, but they do provide useful insights into the actions that physicians and their professional organizations undertook to support the wartime medical effort.

These archival materials and local publications enable us to look beyond the history of the most prominent institutions. They show that Chinese-style physicians had a role to play during the war, an idea not only supported by Chinese medicine's major institutions and spokespeople but also the whole Chinese medical world. However, their eagerness to participate in the wartime medical effort cannot solely be explained by the struggle for legitimacy against Western medicine.[15] In this respect, the discourses of the CINM and grassroot organizations diverge. The former, with important media coverage support, insisted on the threat posed by Western medicine. The latter seemed much more focused on the idea that Chinese medicine and its advancement, through research, publicization, or education, should benefit the whole population. This difference is understandable, since daily practitioners were probably less concerned with the legitimacy of Chinese vs. Western medicine and much more so by their position as physicians in local society.

This chapter will first demonstrate how participating in wartime medical relief was a way for Chinese-style physicians to present themselves as participants in the strengthening of the Chinese nation. For the CINM, but also for smaller organizations of medical practitioners, rescuing the injured or fighting epidemics—and not leaving these tasks to Western medicine alone—contributed to

*Chinese-style physicians and medical relief*     135

increasing their legitimacy in the eyes of the state and the public. A second section will focus on the action and discourse of grassroots organizations whose concern did not necessarily align with that of the CINM. During the war, local associations of physicians became more and more numerous. They undertook medical relief work, supported the advancement of medical knowledge, and forged a professional ethic of serving the people. In so doing, they were certainly motivated by a desire to raise the status of Chinese-style physicians within local society, rather than to defend themselves against the distant threat of Western medicine.

### "National Defense Medicine" or the defense of national medicine

The CINM and its Sichuanese branch was certainly the most visible actor in the Chinese-style medical relief effort. The CINM assisted the population, sometimes collaborating with the Chinese state to strengthen its medical capabilities. However, this agenda was not motivated by patriotic solidarity only, although it certainly played a role. By fighting for the future of the nation against the Japanese threat, supporters of Chinese medicine sought to show that it had a place in modern China.

The CINM carried out actions to support the war effort from 1937 onwards and advertised the usefulness of Chinese medicine, exemplified by "National Defense Medicine." The weekly column was published from early July to early November 1938, when it was apparently discontinued. The CINM sponsored the column and wrote it in collaboration with the Chinese Medicine Relief Hospital (*zhongyi jiuhu yiyuan*). The hospital was founded by Jiao Yitang in 1937 in Nanjing, and moved in 1938 to the district of Beibei, just north of Chongqing, where the wartime siege of the CINM was also located.[16] In 1942 the hospital was reorganized under the name of Beibei Hospital of Chinese Medicine.

An article, entitled "The Long War and the Task of the Chinese Medicine Community," which was included in the first edition of "National Defense Medicine," clearly shows the intimate link between rescuing the Chinese soldiers and protecting Chinese medicine from the threats posed by the advocates of Western science.

136     *The long Second World War, 1931–1953*

> M. Jiao Yitang, director of the Institute of National Medicine, in order to save our country from the crisis, to preserve thousands of years of medical tradition, to gather medical talents from all over the country, to help the country in difficult times and to work for the long-term welfare of the country, has set up the Chinese Medicine Relief Hospital, in order to use Chinese medicine to help our soldiers who have been wounded in the war of resistance for our country, so that after recovering from their diseases, they can return to the battlefield and increase the strength of the war on the front, so that the first ray of life of Chinese medicine is not cut off![17]

In other words, Chinese-style physicians were simultaneously fighting on two fronts: the defense of the Chinese nation against Japan and for the future of Chinese medicine, the "essence of the country" (*jinghua de guocui*).

This article echoes some of the slogans coined during the movement for national medicine. The movement emerged in 1929, uniting Chinese-style physicians against the proposal passed by the Ministry of Health to abolish Chinese medicine. The idea of a "national essence" against Western influence—sometimes framed as "cultural invasion"—was at the center of the protest and one of its most powerful arguments.[18] The defense of national culture in which medicine turned on its head the dismissive qualification of "old medicine" (*jiuyi*) was often used by advocates of Western medicine in opposition to what they promoted as "modern medicine" or just "medicine."[19] This was also how the proposal of 1929, entitled "Abolishing the Old Medicine to Sweep Away the Obstacles to Medicine and Public Health," referred to Chinese medicine.

The proposal's author, Yu Yan (1879–1954), was a Western-style physician trained in Japan and a prolific critic of Chinese medicine. He not only believed that Chinese medicine went against modernity and science but also described it as an "obstacle to medicine and public health." This was no small grievance. His proposal confirmed a change in attitude on the part of the Chinese state, which now relied mainly, if not essentially, on Western medicine. In the same period, the state's intervention in health matters was based on a new theoretical framework. Under the influence of social Darwinism, the idea of a struggle between races that intellectuals such as Yan Fu (1853–1921) and Liang Qichao (1873–1929) promoted, the health of the Chinese population was also tied to the

## Chinese-style physicians and medical relief 137

survival of the Chinese nation. At the end of the nineteenth century, Liang declared: "There are two aspects to preserving the race: one is study in order to preserve its mental power; one is medicine in order to preserve its physical constitution."[20] These considerations were also very present in Yu Yan's mind when he drafted his proposal: he considered Chinese-style physicians unable to "certify the cause of death, classify diseases, or combat epidemics, not to mention engage in eugenics and racial improvement."[21] In other words, only Western medicine was useful to elevate health conditions and thus strengthen the nation. Since the beginning of the twentieth century, the construction of public health institutions had indeed relied on Western medicine.

"National Defense Medicine" was also a response to these attacks. Another article from the column's first edition addressed the education of Chinese-style physicians: "The reason why Chinese medicine and Chinese drugs are suitable for the construction of National Defense Medicine is that Chinese-style doctors are numerous and the production of Chinese drugs abundant. When it comes to treatment, Chinese medical theories and skills have made considerable achievements."[22] The author, Li Ziyou, was the president of the association of Chinese-style physicians of the district of Dazhu, south of Chongqing, and was apparently close to the local School of National Medicine located at the association's address.[23] He admitted that Chinese-style physicians who had already set up their clinics in the province needed further training to fulfil their task of supporting the military and the civil population during those times of hardship. He then spent the rest of the article discussing what this training should be. But he considered that Chinese medicine could be useful to the state and the population, and that it could even have an edge over Western medicine, constrained by the severe lack of a trained workforce. Indeed, in 1935, only 6,470 Western-style physicians in the whole country had been registered by the Ministry of Health, to care for about half a billion inhabitants.[24]

As Li Ziyou's article shows, mobilizing Chinese-style physicians to participate in wartime medical relief also meant training them for this specific task. This concern was obviously shared by the CINM, which presided over the column's publication. During the 1930s, the CINM's Sichuanese branch opened an Academy of National Medicine in Chengdu "to train generalists in medicine following

138 *The long Second World War, 1931–1953*

the program stipulated by the CINM while taking into account the needs of the place and time."[25] In 1938, one year after the beginning of the war, the Academy's curriculum included, among other subjects on Chinese medical theories and techniques and Western scientific knowledge, a course on "military training," which was rather unusual for a school of Chinese medicine, at least before 1937. In Chengdu, a Training Course in National Medicine for the Treatment of Injury opened around the same time. It was affiliated with the Association of National Medicine (separate from the CINM) and its Training Center of National Medicine was founded in 1932 and reopened in 1937.[26] The Center trained both new practitioners of Chinese medicine as well as some who had already set up their practice. Its curriculum was short and included subjects such as surgery, internal medicine, treatment of injuries, hygiene, first aid, and wartime general knowledge.

Local professional organizations of different geographic scale (provincial or local) embraced the idea of participating in wartime medical relief. However, they were not equally successful in fostering individual physicians' involvement in the war effort. Looking at the application for licenses filed by graduates from the Training Course in National Medicine for the Treatment of Injury, it seems that they were rarely involved in medical relief institutions during the war. It is likely that this Training Course was organized primarily to ease its students' licensing. Although the Academy of National Medicine seemed much more committed to modernizing Chinese medical education, its goal was to "train medical generalists following the curriculum prescribed by the Central Institute of National Medicine and taking into account the needs of the time and place."[27] In the course of this research, we were able to identify three graduates from the Academy whose application files were kept in the provincial archives. Among them two were involved in relief activities: one worked in medical relief for the people injured during air raids; the other served in the army as a "military physician" from 1937 to 1939.[28] Although it is difficult to generalize from these few cases, we may assume that the Academy of National Medicine was more inclined to lead its students to engage in wartime medical effort.

The war against Japan opened a space for collaboration between Chinese-style physicians, their professional organizations, and state

*Chinese-style physicians and medical relief* 139

medicine, including military medicine, although most health structures still relied on Western medicine. The conflict generated a huge need for medical treatment, especially for the wounded, as parts of Sichuan were subject to intense bombing. The nationalist government, which had just retreated to its wartime capital, faced many sanitary challenges. Because of the massive destruction that trailed the Japanese army's progress, refugees numbered in the millions—and eventually the tens of millions.[29] Their displacement to China's western provinces, which, like Sichuan, were relatively poor in healthcare infrastructure, posed a major health issue, including preventing epidemics. In 1939, for example, Chongqing was struck by a cholera outbreak, and the fight against it mobilized significant effort from the local health administration.[30] Finally, although the government devoted increasing funding to public health work over the course of the war, its financial capacities were undermined by rampant inflation.

Given all these constraints, and the small number of Western-trained physicians and health workers available at the time, the Chinese government had no choice but to accept the help of Chinese-style practitioners. For instance, the Chinese Medicine Relief Hospital of Chongqing, which sponsored the "National Defense Medicine" column, was financially supported by the CINM and the Ministry of War, as its main purpose was to treat injured soldiers.[31] During the rest of the war, the CINM opened several facilities to treat wounded soldiers, including Chinese medicine clinics in collaboration with the Chongqing Bureau of Public Health and the Honji Hospital in Chongqing sponsored by the National Health Administration (former Ministry of Health) that was so hostile to Chinese medicine before the war.[32]

Interestingly, the efforts of Chinese-style physicians and their institutions also focused on fighting against epidemics and contagious disease, although one of Yu Yan's key arguments in 1928 against Chinese medicine was precisely its ineffectiveness in this domain. The Academy of National Medicine of Chengdu offered a class in "contagious disease" and another in "physiological hygiene." The Chinese term for "hygiene" (*weisheng*) was commonly used for naming public health institutions or the sanitary administration and was increasingly associated with Western science and concern for germs.[33] Contagious disease was also a new

140    *The long Second World War, 1931–1953*

category. And although contagion was part of the Chinese medical tradition, it "was never the only cause of the spread of any disorder."[34] Inclusion of such subjects within Chinese-style medical education certainly showed a willingness to equip future practitioners with skills that would make them useful to state medicine.

Chinese-style physicians' involvement in public health efforts was crucial to avoid marginalization. Since the Manchurian plague of 1910–1911, preventing and fighting epidemic disease had become an increasingly important feature of medical politics. In this regard, the Chinese state's initiative was not new: under the Song dynasty (960–1279), the emperor supported charity infirmaries, circulated formulas for treating diseases, and established "peace and relief wards" (*anjifang*) to isolate the sick and prevent the spread of epidemics.[35] But during the first half of the twentieth century, the fight against epidemic diseases was tailored to Western standards, and Chinese medicine was thus excluded from state medicine. The growing number of public health establishments, such as the health centers found in almost all of Sichuan's 138 districts, employed mainly staff trained in Western medicine.[36]

Popularizing medical knowledge and disseminating medical advice to the public was another way to help the Chinese people face wartime problems. In the "National Defense Medicine" column, Chinese-style physicians published several articles focusing on the prevention and treatment of epidemic disease, especially cholera. For example, in August 1938, the column published a "method for treating cholera," which included a pharmaceutical formula with explanations on its preparation and administration.[37] One month later, an article dealt with cholera, starting with a general presentation that identified Robert Koch's vibrio, and then provided the reader with information regarding its diagnosis and solutions for treatment.[38] In this period, Chongqing was regularly hit by cholera outbreaks, against which the municipality deployed considerable resources.[39] The publication of these articles was thus a way for the authors to contribute to public health work.

Meanwhile, in the district of Shuangliu, the CINM's local branch set up an Epidemic Control Society. According to its accounting books, the society mostly focused on distributing medicines to the population.[40] Locally, Chinese-style physicians or hospitals also tried to gain support from the administration while helping to

## Chinese-style physicians and medical relief    141

fight epidemics. For example, in 1939, a Chinese medical hospital in Chengdu sent a "secret formula" to treat cholera to the local authorities.[41] The letter stated that eminent practitioners from the city had been brought together to research and test the best remedies against this disease that many doctors were still unable to treat properly. They asked for their works' findings to be printed and distributed in the district's towns and villages to propagate this useful knowledge. The administration refused their request because their treatment method "had no scientific basis." Thus, while practitioners of Chinese medicine were useful in caring for the wounded, they remained sidelined in the fight against epidemics.

Participation of Chinese-style physicians in war relief efforts took different forms such as direct support to the military or assistance to civilians by various means. They were guided, of course, by the desire to serve and protect the nation in the face of the Japanese threat and the need to defend Chinese medicine itself as it came under attack from the health administration and promoters of Western medicine. Although histories of Chinese medicine in republican China tend to end in 1937, the case of "National Defense Medicine" shows that the mobilization of Chinese-style physicians for their legitimacy did not stop at the beginning of the war. The need for medical treatment for the wounded soldiers opened a new space for collaboration between Chinese-style physicians and the state and thus opportunities to legitimize the existence of Chinese medicine in a modern Chinese nation. But this strategy also had its limits. Despite their efforts, when facing cholera outbreaks, Chinese-style physicians failed to ward off the critics because of their inability to fight epidemics and contagious disease.

### Medical relief and professional ethics

The CINM's work was the most visible but many local organizations also contributed to medical relief during the war. A new kind of institution, local associations of physicians, brought together practitioners of Chinese medicine in virtually every district in the province. The provision of medical assistance during the conflict was in keeping with a tradition of medical charity and moral exemplarity of physicians dating back to the imperial period. But it was

142        *The long Second World War, 1931–1953*

also the product of the recent emergence of professional organizations, the public associations of physicians, which promoted a discourse of public service.

At the beginning of the twentieth century, there was no such thing as specific medical relief. In Sichuan, like other provinces in China, charitable institutions assisted the poor, orphans, or isolated old persons. They were usually funded by magistrates or the local gentry, with little participation from the state itself.[42] The state's role in supporting medical relief, central under previous dynasties, declined under the Qing dynasty (1636–1912). Merchants who increasingly contributed to finance charity gained some political credit, materialized by the inscription of their names in the local gazetteer compiled by magistrates in every district.[43]

These gazetteers almost systematically listed such institutions in the sections devoted to "buildings" or "good deeds," but provided few details on their activities. We know that they sometimes offered medicines and treatment. The "almhouse" (*jiuji yuan*) in the district of Xindu, north of Chengdu, was responsible for "looking after children, caring for the elderly, lending money and providing medicines."[44] But medical assistance was never charitable institutions' only activity and it was usually associated with other forms of aid.[45] At the beginning of the twentieth century, the "benevolent society" (*cishan hui*) of the district of Dayi "offered medicines and coffins to a substantial number of poor orphans who depended on it."[46] Another institution based in the district of Huayang offered widows and old people "coffins, rice, burial, care and medicine."[47] Thus, medical assistance was just one of a number of services provided by such institutions aimed at supporting the destitute.

The development of professional organizations of physicians, including Chinese-style physicians, brought some significant changes. Through their associations, physicians organized medical relief action themselves, without relying on an external sponsor, asserting their social and professional status. In 1936, with the "Regulation on Chinese-style physicians," a licensing system was established that theoretically restricted the right to practice Chinese medicine to license holders.[48] Physicians formed associations that brought together a growing share of the medical profession. In the 1940s, the Chinese state passed several regulations, including the "Law on physicians" in 1943, which profoundly reorganized this associational

*Chinese-style physicians and medical relief* 143

network.[49] Before this date, different associations gathered Chinese-style physicians in some places, mostly Shanghai, but there was no national system of professional representation. And these first associations of physicians operated outside of state supervision. The law of 1943 led to the creation of "public associations of Chinese-style physicians" in every locality. According to this law, these associations were: (1) mandatory, meaning that every practicing physician should be a member of the local association; (2) unique, only one association per district, city, or province; (3) limited in scope to the management of the profession's internal matters, fixed by the law or by the authorities; and (4) hierarchically organized in accordance with the administrative hierarchy (province, city, district). These "public associations of physicians" (*yishi gonghui*) were officially registered by the Bureau of Social Affairs of the province among other "free professional organizations" (*ziyou zhiye tuanti*), which also included Western-style physicians, journalists, lawyers, and so forth, who were separate from "commercial organizations."[50]

They were also closely linked to the state: at each administrative level, at least in theory, there was a section of the sanitary administration and the corresponding association of physicians. Some responsibilities were delegated to these organizations regarding the profession's affairs. For example, they provided the administration with up-to-date statistical information on practitioners established in the locality.[51] Associations of Chinese-style physicians also participated in the qualification committees responsible for organizing exams for future practitioners. This link between the state, professional associations, and the participation of physicians in wartime medical relief is well illustrated by the following statement reported by the *Xinan ribao* in early September 1938:

> In view of the recent explosion of the population in our city [Chongqing], the misery of the refugees, many of whom are sick and living on the streets, and the displacement of the national government, the city's Party headquarters intends to order the members of the Western- and Chinese-style physicians associations to give free medical consultations at fixed times every day.[52]

Associations of physicians were thus responsible for mobilizing their members to participate in relief efforts and serve the nation, whose interests were represented by the state. This call was also a

144    *The long Second World War, 1931–1953*

way for the nationalist government to allocate more resources to public health and war medicine by delegating civil daily healthcare for those in need to private actors.

Conversely, it seems that physicians who engaged in medical relief were also active in their professional association. Two physicians in the district of Dazhu worked for the local branch of the Red Cross Society. Interestingly, both seem to have had some ties with the district's School of National Medicine, since one graduated from this school, and the other was a disciple of the school's former director.[53] This school was linked to the local Association of Chinese physicians—they shared the same address—and many of the school's directors also assumed the position of president of the association.[54] In the district of Hechuan, one Chinese-style physician worked successively in the district's almshouse, the dispensary affiliated with CINM's local branch, the "Volunteer ambulance team," and the Chinese National Medicine Association's local branch.[55]

Although the information that we have does not allow for a quantitative analysis of this trend, these examples tend to indicate a connection between the engagement of individual physicians in relief work and participating in professional organizations, either branches of the CINM or other local associations of practitioners of Chinese medicine.

The associations of physicians' discourse and actions may show the emergence of a shared professional ethic, shifting the focus from individual moral exemplarity to collective engagement in medical relief. Participation of Chinese-style physicians in the war effort was part of this evolution, perhaps even accelerating it. To measure the extent of this change, we first return to sources from the early twentieth century. They point toward a moral responsibility for physicians not only to provide effective and unharmful treatment to their patients but also to make sure they are also accessible even to the poorest civilians. Such obligations were individual, with good and charitable doctors being awarded public recognition.

Local gazetteers give an idea of the moral values to which physicians had to abide. They contain, among many other pieces of information, biographies of individuals deemed either important or admirable enough to be remembered. According to Volker Scheid, three criteria could justify including their biography in the local gazetteers: intellectual stature, the effectiveness of their treatment, and

## Chinese-style physicians and medical relief    145

moral exemplarity.[56] Selflessness, charity, and filial piety were moral qualities often present in these biographies.[57] A physician's generosity and selflessness were demonstrated by providing free care to the poor, but acts of charity were not limited to the medical sphere: doctors could also distinguish themselves by distributing food to the destitute, for instance. But obviously, all did not necessarily observe such moral values. In his *Overview of Chengdu* published in 1909, columnist Fu Chongju condemned the greed and dishonesty of some of the city's practitioners. Those he named the "doctors in sedan chair" (*zuojiao*) usually waited a day or two after being called to see a patient, pretending to be particularly busy to give the impression that they had a large clientele and justify exorbitant prices.[58] They did not care about the poor and only treated well-off clients: "the poor would go broke with every illness, so the sick would rather die than go to these or other doctors." Fu had more regard for "street doctors" (*paojie*) or "stall doctors" (*baitan*) whose prices were much more reasonable, especially for the more modest, and who sometimes agreed to treat the needy free of charge. This literature insisted heavily on the individual duty to lend aid to the poor.

The professionalization of physicians and the rise of associations of medical practitioners brought about a significant shift: moral duties took on a more collective shape, and charitable actions were now directed to the poorest and also to the "nation" as a whole. This change appears clearly in the "National Defense Medicine" column and in the documents produced by local associations of Chinese-style physicians. In its statutes, the Association of Chinese-style physicians of Sichuan (created in 1945) stated that its purpose was "to improve medical research" and "to promote the medical knowledge of the people and public welfare (*gonggong fuli*)."[59] By invoking the notion of the "public" (*gong*), these professional organizations situated themselves in an intermediary social space between the official domain belonging to the state (*guan*) and the private (*si*).[60] They also framed medical knowledge as a matter of "the people," a common good that belonged not only to erudite elites or specialists but also to the nation as a whole. In this perspective, the advancement of medical research was not merely the concern of Chinese-style physicians because it benefited the entire country. Finally, this attitude echoed the growing concern for a healthy nation, or even the rise of a form of "hygienic modernity."[61]

146    *The long Second World War, 1931–1953*

Just like the state-supported public health work based on Western medicine, Chinese-style physicians claimed that their medical and research activities contributed to "public welfare."

Such a discourse was also present at the most local level, in the physicians' associations in the districts. The statutes of the association of Guanghan district (created in 1942) stated that it worked "to improve medical research" and "to the advancement of the nation's health and medical affairs."[62] In 1939, a report on the province's professional associations detailed the concrete work of these district associations.[63] The association of Hechuan district, for example, declared in 1939 that it had "[offered] free consultation, distributed free medicines and [organized] academic discussion." In concrete terms, the association supported the publication of Chinese medical journals, the organization of seminars, specialized libraries, and dispensaries offering care to people in need. Traditionally, it was members of the local gentry who sponsored charitable institutions to provide help to the poor.[64] That medical professional organizations took on this task may show evidence of their will to enhance the social status of Chinese-style physicians, positioning them as members of the local elite.

Some associations of physicians' activities echoed the good deeds undertaken by individual doctors at the beginning of the twentieth century, for example, treating the poor for free. Others, such as those aiming to enhance the people's medical education, were few in number. Finally, the discourse underlying the medical work carried out during the war was quite different from that of gazetteers depicting the qualities of virtuous physicians. Associations of Chinese-style physicians were not only concerned with the poor but also and more generally with the "health of the people" (*renqun de jiankang*). They focused on collective and impersonal endeavors such as the advancement of medical knowledge, public welfare, and the nation's health instead of praising the moral qualities of individual practitioners.

### Conclusion

The mobilization of practitioners of Chinese medicine during the Second World War lies at the intersection of different historical trends. Beyond individual decisions motivated by patriotism, their collective participation in wartime medical relief took on a professional

## Chinese-style physicians and medical relief 147

dimension. The dire need for a medical workforce to alleviate the suffering caused by combat and bombings provided Chinese-style physicians with the opportunity to collaborate with the Chinese state and to strengthen the legitimacy of their profession. And the discourse of associations of Chinese-style physicians built the idea that the profession should put itself in the service of the people, an idea that would gain strength under Mao Zedong's regime.

In claiming that Chinese medicine was best suited to become "National Defense Medicine," its spokespersons such as the CINM fought against the government's hostile attitude toward Chinese medicine, especially the Ministry of Health. They aimed to show that Chinese medicine was useful if not indispensable to the future of the Chinese nation. The mobilization of Chinese-style physicians to help fight disease and rescue injured or displaced people proved they had a role to play in modern China.

Moreover, the mobilization of Chinese-style physicians articulated ongoing changes in their own profession and the organization of medical relief. Indeed, the rise of professional medical organizations, fostered by regulations issued by the nationalist government associations of Chinese-style physicians, came to play an important role in providing medical support to the population. Since the end of the Qing dynasty, medical assistance to the most vulnerable was mainly the task of the gentry, who financed charitable institutions in towns and districts. In the 1930s to 1940s, physicians, through their local associations, played a more active part in relief work, which was probably a way for them to strengthen their social status. For its part, the state could continue to delegate parts of the relief effort to focus its resources on what were deemed the most crucial medical activities, among which was treating soldiers and preventing epidemics. This focus was not new. Since imperial times, disaster relief had been organized with the help of non-state actors. Nor was its reliance on associations (*gonghui*) specific to the field of medicine and health: for instance, in rural areas some of the village's affairs were dealt with by the villagers' association.[65]

These changes were not without consequences for both the medical profession and the medical relief system. Whereas ancient charitable institutions provided a variety of services to people in need, it seems that associations of physicians now focused on strictly medical relief work. For Chinese-style physicians, such work showcased a new professional ethics. Indeed, although the medical relief they

148    *The long Second World War, 1931–1953*

provided was quite similar to that of previous charitable institutions, it was framed in a new discourse emphasizing public welfare and not merely assistance to the poor.

Although the progress of Chinese-style physicians during the war was modest, endeavors to strengthen the profession did not stop during the conflict. Of course, the Japanese invasion did disrupt the life of many institutions that had championed the cause of Chinese medicine. The war forced schools or journals of Chinese medicine, for example, to cease their activities.[66] But this observation mostly applies to certain areas that have received particular attention in historiography. This is especially the case for Shanghai, where intellectual growth was abruptly interrupted. Looking at the wartime period from the viewpoint of Sichuan offers a different picture. The CINM continued working to promote Chinese medicine, creating new schools such as the Academy of National Medicine of Chengdu. And the profession continued to structure itself, as public associations of physicians sprung up in almost every district. They organized dispensaries, distributed medicines, and created their own journals to advance Chinese medical knowledge or to make it available to a wider audience.

Under the communist regime, the Chinese government's attitude toward Chinese medicine radically changed. Although in the 1940s Mao Zedong expressed a certain mistrust about the "old medicine," from the 1950s onward the achievements of Chinese medicine, now called Traditional Chinese Medicine (TCM), became a source of national pride. The movement "doctors of Western medicine study Chinese medicine," which required modern physicians to be trained in TCM, illustrates this shift in favor of Chinese medicine.[67] During the 1960s, when official propaganda emphasized to "be prepared for war, be prepared for natural disasters, and serve the people whole-heartedly," authorities promoted the use of Chinese herbal medicine, since it was the most accessible therapeutic solution.[68]

## Notes

1 Sean Hsiang-lin Lei, *Neither Donkey nor Horse: Medicine in the Struggle Over China's Modernity* (Chicago, IL: The University of Chicago Press, 2014), pp. 142–147.

## Chinese-style physicians and medical relief 149

2 Xiang Wen, "Jiao Yitang yu zhongyiyao shiye" [Jiao Yitang and the Cause of Chinese Medicine], *Nanjing yike daxue xuebao*, 1 (2003), 51–55.

3 Hsiang-lin Lei, *Neither Donkey nor Horse*, pp. 113–117.

4 Ka-che Yip, *Health and National Reconstruction in Nationalist China: The Development of Modern Health Services, 1928–1937* (Ann Arbor, MI: Association for Asian Studies, 1995), pp. 100–131.

5 Robert A. Kapp, *Szechwan and the Chinese Republic: Provincial Militarism and Central Power, 1911–1938* (New Haven, CT: Yale University Press, 1973), p. 3.

6 Xavier Paulès, *La République de Chine: Histoire Générale de La Chine (1912–1949)* (Paris: Les Belles Lettres, 2019), p. 141.

7 Ling Zhang, "kangzhan shiqi Sichuan de gonggong weisheng guanli" [Public Health Management in Sichuan during the War], *Chongqing shifan daxue xuebao*, 3 (2015), 28–35.

8 Robert P. Hymes, "Not Quite Gentlemen? Doctors in Song and Yuan," *Chinese Science*, 8 (1987), 9–76; Yüan-ling.Chao, *Medicine and Society in Late Imperial China: A Study of Physicians in Suzhou, 1600–1850* (New York: Peter Lang, 2009); Florence Bretelle-Establet, "Chinese Biographies of Experts in Medicine: What Uses Can We Make of Them?" *East Asian Science, Technology and Society*, 3:4 (2009), 421–451.

9 Florence Bretelle-Establet, "Is the Lower Yangzi River Region the Only Seat of Medical Knowledge in Late Imperial China? A Glance at the Far South Region and at Its Medical Documents," in Florence Bretelle-Establet (ed.), *Looking at It from Asia: The Processes That Shaped the Sources of History of Science* (Dordrecht: Springer, 2010), pp. 331–369.

10 Bridie Andrews, *The Making of Modern Chinese Medicine, 1850–1960* (Vancouver: University of British Columbia Press, 2014); Lei, *Neither Donkey nor Horse*.

11 Nicole E. Barnes, "Protecting the National Body: Gender, Public Health and Medicine in Southwest China during the War of Resistance against Japan, 1937–1945" (PhD dissertation, University of California, 2012), p. 29.

12 John R. Watt, *Saving Lives in Wartime China: How Medical Reformers Built Modern Healthcare Systems amid War and Epidemics, 1928–1945* (Leiden: Brill, 2014); Michael Shiyung Liu, "Epidemic Control and Wars in Republican China (1935–1955)," *Extrême-Orient, Extrême-Occident*, 37, (2014), 111–139.

13 It should be noted, however, that Nicole Barnes devoted an entire chapter of her doctoral thesis to exchanges between Chinese and

150  *The long Second World War, 1931–1953*

Western medicine in wartime Chongqing, showing how the central government and local authorities integrated to some extent Chinese medicine in their medical relief system. Barnes, "Protecting the National Body," chap. 7.

14 Besides these archival materials, the present chapter also uses documents consulted in the archival centre of the district of Shuangliu (SDA), in the periphery of Chengdu.

15 Paul Unschuld, "Epistemological Issues and Changing Legitimation: Traditional Chinese Medicine in the Twentieth Century," in Charles M. Leslie and Allan Young (eds), *Paths to Asian Medical Knowledge* (Berkeley, CA: University of California Press, 1992), pp. 44–61.

16 Kuo-li Pi, "Zhanzheng de qishi: Zhongguo yixue wai shang xueke de zhishi zhuanxing (1937–1949)" [The Enlightenment of War: Knowledge Transformation in Traditional Chinese Surgery and Traumatology, 1937–1949], *Guoshi Guan Guankan*, 63 (2020), 89–91, 93–126.

17 "Changqi kangzhan yu zhong yiyao jie de renwu" [The Long War and the Task of the Chinese Medicine Community], *Xinan Ribao* (July 1, 1938), p. 4.

18 Xiaoqun Xu, ' "National Essence' vs'Science': Chinese Native Physicians' Fight for Legitimacy, 1912–37," *Modern Asian Studies*, 31:4 (1997), 847–877.

19 Andrews, *The Making of Modern Chinese Medicine, 1850–1960*, p. 9.

20 Ralph C. Croizier, *Traditional Medicine in Modern China: Science, Nationalism, and the Tensions of Cultural Change* (Cambridge: Harvard University Press, 1968), p. 59.

21 Lei, *Neither Donkey nor Horse*, pp. 112–113.

22 "Zenme xunlian zhongyi" [How to Train Chinese-Style Physicians], *Xinan Ribao* (July 1, 1938), p. 4.

23 SPA, 186-02-3131, "Renmin tuanti zhuce bu" [Register of People's Organisations], vol. 3, c. 1949.

24 *Annuaire Statistique Du Ministère de l'Intérieur (Neizheng Bu Nianjian* 内政部年鑒*)* (Shanghai: Shangwu yinshuguan, 1936).

25 Shuangliu District Archives (hereafter SDA), 42-01-364, "Guoyi xueyuan jianzhang" [Shortened Statutes of the Academy of National Medicine], 1936.

26 Qing Cai, "Cong 'guoyi gonghui' dao 'zhongyi gonghui': minguo shiqi Chengdu zhongyi zhiye tuanti de xingshuai zhuanbian" [From 'Associations of National Medicine' to 'Associations of Chinese-Style Physicians': The Rise and Fall of Professional Organizations of Chinese Medicine in Chengdu during the Republic], *Xinan minzu daxue xuebao*, 9:38 (2017), 207–213.

## Chinese-style physicians and medical relief    151

27  SDA, 42-01-364, "Guoyi xueyuan jianzhang" [Shortened Statutes of the Academy of National Medicine], 1936.

28  SPA, 113-01-0341, "Qingling zhongyi zhengshu lülishu" [Curriculum Vitae for Application for a Certificate of Chinese-Style Physician], 1941; SPA, 113-01-2336, "Qingling zhongyi zhengshu lülishu" [Curriculum Vitae for Application for a Certificate of Chinese-Style Physician], 1939.

29  Harriet Zurndorfer, "Wartime Refugee Relief in Chinese Cities and Women's Political Activism, 1937–1940," in Billy K. L. So and Madeleine Zelin (eds), *New Narratives of Urban Space in Republican Chinese Cities: Emerging Social, Legal and Governance Orders* (Leiden: Brill, 2013), pp. 65–91.

30  Barnes, "Protecting the National Body," p. 103.

31  Pi, "Zhanzheng de qishi."

32  Barnes, "Protecting the National Body," pp. 318–321.

33  Ruth Rogaski, *Hygienic Modernity: Meanings of Health and Disease in Treaty-Port China* (Berkeley, CA: University of California Press, 2004), p. 304.

34  Angela Ki-che Leung, "The Evolution of the Idea of Chuanran Contagion in Imperial China," in Qizi Liang and Charlotte Furth (eds), *Health and Hygiene in Chinese East Asia: Policies and Publics in the Long Twentieth Century* (Durham. NC: Duke University Press, 2010), pp. 25–50, at p. 44.

35  Angela Ki-che Leung, "Organized Medicine in Ming-Qing China: State and Private Medical Institutions in the Lower Yangzi Region," *Late Imperial China*, 8:1 (1987), 134–166.

36  SPA, 113-01-0766, "Sichuansheng gexian weishengyuan zuzhi jihua" [Organization Plan for Health Centers in the Districts of the Province of Sichuan], 1939.

37  "Huoluan ban zhifa" [Method for Treating Cholera], *Xinan Ribao* (12 August 1938), p. 4, continued in *Xinan Ribao* (August 26, 1938), p. 4.

38  "Zhenxing huoluan zhi yanjiu ji zhifa" [Research and Treatment of True Cholera], *Xinan Ribao* (September 23, 1938), p. 4.

39  Barnes, "Protecting the National Body," ' p. 66.

40  SDA, 42-01-364, "Shuangliu xian fangyi hui jingshou zhangmu qingce" [Accounts of the Society for the Prevention of Disease of the District of Shuangliu], 1933.

41  SDA, 42-01-364, "Shuangliu xian fangyi hui jingshou zhangmu qingce" [Accounts of the Society for the Prevention of Disease of the District of Shuangliu], 1933.

42  Tongzu Qu, *Local Government in China under the Ch'ing* (Cambridge: Council on East Asian Studies, 1962), pp. 182–183.

152   *The long Second World War, 1931–1953*

43 Leung, "Organized Medicine in Ming-Qing China."
44 *Xindu xianzhi* [Gazetteer of the District of Xindu], 1929. Local gazetteers cited in this chapter are drawn from Weixin Wang, *Zhongguo di fang zhi ji cheng: Sichuan fu xian zhi ji* [Collection of China's Local Gazetteers: Gazetteers of Prefectures and Districts of Sichuan] (Chengdu: Ba Shu shushe, 1992), juan 2.
45 Florence Bretelle-Establet, *La Santé En Chine Du Sud, 1898–1928* (Paris: CNRS, 2002), pp. 16–20.
46 *Dayi xianzhi* [Gazetteer of the District of Dayi], 1930, juan 3.
47 *Huayang xianzhi* [Gazetteer of the District of Huayang], 1930, juan 3.
48 Xiang Wen, "Nanjing guomin zhengfu 'zhongyi tiaoli' shuping" [Analysis of the 'Regulation on Chinese-Style Physicians' of the Nationalist Government of Nanjing], *Minguo Dangan*, 4 (2004), 82–86.
49 Reproduced in Qihui Wang, *Minguo yishi falü yanjiu* [Research on Law of Physicians during the Republic of China] (Nanjing: Nanjing University, 2015), pp. 213–216.
50 SPA, 186-02-3131, 3132, 3135, "Renmin tuanti zhuce bu" [Register of People's Organisations], vol. 1–3, c. 1949.
51 SPA, 113-01-2094, "Sichuan sheng Zhong yishi gonghui zhangcheng" [Statutes of the Association of Chinese-Style Physicians of the Province of Sichuan], 1935.
52 *Xinan ribao* (September 8, 1938), p. 3.
53 SPA, 113-01-0358, "Qingling zhongyi zhengshu lülishu" [Curriculum Vitae for Application for a Certificate of Chinese-Style Physician], 1942.
54 SPA, 186-02-3131, "Renmin tuanti zhuce bu" (Register of People's Organisations), vol. 1, c. 1949, p. 95.
55 SPA, 113-01-0799, "Qingling zhongyi zhengshu lülishu" [Curriculum Vitae for Application for a Certificate of Chinese-Style Physician], 1941.
56 Volker Scheid, *Currents of Tradition in Chinese Medicine, 1626–2006* (Seattle, WA: Eastland Press, 2007), p. 56.
57 Bretelle-Establet, *La Santé En Chine Du Sud, 1898–1928*, p. 90.
58 Chongju Fu, *Chengdu Tonglan* [Comprehensive Guide to Chengdu], 2 vols (Chengdu: Bashu shushe, 1987), p. 195; originally published in 1909–1911.
59 SPA, 113-01-2094, "Sichuan sheng Zhong yishi gonghui zhangcheng" [Statutes of the Association of Chinese-Style Physicians of the Province of Sichuan], 1935.
60 William T. Rowe, "The Public Sphere in Modern China," *Modern China*, 16:3 (1990), 309–329.
61 Rogaski, *Hygienic Modernity*.

## Chinese-style physicians and medical relief   153

62 SPA, 186-01-1739, "Guanghan zhongyi gonghui huizhang" [Statutes of the Association of Chinese-Style Physicians of Guanghan], 1942.

63 SPA, 186-02-3140, "Sichuan sheng ziyou zhiye tuanti zong baogao" [General Report on Free Professional Organizations of Sichuan Province], 1939.

64 Pierre Fuller, *Modern Erasures: Revolution, the Civilizing Mission, and the Shaping of China's Past* (Cambridge and New York: Cambridge University Press, 2022), pp. 40–41.

65 Prasenjit Duara, *Culture, Power, and the State: Rural North China, 1900–1942* (Stanford, CA: Stanford University Press, 2000), p. 195.

66 Kim Taylor, *Chinese Medicine in Early Communist China, 1945–1963: A Medicine of Revolution* (London: Routledge, 2005), p. 8.

67 *Ibid.*, p. 75.

68 Xiaoping Fang, *Barefoot Doctors and Western Medicine in China* (Rochester, NY: University of Rochester Press, 2012), pp. 85–86.

# 6

# 'There is no enemy here!' Humanitarian rhetoric in South America during the Second World War: Peru/Ecuador

*François Bignon*

In August 1941, a Peruvian captain arrived at a hospital in southern Ecuador, recently occupied by the Peruvian armed forces, and reprimanded the nuns for fleeing instead of caring for their patients. Alerted by rumours of Peruvian abuses spread by civilians and Ecuadorian soldiers on the run, the hospital staff had indeed taken fright. The captain and the nuns are believed to have had the following conversation:

- Captain Odría: How is that possible, Mother? You have left the wounded and the sick alone.
- Sister Apolina: You must understand ... we were told that you were close and ... in war ...
- Captain Odría: Mother, you have nothing to fear, our army is respectful and respectable.[1]

Even if the exact circumstances of this encounter reported by another Peruvian officer remain unclear, the alleged attitude of Captain Manuel Odría, later to became dictator of Peru, reveals that the fate of the wounded and civilians was the subject of disinformation and false pretenses in the war between Peru and Ecuador in 1941–1942.[2] This chapter explores why this was the case, examining how the treatment of the wounded became a matter of public concern and an important political issue during this conflict. It compares how the Peruvian and Ecuadorian medical services were politicised during the war and considers how far medical aid was used to promote the status of both states in international affairs. It finally analyses the humanitarian intervention of foreign powers, especially the United States. In doing so, it reflects on the broader

*Humanitarian rhetoric in South America* 155

specificities of Latin American humanitarian rhetoric during the Second World War.

The conflict between Peru and Ecuador provides a fascinating case study to analyse humanitarian propaganda because communication played an essential role in delegitimising the adversary and attracting new and powerful sympathies. The peculiarity of this South American war lies in its interlocking nature amid the world conflict. At its heart laid a conflict for vast territories located between the Pacific coast and the Amazon forest, which started at the beginning of the nineteenth century. After a period of calm in the 1920s, the situation gradually degraded in the 1930s as a result of bilateral diplomatic talks reaching a dead end and as a consequence of the general atmosphere of international tension. Amid growing tensions, the United States, Brazil and Argentina, joined afterwards by Chile, acted as mediators from May 1941. Washington tried to settle the dispute once and for all to prevent a bellicose situation on the South American continent from becoming a new front in the world war. Some high-ranking members of the Peruvian army, convinced that a purely diplomatic settlement would be unfavourable to Peru's territorial claims, launched a military operation at the beginning of July 1941, responding, according to the official account, to an Ecuadorian attack. After a week of land, naval and air operations, which confirmed Peru's overwhelming military superiority, the Ecuadorian army was routed and a southern part of the country was occupied for several months, bringing Peruvian military and Ecuadorian civilians into contact. Following the ceasefire that came into effect on 31 July, an agreement was signed in the Peruvian port of Talara. It recognised the temporary occupation of southern Ecuador and established a large, demilitarised zone between Peruvian and Ecuadorian military positions, under the control of 'military observers' from mediating countries. The diplomatic settlement of the conflict was reached in January 1942 in Rio de Janeiro, within the context of the preparation of the Western Hemisphere for the war against the Axis powers, following the attack on Pearl Harbor. The need to present a united front was considered of the utmost importance and thus there was a need to put an end to internal conflicts in the Americas. That is why some Ecuadorians presented the Rio agreement as an unfair diplomatic sacrifice on the altar of peace, an 'American Munich'.[3]

156　　*The long Second World War, 1931–1953*

Although humanitarian rhetoric has been analysed in relation to the efforts of neutral countries in other conflicts, the humanitarian discourse of Andean countries at war during the Second World War remains to be studied.[4] The 1941 global and intrusive context of raging war in Europe and Asia and the growing tensions in the Pacific led, in this part of the world, to the enemy's actions being carefully watched in order to publicly disqualify them.[5] During the war, Peruvians and Ecuadorians accused each other of sympathy for the Axis powers in order to attract the support of the continental community. This situation impacted Peru and Ecuador's humanitarian management. If one defines humanitarianism by the treatment of civilians and prisoners during the war, by the debates on *jus in bello* rather than *jus ad bello*, then the 1941 conflict was perceived rather through the prism of the second one. Ecuadorian national memory generally refers to the events as a Peruvian 'aggression', as Bryce Wood's work reminds us.[6] Like the historiographical debates about the origins of the First World War, historiographical debates on this Andean conflict initially focused on the responsibility for the outbreak of the war rather than on the behaviour of the troops once the conflict had begun.[7] The fact that the fighting lasted for at most a few weeks probably explains this historiographical gap. The lack of historical works on the humanitarian aspects of the conflict also stems from the scarcity of sources available to historians, consisting mainly of rare bulletins from the Ecuadorian/Peruvian national Red Cross committees, propaganda works, and scattered correspondence involving military officers and diplomats. This fragmented archival record nevertheless points towards new directions for future research in the field, raising key questions about the humanitarian efforts undertaken by each country in terms of their organisational structure, scope and financing and paving the way for a more systematic comparison between the two belligerent countries. Drawing on this already available source material, this chapter sheds light on the general intention of these actions and the media strategies that accompanied them.

## Mobilising national Red Cross Committees

When war broke out in July 1941, the two belligerents proclaimed their adherence to the great humanitarian principles and organised their national Red Cross committees while refusing the diplomatic

*Humanitarian rhetoric in South America*     157

interference of the International Committee of the Red Cross (ICRC) in Geneva. Peru boasted about having been the first on the American continent to accede in 1879 to the Geneva Convention of 1864 (on the improvement of the fate of wounded soldiers in armies on campaign). This accession took place during the War of the Pacific led against Chile (1879–1884) and was confirmed by the Swiss Federal Council on 30 April 1880.[8] On 6 July 1906, Peru signed but never ratified the 1906 Geneva Convention on Wounded and Sick. It did ratify, however, the 1929 Geneva Convention on Wounded and Sick on 10 March 1933. Signing but not ratifying international instruments was a common practice among the Andean countries at that time, and was the result of political and practical considerations. Diplomatic representatives were happy to sign innovative texts, often European, in order to remain aligned with a West to which the elites wanted to belong. But national parliaments, which, following the American model, generally had to confirm these commitments, remained much more cautious. Domestic political instability and the practical consequences of applying these texts made them highly perilous. This meant they were often left unimplemented for years or never implemented. Ecuador, for example, had signed the founding pact of the League of Nations in 1919 but did not fully join until September 1934.[9] However, the fact that Peru had not ratified certain agreements did not mean that it was directly opposed to humanitarian principles, as Peru had been at the forefront of humanitarian efforts in the region. Peru's diplomacy in the early twentieth century had made the peaceful resolution of disputes through arbitration and collective proceedings its trademark, and humanitarian law was no exception. Support for the national committee was along the same lines.

By 1941, a national Red Cross Society was already well established in Peru. A small 'civil ambulance service of the Red Cross in Peru' had been formed as early as the war of the Pacific and later transformed into a national committee. In 1939, the national committee had commemorated its sixtieth anniversary and inaugurated a new social center intended for the middle and popular classes in the capital.[10] Lima liked to present itself at the vanguard of health and humanitarian progress on the continent. On the occasion of the Pan-American Conference of 1941, held in the Peruvian capital, it was President Prado himself who instituted by decree the 'Pan-American Health Day'.[11]

158     *The long Second World War, 1931–1953*

By contrast, the Ecuadorian Republic joined the Red Cross Movement later. It was not until 3 August 1907 that Ecuador adhered to the Geneva Convention of 22 August 1864, and not until 13 April 1923 that it adhered to the 1906 Convention on Wounded and Sick.[12] For a long time, the Ecuadorian government turned a deaf ear to international humanitarian law and to the effective organisation of a national society. This Ecuadorian delay can seem paradoxical in the light of the presence of the Liberals, which had held power since 1895 and always seemed ready to import the latest European novelties to modernise the nation.[13] Diplomatic issues were certainly the biggest obstacle, even if national committees could still develop without subscribing to international texts. The government of Quito was usually reluctant to subscribe to any international text, perceived as instruments favourable to the Peruvian side, in their territorial controversy. In 1910, Ecuador had been on the brink of war after refusing the territorial arbitration that the Spanish crown had been preparing for decades. This situation was unblocked in the 1920s. Ecuador made a 180-degree turn on international issues and finally joined major international institutions, such as the League of Nations in 1934. International conventions, hitherto viewed with some mistrust by diplomats in Quito, were now mobilised to destabilise neighbouring Peru, which at that time controlled large swathes of border territory by military force alone, backed by authoritarian governments. The Ecuadorians now viewed humanitarian diplomacy as a weapon they could wave in their favour and, for consistency's sake, they needed to have a functioning national committee.

The Ecuadorian Red Cross Society was created by decree in 1910, but did not receive its articles of association until 1922, becoming operational only in 1923.[14] In 1925, it had 19 life-time members, 340 honorary members, and 4,173 annual members, as well as 1,021 members of the Red Cross Youth.[15] Several factors explain this rapid development. No doubt personal ties with European diplomacy forged by the first president of the national committee, Luis Robalino Davila, helped launch a national organisation. Davila resigned from the presidency of the Ecuadorian Red Cross when he was appointed Ecuador's diplomatic representative in Switzerland in 1924. In the 1930s, he was replaced as president by Army General Ángel Isaac Chiriboga, a key man in the

Ecuadorian military system and in the preparations for the war. The 1922 decree set the Ecuadorian Red Cross Society as an auxiliary institution to the army health service.[16] The society therefore maintained a close relationship with the military at a time when captains, the middle managers of the martial institution, held considerable power following the Julian Revolution of 1925. Its scope of operations focused initially on providing assistance to victims of the numerous earthquakes in the region (Machachi in 1923, Tulcan in 1925), making the fight against natural disasters the society's primary task, similar to what had happened in the United States.[17] Its activities rapidly expanded and reached other vulnerable populations. The Ecuadorian Red Cross Society established the distribution of milk to children, created a kindergarten for hospitalised children, sent donations to the victims of the Spanish Civil War and established an ambulance service.[18]

Both Ecuador and Peru had therefore operative national Red Cross societies and good relationships with the International Committee in Geneva when war broke out. This situation may explain why in July 1941, the ICRC proposed to both countries its diplomatic intervention as a 'neutral intermediary', just a few days after the Peruvian offensive had begun. Two days later, the Ecuadorian government, on behalf of the national society of the Red Cross, responded by saying that the situation was calmer and that the Genevan institution's services were not required.[19] This answer was all the more disturbing because that same day the great Peruvian offensive began, leading to the capture of part of the Ecuadorian territory. The Peruvian response was even more laconic. On 19 August, several weeks after the message of Geneva, they answered with a lapidary sentence in which they 'thanked' the offer but stated that Peru 'was not currently in a war'.[20] This was partially true. By this date, the offensive had come to a halt on the Pacific front, but Peruvians occupied an Ecuadorian province and operations continued in Amazonia.

On both sides, political authorities were reluctant to accept the intervention of the Swiss institution in the Andean conflict. On the Peruvian side, it was not surprising. Despite its traditional call for collective diplomatic solutions, its strong position on the ground led Peru to reject any external intervention and to favour purely bilateral discussions with a weakened Ecuador. This rejection would also

160    *The long Second World War, 1931–1953*

include the Swiss organisation. On the Ecuadorian side, one could have expected a greater eagerness to resort to the services of the Red Cross once the country was defeated and occupied, especially since the main diplomatic objective of the Ecuadorian chancellery, since 1939, had been to invite international allies to the negotiating table so as to not find themselves face-to-face with its powerful Peruvian neighbour. It was perhaps the Geneva Committee's offer to be an 'intermediary', which could be interpreted as a diplomatic or political role rather than a humanitarian one, that precipitated this refusal. In any case, this refusal did not prevent the humanitarian deployment of national societies on the ground to respond to the consequences of the war.

## Prisoners of war: a very political treatment

Humanitarian action and media coverage of victims, prisoners of war and civilians, as well as of those providing medical care, highlighted the prevalence of political considerations over technical ones. On the ground, the symbols of the Red Cross were displayed very early in the conflict. The Red Cross emblem, for example, was deployed from the onset of the war. Ecuadorian soldiers reportedly waved the Red Cross flag and a white flag to call for a truce during the first day of combat, but the Peruvians, shocked earlier that day by a manoeuvre in which the Ecuadorians took advantage of the truce to open fire, fired back.[21] This initial skirmish, similar to dozens of border clashes in the region over the previous decade, was followed by an escalation and eventually led to a full-scale war between the two countries. This episode meant not only the misuse of humanitarian symbols in the field of operations but also the failures to contain the conflict.

Despite this dreadful start, national Red Cross committees were very active, especially regarding prisoners of war. However, their involvement was framed by diplomatic considerations. On the Ecuadorian side, the chancellery stated that spontaneous donations had quickly flowed to the Red Cross to demonstrate the unity of the nation in this ordeal.[22] The stakes were higher for the Peruvians, who occupied Ecuadorian territory and captured around a hundred soldiers and several hundred civilians considered suspicious.

## Humanitarian rhetoric in South America    161

They were placed in a 'concentration camp' in the vicinity of the Peruvian city of Piura, where they were cared for by national and local Red Cross committees, which also provided medicine, care and food for wounded Peruvian soldiers.[23] Ecuadorian soldiers who were prisoners in Piura and Iquitos (around fifty military and civilian prisoners in this Amazonian location) received subsidies (objects and money in dollars) sent by the Ecuadorian Red Cross, which handed them over to the Peruvian Red Cross by sending them from the Ecuadorian main harbour Guayaquil to the Peruvian main one, Callao.[24] The national societies of the two warring nations therefore cooperated.

This cooperation was backed by public propaganda in favour of humanitarian actions. Throughout the conflict and beyond, Peruvians were keen to publicly demonstrate their support for the (national) Red Cross and their dignified treatment of prisoners of war. The President of Peru ostensibly lent his personal car to the director of the Peruvian Red Cross to travel to the front, even travelling in his company with his entire family.[25] The Army also deployed a discourse that highlighted its positive treatment of prisoners by its specialised military police service (*prebostazgo*). In his memoirs some years after the war, the general in charge of the Peruvian operations praised the 'humane' treatment that these prisoners of war received.[26] General Ureta emphasised the fact that they were given clothes and care. Correspondence with their families in Ecuador was allowed and facilitated. Some prisoners even received between 3 and 6 dollars from the Peruvian Military Health Service, probably to provide for their basic needs.

General Ureta's insistence on this matter was due to Ecuadorians conducting a relentless propaganda campaign, accusing the Peruvians of being the armed wing of the Axis in the region, condemning the presence of communities of Germans, Italians and Japanese as likely 'fifth columnists'. Peruvians had also accused the Ecuadorian government of playing into the hands of Berlin and Rome. However, Peru's victory in the war had put it on the receiving end of these type of opprobrium. Although the Ecuadorian accusation was supported by widely known facts, such as the presence of immigrant populations from Axis countries, it did not stand up to scrutiny. The influence of Germany and fascist Italy was no less important in Ecuador, whose army had been trained by German and Italian instructors, unlike the

162    *The long Second World War, 1931–1953*

Peruvian army who had relied on the French army. During operations, Ecuadorian officers flew to the front line in aircraft belonging to Sociedad Ecuatoriana de Transportes Aéreos (SEDTA), a German-owned civil aviation company. The United States was concerned about this influence in both countries. Due to American pressure, Italian and German economic assets were banned from these countries at the beginning of the war, as happened in most of the Western Hemisphere. In Ecuador, the government expropriated SEDTA after lengthy discussions in August 1941, and replaced it with Panagra of the United States, which bought SEDTA facilities.[27] In Peru, the Lufthansa contract (another German-owned company) had been cancelled as early as March 1941.[28] The ethnic Japanese population, settled in Peru at the turn of the century, became an easy target in a country where their economic success had fuelled resentment, and became the object of riots and discrimination, leaving a bitter memory for the populous Japanese-Peruvians.[29] Between 1942 and 1945, around 1,800 of the community's 25,000 members were arrested and deported by boat to camps in New Mexico and Texas, as a result of cooperation between the Peruvian government and police, American diplomacy and the Federal Bureau of Investigation.[30]

Ecuadorian accusations were, therefore, nothing more than propaganda, especially when the government in Quito denounced the (imaginary) presence of soldiers from the Japanese Empire alongside Peruvian troops. Even military observers sent after the fighting ended by the mediating powers (United States, Brazil, Argentina and Chile) rightly complained about 'unfounded denunciations propagated by Ecuadorian journalists'.[31] Nevertheless, the Peruvian army was worried about these assertions, which threatened to cast shame on the behaviour of its troops and risked unfavorable diplomatic consequences. It therefore became necessary to contradict these rumours and show, as much as possible, that prisoners of war were being well treated. This explains why Ecuadorian prisoners of war appeared several times in the propaganda film *Alerta en la frontera*, both as trophies, testament to Peru's victory, and as proof that they were being well treated. The Peruvian government's efforts on this matter were likely aimed at the international community, which had long been sensitive to the plight of prisoners of war, but also at its own citizens, who received from their government a positive discourse on the role of humanitarian actors during the war.

*Humanitarian rhetoric in South America*     163

## Close-up on caregivers

In addition to focusing on the victims of the war, Peruvian propaganda highlighted the patriotic work carried out by caregivers, both doctors and nurses. While we lack sources to examine the visual strategies of the Ecuadorian side, it is interesting to study the way in which caregivers were presented by Peruvians on the front line and in the rear, and to compare it with the humanitarian imagery deployed elsewhere.

An interesting example is the propaganda film *Alerta en la frontera (Border Alert)*, a film produced by the private German director Kurt Hermann, but filmed with the logistical help of the Peruvian army on the battlefield, in which paramedics and nursing staff are presented in an heroic light. Its overly triumphalist content caused it to be banned by the Lima government and never shown until the twenty-first century.[32] This film lasted a little less than one hour and gave a prominent place to infirmary services, placing them on equal footing with the navy, for example. Their vehicles marked with recognisable crosses appeared several times between the story of the fighting and the display of weapons. The entire logistical chain of the medical services was represented, from the arrival of the ambulances on the front line to the pouring in of the military nurses, who went to pick up the wounded on stretchers at the risk of their lives, before evacuating them on the back lines where modern facilities awaited. The film's insistence on the heroic figure of caregivers, whose sacrifice was equal to or even larger than that of the victims (or soldiers) was not specific to this conflict. It was consistent with the shift in the focus of humanitarian photography from the suffering body to medical staff that could be seen in other major humanitarian organisations of the time.[33] In a way, the film even anticipated this phenomenon, which came to the fore in the postwar period, and it can be explained here by the fact that the film was produced by one of the belligerents and not by an organisation from outside the conflict.

The film also reflected a gendered division of healthcare work, with men working on the front line and women at the rear. Female nurses only appeared in facilities far away from the front lines, long after the doctors and stretcher-bearers had done so. The coverage of the wife and daughter of the Peruvian president, Enriqueta Garland

164     *The long Second World War, 1931–1953*

de Prado and Rosita Garland Prado, was also highly gendered, the latter appearing in a role that could be described as that of the nurse of the nation. During operations, both the mother and daughter went to the front to raise the morale of the troops and distribute food rations, remaining confined to performing acceptable work for women in a war zone. The daughter of the president occasionally wore a uniform of auxiliary nurse. On their return to Lima, they were welcomed as heroines of the war and received numerous official tributes on behalf of the army and the parliament. During a public ceremony, a Catholic chaplain praised in a poem the actions of the mother who, 'with maternal eagerness', had brought 'holy and tender relief', and those of the girl who, alongside with her mother as 'noble nurses', gave 'consolation in bitterness'. He specified that both 'gave comfort to all the wounded/and the heroes offered their prayer/and even arriving in the opposite region/consoled the poor and afflicted'.[34]

Stressing women's compassion and their role as mothers and carers while at the same time placing them in the background was a common feature of humanitarian iconography and films.[35] A parallel can be drawn between the media treatment of First Lady Enriqueta Garland de Prado, who appears in the film *Alerta en la frontera* distributing food rations to soldiers, and that of the surgeon María Gómez Álvarez in the Varsovia Hospital in Toulouse a few years later, since in both cases the humanitarian actions of these women were commented on and therefore interpreted (or even played down) by a male voiceover.[36] As is usually the case, we do not have the direct testimony of the president's mother and daughter and can only suggest what they thought. We can, however, note that they were fully in line with the practices of this category of upper-class women who were able to use the ambiguous discourse of these 'women humanitarians' to enter political and media spaces that were otherwise off-limit to them.[37] The specificity of this gendered communication lay in the link between humanitarian action and Catholicism, underlined by the presence of the chaplain, and places Peru within the Iberian humanitarian tradition, present in Spain since the nineteenth century.[38]

The figure of the patriotic nurse who helps her wounded compatriots was predominant, but this care could also be extended towards the enemy. Not only did the First Lady and her daughter console the Peruvian soldiers, but the chaplain's poem also indicated that

## Humanitarian rhetoric in South America 165

they would have assisted the civilians and prisoners of the opposing nation, thus respecting the Geneva Convention of 1864 and its successive versions (1906, 1929). The film also heavily highlighted the care given to the Ecuadorian enemy soldiers in Peruvian hospitals, where 'the wards are occupied by wounded from both sides. Peruvians, Ecuadorians, without differences, mixed, together, receive attention with the same will and the same zeal'. 'There is no enemy here!',[39] the voiceover emphatically stated as the film showed what appeared to be an Ecuadorian soldier being treated by a Peruvian medical team. How can we explain the centrality of caregivers, both for compatriots but also enemies, in the Peruvian discourse? One can underline the continuity with the traditionally pacifist discourse of the South American nations of the time, which considered the American continent as the continent of peace, as opposed to the warmongering Europe.[40] This American mythology of peace was reflected in the 1930s in the proliferation of legal instruments to limit conflicts between the American 'sister republics', largely within the framework of the pan-American relationships, although their effective scope was limited. The American states had to present themselves as 'respectable', as Odría said to the nun, adopting the main advancements of the international community, foremost among which was the safeguarding of peace and the dignified behaviour of the country's representatives towards foreign interests. To this ideological cause, we should probably add a more trivial reason related to the conditions of filming and journalistic follow-up of a political move: it was easier (and maybe reassuring) to film and report on the nurses and wounded in the rear than the fighting on the front line. In any case, the focus on Peruvian caregivers enabled Peruvian authorities to sanitise the war and downplay the violence of the fighting by referring from the outset to the Ecuadorian victims of the conflict, soldiers and civilians alike, through the reassuring prism of Peruvian charity, a tendency that was confirmed during the occupation that followed the fighting.

### Dealing with civilians under occupation

Between August 1941 and February 1942, the Peruvians had to manage the unprecedented situation of having to administer a foreign province and its civilian population, estimated at nearly seventy

**166**    *The long Second World War, 1931–1953*

thousand before the fighting. This led the army in charge of the region to present itself as a 'humanitarian' army, a self-fashioning process ultimately motivated by geopolitical necessities.

This 'humanitarian army' faced many difficulties on the ground. The first was to feed the population and revive the local economy while the traditional supply channels were interrupted. General Ureta initially planned to provide supplies and subsidies from Peru and then present the bill to the Ecuadorian government.[41] The Peruvian prefect of Tumbes, the civil authority of the region bordering Ecuador, proposed instead that they should buy Ecuadorian products and their harvest of tobacco to kickstart the local economy and win their hearts and minds.[42]

The results on the ground did not meet the Peruvian ambitions. Both the economy and the administrative management of the region were seriously undermined. The herds abandoned by their masters were quickly reduced to feed the troops or stolen by starving residents. The Peruvian army had to organise in haste a service of 'gathering and exploitation of the cattle', and the Peruvian police force, specially sent on site, investigated the thefts without success. A great part of the tobacco harvest was lost because of the 'lack of arms'. The limited earthworks did not improve the road network in the medium term, and overall the civil administration, set up by the Peruvian army, was no more efficient than the previous Ecuadorian administration.[43] The Peruvian army's failure was predictable. To be sure, Peruvians did not plunder the resources of the Ecuadorians, but their efforts at reviving the productive apparatus served essentially their own national interest. This is one of the reasons for the terrible reputation that the Peruvian army left in the region.

The other actual result of the presence of the Peruvian army on Ecuadorian ground was the constant accusations of exactions and bad behaviour, sometimes false as noted by neutral observers,[44] made by the government in Quito. This propaganda war about the attitude of Peruvian soldiers focused on a few specific events. For example, according to Quito, the Peruvians were responsible for the pillage of the region and for the fire in one of its most important cities, Santa Rosa, whose centre burned entirely except for the church. The Ecuadorian press, quoted by the Peruvian government, published stories accusing Peruvian troops of having whipped and shaved the head and eyebrows of captured Ecuadorian men,[45] a practice that would be found to be perpetrated against women

# Humanitarian rhetoric in South America 167

during the liberation of France just three years later. The Peruvian army and government contested those accusations. Peruvian officers, compared explicitly by Ecuadorian newspapers to the Nazis, considered themselves victims of a smear campaign. They were anxious to dissociate themselves from the atrocities that were committed on the European continent, asking their diplomats to respond. The Peruvian Minister for War sent a telegram to the victorious General Ureta expressing his concern: 'Several Ecuadorian newspapers arriving by plane give news Peru established Nazi-style concentration camps for Ecuadorian civilian prisoners. In order for Chancellery to deny tendentious news, please inform where and how Ecuadorian civilian prisoners are concentrated this region.'[46] The Peruvian government financed an important work of counter-propaganda which resulted in the printing of thousands of leaflets presenting their version of the facts, sometimes translated into English and distributed in Washington, DC.[47] These leaflets aimed to exonerate Peru from the fire of Santa Rosa. To do so, the Peruvians dispatched their civil police to carry out an investigation, which logically led to the conclusion that it was the Ecuadorian troops who had plundered, burned and mistreated the local populations as they retreated.[48]

Not only did the Peruvian propaganda take it upon itself to assert that it was not responsible for any abuses but it went even further by emphasising the positive role of its presence in the occupied region. The above-mentioned film, *Alerta en la frontera*, affirmed clearly that the Peruvian troops not only respected but also put in order and modernised the region. Over images showing Peruvian soldiers installing communication lines and clearing roads and rubble, the voiceover exclaimed that

> The Peruvian soldiers, with the generosity and the honesty that characterise them, respect the foreign society as their own. ... It is also necessary to assure the life of the inhabitants of the occupied zone, the civil guards gather the dispersed cattle. Thus, they guarantee the property of the inhabitants, preserving their plantations and their abandoned seedlings. ... Protected by respect and law, trade and industry are re-established, the railroads are functioning again and the traffic on the rivers and roads becomes normal. ... Ecuadorian families that had abandoned their towns return to their homes upon hearing the news spread beyond the border that Peru, that knows how to be respected, also respects life and foreign property.[49]

168 *The long Second World War, 1931–1953*

The Peruvians also had to answer to the very specific accusation of having attacked a hospital. While several testimonies collected in the twenty-first century claim that the Peruvians did indeed destroy a hospital and kill patients,[50] military and diplomatic documents from Peru and Ecuador have not been able to confirm this fact. On the contrary, the Peruvian army presented itself as the protector of these places. For example, the hospital run by Catholic Sisters in Santa Rosa continued to function with the support of Peruvian officers. The collaboration between nuns and officers was so compromising that the nuns would have decided to leave for Peru with the Peruvian troops during the evacuation of the region.[51] While it does not seem that Peru did target a hospital during the aerial bombardments, this accusation was part of a set of practices attributed to the Peruvians, constructed from facts or from the collective memory (such as summary executions, rapes, looting and use of Japanese troops). This underlines that an attack on a hospital has since been considered by both Peruvian and Ecuadorian memory as an intolerable infringement of the customs of war.

In the end, forced by the Ecuadorian accusations that designated the anti-humanitarian practices of the Axis powers as a counter-model, the Peruvians, even if there was a gap between reality and their intentions, developed a humanitarian discourse aimed at the local populations and the international community. This can be explained by the need not to be sanctioned by the diplomacy of the continent, but it was also the result of Peruvian war effort planning. Some Peruvians officers intended to annex the occupied Ecuadorian region, and humanitarian work had to support this objective. In spite of this hidden goal, the Peruvian army was forced to evacuate the occupied territories after the signing of the border agreements in January 1942. The humanitarian rhetoric was then taken up by outside powers.

### Neutrals and the United States: a humanitarian example of pan-American cooperation

Finally, it is important to note that this occupation was a humanitarian issue not only for the two belligerent states but also for the international community and in particular the United States, which

## Humanitarian rhetoric in South America 169

used the aftermath of the conflict as a laboratory and showcase for humanitarian aid.

The humanitarian concerns of the powers in the region were enhanced by the Talara agreement, which established a demilitarised strip around 30 km wide between the Peruvian and Ecuadorian positions, where only Ecuadorian civilian police maintained order under the supervision of foreign military observers. The four mediating powers, the United States, Brazil, Argentina and Chile, sent officers to the area, inventing an almost new way of dealing with armed conflicts on the continent. The novelty of the exercise became apparent to the members of this mission when they came to establishing the nature of the hierarchical relationship between them and the tone of their dialogue with the two warring governments, as well as defining the modus operandi of the investigation on the ground. The officers gradually organised themselves by inventing a new profession, that of military intervention force, prefiguring the Blue Helmets. The Talara agreement gave these observers a security role. The aim was to prevent the resumption of armed hostilities. However, the group's functions were rapidly expanded as the territories concerned became more disorganised, and it began to administrate local authorities and gather information of a humanitarian nature. Its members organised the police and the administration in the demilitarised zone, and circulated in the occupied zone to gather information on the sanitary state of the populations, documenting possible Peruvian exactions. For this reason, they were not welcomed by Peruvian officers, who were 'cold' towards them.[52] In spite of the technical difficulty of their work, they concluded that the majority of accusations of exactions were invented by the Ecuadorian press. Only during the definitive departure of the Peruvian troops did they plunder the region.[53] The foreign officers had therefore fulfilled, or even invented, a humanitarian information mission.

After their departure, humanitarian needs did not diminish. As Monica Rankin has demonstrated, Americans deployed an important fund to reconstruct the area, as part of the 'emergency reconstruction diplomacy' that was organised in the El Oro region by the Office of the Coordinator of Inter-American Affairs (OIAA).[54] This organisation's aim was to bring the peoples of the Americas closer together in a perspective of continental solidarity in times of war. It is particularly known for its cultural action in the fields

170    *The long Second World War, 1931–1953*

of cinema and radio, for example, but it embraced a very broad spectrum of activities including reconstruction.[55] Assistance in this area to the El Oro region was one of the measures designed to facilitate the acceptance of the peace protocol by the Ecuadorians. The experts from the United States and other countries of the continent arrived very quickly after the withdrawal of the Peruvian troops. They were very ambitious for the region. It was not only a question of helping the region to recover from the military invasion but also of bringing modernity to a region considered as the archetype of South American underdevelopment. Construction of infrastructure, drainage, vaccination campaigns, infant feeding: it was about making the region a model for the rest of the continent.

It is interesting to note that these continental experts' efforts were in perfect continuity with that of their predecessors from the newly evacuated occupying army. Winners, losers and neutrals shared a vision of humanitarian aid that would potentially provide poor regions with new and unexpected opportunities. But just as the Peruvians had failed, the American mission did not deliver the expected results, despite the substantial investment. As Monica Rankin has shown, the mission suffered from many contradictions. The experts sent were far from being the most competent, as the latter were reserved for the US war effort in the Pacific. Coordination with local authorities was weak to such an extent that one wonders whether there were any exchanges between the aforementioned military observers who had established regular contact with these authorities and the experts who disembarked after the evacuation. The objectives for humanitarian aid to the inhabitants and the needs of continental defence could also be contradictory, with the latter sometimes being prioritised and directing the programmes in another direction. Finally, the initial plans were revised downwards because of their cost until the mission ended in 1944.[56]

The El Oro experience raises the question of its place in the development of American humanitarian action during the long Second World War, and more broadly in the twentieth century, both before and after the war between Peru and Ecuador. In the case of the United States, we can detect a continuity with the humanitarian impulse – highlighted by Branden Little[57] – that arose during the First World War and was then mobilised in its 'catastrophic diplomacy' studied by Julia Irwin.[58] The example of the Andean War of 1941

## Humanitarian rhetoric in South America 171

shows that there could still be a humanitarian interest in conflicts outside the United States, which could coincide with a diplomatic objective of displaying effective solidarity between the northern and southern parts of the hemisphere in order to maintain the neutrality of the Latin American states in the global conflict. The intervention in Ecuador was therefore part of a long-standing process, reactivated by the aftermath of the Second World War, and may also have had repercussions after the event. Although the experience was not crowned with total success, it could constitute an important precedent for Washington's strategy in the Latin American region thereafter. Indeed, development through modernisation was one of the main ways of fighting against the Soviet influence during the Cold War.[59] The Ecuadorian post-war management can therefore be seen as an early step towards the international implementation of this doctrine formulated in American agencies during the Great Depression and clarified during the Second World War around the Atlantic Charter of 1941, as Elizabeth Borgwardt has shown.[60] However, the mission's legacy is uncertain. Only by analysing more archives could we shed light on the lessons learned from this experience by the American government and the continent's humanitarian organisations based on their actions during the second half of the twentieth century. In view of the mission's mixed results, it is likely that the deployment of humanitarian aid in the El Oro region was more of a temporary showcase than a real laboratory for the future.

## Conclusion

Over and above the discrepancy between rhetoric and action, which always exists in this type of situation, we have highlighted in this chapter two different strategies in the instrumentalisation of humanitarian aid for propaganda purposes. The first, implemented by Ecuador, could be described as offensive and opportunistic. The Ecuadorian government mainly used humanitarian rhetoric to make accusations against its Peruvian neighbour, disregarding the fact that Quito had long been reluctant to commit itself fully to humanitarian action and that, as a consequence, its facilities were limited. By contrast, Peru's attitude appears to have been defensive but nevertheless more far-reaching. Although it aimed to exonerate

## 172    *The long Second World War, 1931–1953*

itself, Lima was able to rely on a long tradition and well-established infrastructure dedicated to humanitarian action. Even within two countries that were culturally quite similar, humanitarian rhetoric and practice were not homogeneous. Local issues and traditions continued to shape the reception of the humanitarian spirit.

The analysis has also revealed certain attitudes to humanitarian issues which were common among the two Andean countries, and even in the nations of the American continent involved in the conflict. For Peru and Ecuador, humanitarian action and the communication efforts that had to highlight it were more of a moral duty essential for gaining international respectability than a legal commitment based on treaties. It had to be carried out in the name of a certain continental idea associated with the concepts of peace, fraternity and development. This idea was clearly imposed as a constraint by the prevailing pan-Americanism and the diplomatic weight of the United States, but could also be rooted in the historical and cultural ties that bound the countries that had emerged from the former Spanish Empire, where the neighbour could not be the 'enemy'. This conflict highlights the depth of the penetration of humanitarian sentiment in the American continent, both in the North and in the South, and the belief, not stated but implicit, that humanitarianism was a typical value of the American continent, much more so than of Europe, which was once again sinking into barbarism. Finally, humanitarian action and discourse were directed towards their neighbour rather than towards distant territories and peoples, which could underline a certain localism in humanitarian action in the region. The specificity of this goal should be verified over the long term by conducting studies on the history of humanitarian action, which have hitherto focused on other parts of the world.

### Notes

1 '¿Cómo es posible Madre? Dejaron ustedes abandonados a sus heridos y enfermos. Sor Apolina: Usted comprenderá … nos avisaron que estaban cerca y … en la guerra … Odría: Madre no tenían ustedes nada que temer, nuestro ejército es respetuoso y respetable'. Original quotations appear as endnotes only when they are of significant length

# Humanitarian rhetoric in South America 173

or when their translation is open to interpretation. All translations are by the chapter's author. Salvador Mariátegui y Cisneros, *Conflicto Peruano-Ecuatoriano: 1941* (Lima: Editorial Minerva, 1968), p. 135.

2 It is unclear how humanitarian issues during this conflict influenced Manuel Odría's populist government of Peru. Odría only referred to the conflict to emphasise his role in the 'great victory'.

3 Pío Jaramillo Alvarado, *La Guerra de Conquista en América* (Guayaquil: Editorial Jouvin, 1941).

4 Cédric Cotter and Irène Herrmann, 'The Dynamics of Humanitarian Rhetorics: Switzerland, the United States and other Neutral Countries', *Relations internationales*, 159:3 (2014), 49–67; on neutrals during the Second World War, see Neville Wylie, *European Neutrals and Non-Belligerents during the Second World War* (Cambridge: Cambridge University Press, 2010).

5 For a broader view of the relationship between the Second World War and the American continent, see Robert A. Humphreys, *Latin America and the Second World War* (London: Athlone, 1981) and Thomas M. Leonard and John F. Bratzel, *Latin America during World War II* (Lanham, MD: Rowman & Littlefield Publishers, 2007)

6 Bryce Wood, *Aggression and History: The Case of Ecuador and Perú* (New York: Columbia University, 1978).

7 Within a broad literature on the origins of the First World War, see Émile Durkheim and Ernest Denis, *Qui a voulu la guerre? Les origines de la guerre d'après les documents diplomatiques* (Paris: Librairie Armand Colin, 1915); Pierre Renouvin, *Les origines immédiates de la guerre (28 juin-4 août 1914)* (Paris: A. Costes, 1925); Fritz Fischer, *Griff nach der Weltmacht: die Kriegszielpolitik des kaiserlichen Deutschland 1914/18* (Düsseldorf: Droste, 1961).

8 *Bulletin international de la Croix Rouge* (hereafter *BICR*), 43 (July 1880), pp. 128–129.

9 Yannick Wehrli, 'États latino-américains, organismes multilatéraux et défense de la souveraineté: Entre Société des Nations et espace continental panaméricain (1919–1939)' (PhD dissertation, Geneva University, 2016), pp. 148–152.

10 *BICR*, 249 (September 1939), p. 786.

11 *BICR*, 266 (March 1941), p. 160.

12 *BICR*, 52 (April 1923), pp. 429–441; *BICR*, 53 (May 1923), pp. 541–542.

13 Françoise Martinez, Emmanuelle Sinardet and Lissell Quiroz (eds), *'Race' et Citoyenneté dans Les Andes: Bolivie-Équateur-Pérou. 1880–1925* (Paris: Atlande, 2021).

14 *BICR*, 52 (April 1923), pp. 429–432.

174    *The long Second World War, 1931–1953*

15 *BICR*, 81 (September 1925), p. 784.

16 *BICR*, 52 (April 1923), p. 431.

17 Julia F. Irwin, *Making the World Safe: The American Red Cross and a Nation's Humanitarian Awakening* (Oxford: Oxford University Press, 2013); Julia F. Irwin, *Catastrophic Diplomacy: US Foreign Disaster Assistance in the American Century* (Chapel Hill, NC: The University of North Carolina Press, 2024).

18 *BICR*, 226 (October 1937), p. 1015.

19 Archives of the International Committee of the Red Cross: B.G.85, Sociétés nationales; Pérou; Équateur.

20 'Peru no encuentrase estado guerra', *Ibid.*

21 Centro de Estudios Histórico-militares del Perú (hereafeter CEHMP): Gabinete militar, Oficios remitidos 1941. MG-1941, 166. The minister of war to the minister of foreign relations, 16 July 1941.

22 Archivo histórico del Ministerio de Relaciones Exteriores, Quito (hereafter AHMRE): Q.2.1. 'Circular reservada n°12-B-12, Los últimos incidentes en la frontera sur', 11 July 1941.

23 Eloy G. Ureta, *Apuntes Sobre Una Campaña (1941)* (Madrid: Editorial Antorcha, 1953), p. 386.

24 'Atenciones prestadas a los prisioneros ecuatorianos', *Revista de la Cruz Roja Peruana*, tercera época, 19 (1941), p. 54.

25 'Visita del presidente de la Cruz Roja peruana a los comités del Norte', *Revista de la Cruz Roja Peruana*, tercera época, 19 (1941), pp. 5–10.

26 Ureta, *Apuntes*, pp. 191–194.

27 *Foreign Relations of the United States, 1941, vol. VII*, pp. 284–290.

28 *Foreign Relations of the United States, 1941, vol. VII*, p. 503.

29 Isabelle Lausent-Herrera, 'Le parcours difficile de la communauté japonaise au Pérou', *Problèmes d'Amérique Latine*, 97(1990), 27–49.

30 Daniel M. Masterson and Jorge Ortiz Sotelo, 'Peru: International Developments and Local Realities', in Leonard and Bratzel (eds), *Latin America during World War II*, pp. 135–138.

31 AHMRE: T.5.3.1.7., 'Informe general de los observadores militares del lado ecuatoriano desde la iniciación de las hostilidades hasta la ratificación del Protocolo de Paz, Amistad y límites, firmado en Rio de Janeiro entre Ecuador y Perú, en el período comprendido entre 10 de mayo de 1941 y 28 de febrero de 1942', 15 March 1942.

32 Kurt Hermann, *Alerta en la frontera*, 53 minutes, 1941. Production: Federico Uranga; Photography: Manuel Trullen; Sound: Bertalan Petrick; Narration: Ricardo Villarán; Voice: Gustavo Montoya; Assistants: Pedro Valdivieso, Cesar Chugo and Jorge Torrico; Music: 'Zarumilla' March and Richard Wagner's 'Ride of the Valkyries'.

# Humanitarian rhetoric in South America 175

33 Davide Rodogno and Thomas David, 'All the World Loves a Picture: The World Health Organization's Visual Politics', in Heide Fehrenbach and Davide Rodogno (eds), *Humanitarian Photography: A History* (Cambridge: Cambridge University Press, 2015), pp. 223–248.

34 'Con afán materno', 'Alivio santo y tierno', 'nobles enfermeras', 'consolación en la amargura', 'dieron consuelo a todos los heridos/A los héroes brindaron su plegaria/y aun llegando a la región contraria/consolaron a pobres y afligidos'. Claudia Rosas Lauro (ed.), *Mujeres de Armas Tomar. La Participación de Las Mujeres En Las Guerras Del Perú Republicano* (Lima: Ministerio de Defensa, 2021), pp. 322–323.

35 Esther Möller, Johannes Paulmann and Katharina Stornig (eds), *Gendering Global Humanitarianism in the Twentieth Century: Practice, Politics and the Power of Representation* (Cham: Palgrave Macmillan, 2020); Dolores Martín-Moruno, Brenda Lynn Edgar and Marie Leyder, 'Feminist Perspectives on the History of Humanitarian Relief (1870–1945)', *Medicine, Conflict and Survival*, 36:1 (2020), 2–18.

36 Àlvar Martínez-Vidal, 'The Powers of Masculinization in Humanitarian Storytelling: The Case of the Surgeon María Gómez Álvarez in the Varsovia Hospital (Toulouse, 1944–1950)', *Medicine, Conflict and Survival*, 36:1 (2020), 103–121.

37 Martín-Moruno, Edgar and Leyder, 'Feminist Perspectives', pp. 3 and 5. The expression 'women humanitarians' is due to Sybil Oldfield.

38 Jon Arrizabalaga, 'The "Merciful and Loving Sex": Concepción Arenal's Narratives on Spanish Red Cross Women's War Relief Work in the 1870s', *Medicine, Conflict and Survival*, 36:1 (2020), 41–60.

39 'Sus salas son ocupadas por heridos de ambos bandos. Peruanos y Ecuatorianos, sin diferencias, mezclados, confundidos, reciben atención con la misma voluntad y el mismo celo. Aquí no hay enemigo.' Hermann, *Alerta en la frontera*.

40 Olivier Compagnon, *L'adieu à l'Europe: L'Amérique Latine et La Grande Guerre: Argentine et Brésil, 1914–1939* (Paris: Fayard, 2013).

41 CEHMP: Gabinete militar, Oficios remitidos 1941, MG-1941, 166. The minister of war to the minister of development, 16 August 1941. Ureta's original message is dated 11 August 1941.

42 CEHMP: Gabinete militar, Oficios remitidos 1941, MG-1941, 166. The minister of war to the minister of finance and trade, 22 August 1941.

43 Comisión catalogadora del centro de Estudios Histórico-Militares del Perú, *Colección Documental Del Conflicto y Campaña Militar Con El Ecuador En 1941*, vol. 4, 1036 (Lima, 1978).

176 *The long Second World War, 1931–1953*

44 AHMRE: T.5.3.1.7., 'Informe general de los observadores militares'.

45 *La Ocupación de la Provincia de El Oro por las Fuerzas Peruanas* (Lima: Oficina de prensa del ministerio de relaciones exteriores del Perú, 1941), p. 5. The Peruvian document probably referred to the newspaper *El Telégrafo de Guayaquil*.

46 'Varios diarios Ecuador llegados avión dan noticias Perú establecido campos concentración a la manera nazi, para prisioneros civiles ecuatorianos. Fin Cancillería desmienta esa tendenciosa noticia, sírvase informar lugares y forma encuéntranse concentrados prisioneros civiles ecuatorianos esa región.' CEHMP: Gabinete militar. Oficios remitidos 1941, MG-1941, 166. The minister of war to General Ureta, 29 October 1941.

47 *La Ocupación de la Provincia de El Oro* was translated to English and distributed under the title *The Occupation of the Ecuadorean Province of 'el Oro' by Peruvian troops* (Lima: Press Office of the Ministry of Foreign Affairs of Peru, 1941).

48 CEHMP: Gabinete militar, Oficios remitidos 1941, MG-1941, 166. Colonel Luis E. Vinatea, commander of the 1st light division, to general Ureta, 5 August 1941.

49 'Los soldados peruanos, con la generosidad y la honradez que los caracterizan, respetan la sociedad ajena como la suya propia. ... También hay que asegurar la vida de los habitantes de la zona ocupada, los guardias civiles recogen el ganado disperso Asimismo, garantizan la propiedad de los naturales, resguardado sus plantaciones y sembríos abandonados. ... Al amparo del respecto y el orden, se restablece el comercio y la industria. Los ferrocarriles funcionan nuevamente y el tráfico en los ríos y caminos se normaliza. ... Familias ecuatorianas que habían abandonado sus poblaciones, regresan a sus hogares, ante la noticia difundida más allá de la frontera de que el Perú, que sabe hacerse respetar, respeta igualmente la vida y la propiedad ajena.' Hermann, *Alerta en la frontera*.

50 Interview with Ustiniano Salazar Zelada, Peruvian voluntary soldier, 17 February 2015; interview with Catalina Vélez Romero, a civilian from El Oro region, 16 September 2016.

51 Mariátegui y Cisneros, *Conflicto Peruano-Ecuatoriano: 1941*, p. 135.

52 AHMRE, T.5.3.1.7., 'Informe general de los observadores militares'.

53 *Ibid.*

54 Monica Rankin, 'The United States in El Oro: The OCIAA and the Diplomacy of Emergency Rehabilitation during WWII', *The Latin Americanist*, 63:2 (2019), 163–188.

55 Darlene J. Sadlier, *Americans All: Good Neighbor Cultural Diplomacy in World War II* (Austin, TX: University of Texas Press, 2013).

*Humanitarian rhetoric in South America* 177

56 Rankin, 'The United States in El Oro'.
57 Branden Little, 'Band of Crusaders: American Humanitarians, the Great War, and the remaking of the World' (PhD dissertation, University of California, 2009).
58 Irwin, *Catastrophic Diplomacy.*
59 David Ekbladh, *The Great American Mission: Modernization and the Construction of an American World Order* (Princeton, NJ: Princeton University Press, 2011).
60 Elizabeth Borgwardt, *A New Deal for the World: America's Vision for Human Rights* (Cambridge, MA: The Belknap Press of Harvard University Press, 2005).

# 7

# Unitarian Service Committee's activities with refugee populations and the Resistance in France during and after the Second World War

*Jon Arrizabalaga and Àlvar Martínez-Vidal*

> Back then they all consumed by one wish: to leave. And they were all afraid of one thing: being left behind.
>
> (Anna Seghers, *Transit* [1944], Berlin: Aufbau-Verlag GmbH, 2012, p. 6, I)

The Unitarian Service Committee (USC) was founded in Boston, in May 1940, as a non-profit, non-sectarian associate member organisation of the American Unitarian Association (hereafter AUA), to assist European refugees threatened by Nazi persecution.[1] Its organisation was similar to that of the Quakers' American Friends Service Committee, but unlike the Friends' Service Committee, which was neutral, they openly supported the Allied cause. Soon after the Nazis invaded France and occupied Paris, the USC established its first European office in Lisbon in order to aid refugees in their transit to the Americas across the Pyrenees and Spain. Lisbon was primarily chosen for geostrategic reasons, as the capital of a neutral country Portugal, and one of the few important non-military harbours in continental Europe that was still in operation.

After the Armistice and the establishment of the Vichy regime, French authorities created new internment camps to accommodate thousands of refugees from different parts of Europe, including soldiers from the Spanish Republican army and their families, members of the International Brigades, central European Jews, Czech and Polish resistants, or fugitives from the Nazis and their allied regimes for ethnic, ideological or religious reasons.[2] The camps'

*Unitarian Service Committee's activities*     179

barracks were crowded with 'democratic politicians and statesmen, scientists and students, businessmen and trade unionists, aged men and women and adolescents'.[3] These camps also hosted French Jews, most of whom were later deported to Nazi concentration camps. Living conditions in the camps – including the so-called hospital camps – rapidly declined as the war went on due to the lack of clothes, food and medicine, in addition to human overcrowding and the poor physical state of the barracks.[4]

Largely due to the legal obstacles to emigration put in place by Vichy authorities and the high cost and risk of helping refugees to get out of Europe,[5] the USC's Boston general headquarters changed their strategy. While they had initially hoped to help them escape the old continent, they soon prioritised direct humanitarian aid for people in French internment camps and other reclusion spaces. They believed that the collective situation of the most in need refugees could be in this way substantially improved by means of food, clothing, footwear, medicine and sanitary material. With this in mind, they opened a second USC European office in Marseille to coordinate this new relief policy across France. In June 1942, anticipating the worsening of circumstances in France, the USC transferred its Marseille office to Geneva, where the European headquarters settled from 1943 to the end of the Second World War. After the Liberation of France, the USC's French headquarters were moved to Paris, and in January 1945 a new office was opened in Toulouse.

While other relief organisations, such as British and American Quakers, remained predominantly focused on delivering general aid such as clothes, food and writing tools, the USC became increasingly more interested in providing specialised medical care to refugees. Between 1943 and 1946, the USC developed medical and social relief programmes of about $365,000 in different European countries (France, Italy, Switzerland, Germany, Hungary, Netherlands, Czechoslovakia, Austria, Portugal, Poland, 'The Balkans' and Spain).[6] This chapter examines USC activities with refugee populations in France from its establishment to the late 1940s through a study of two major medical care institutions, namely the medico-social dispensary known as the Marseille Clinic and the so-called Varsovie Hospital at Toulouse. By focusing on USC's activities, actors, including its recipients of aid, and intervention spaces, this chapter sheds new light onto the entanglements between humanitarian aid and the

180     *The long Second World War, 1931–1953*

Resistance against fascism and Nazism. It also reveals understudied aspects of medical relief work for Spanish Republican refugees during the long Second World War.

## USC's founding and its setting in Europe

The creation of the USC was a result of both an increased awareness that citizens from Nazi-occupied European countries were being persecuted for their political or religious beliefs and a reaction against the prevailing apathy in US public opinion towards refugees in Europe.[7] Its founding executive director, Robert Dexter (1887–1955), was a North American social worker who had been continuously involved in humanitarian efforts since the First World War and had participated in the international and social engagement of the American Unitarian Association (AUA) since 1927.[8]

The USC's founding coincided with, and was indeed prompted by, the Nazi military invasion of northern and western France. The occupation of Paris led to the Armistice on 22 June 1940 and the establishment of the Vichy regime. At this point, thousands of foreign refugees, along with French citizens displaced from Alsace, Lorraine and other war zones, poured into unoccupied southern France, where they met a large number of Spanish Republican exiles, who had fled there after the defeat of the Spanish Republic in 1939, as well as Italian refugees having escaped from Mussolini's fascist regime.[9] The concentration of this mixed refugee population created specific humanitarian challenges and huge medico-social demands. Marseille and its surroundings became the last hope for tens of thousands of refugees wanting to escape from Europe by sea.[10]

In late June 1940, Unitarian Reverend Waitstill H. Sharp (1902–1983) and his wife Martha (1905–1999) arrived in Lisbon, where they took on the mission of coordinating the USC's relief work in France that was mostly focused on promoting the rescue and migration to the Americas of Jewish, anti-fascist and leftist refugees.[11] In mid-September 1940, Unitarian Reverend Charles R. Joy (1885–1978) replaced the Sharps as the head of Lisbon USC office. In about January 1941, after having succeeded to convince Dexter that the

## Unitarian Service Committee's activities 181

USC should shift its humanitarian relief priorities in Europe, Joy opened in Marseille the USC's second office in Europe. In this populous French port city, refugees from all over Europe were waiting for weeks or even months for the indispensable visas to be allowed to embark and get out of Europe.

As the USC's director in France and the head of its Marseille office, Joy appointed Noel Field (1904–1970), a multilingual American Quaker with a Harvard degree in international relations (1924) and a one-year medical social-service diploma at the Boston School for Social Work, to help him coordinate medical work with refugees in the camps. Field had developed social work in collaboration with colleagues from the Massachusetts' prison system (1925–1926) before joining the American Foreign Service (1925–1930) and working as a drafting officer in the Department of State (1930–1935). Later, he was a member of the League of Nations' Disarmament Section (May 1936–1940) and one of its commissioners in Spain (1938–1939). As part of this role, he organised an 'orderly repatriation' of the International Brigades after the Non-Intervention Committee requested their withdrawal.[12]

Field had been recommended to Joy by Donald A. Lowrie (1889–1974), who worked in the YMCA offices in Geneva to provide relief for war prisoners. Lowrie was the promoter and chairman of the Comité de Coordination pour l'Assistance dans les Camps (Coordination Committee for Relief Work in Internment Camps), better known as the Nimes Committee.[13] Throughout the course of the Second World War, Joy and Field oversaw USC's emigration, social relief and healthcare programmes for refugees being persecuted by the Nazis and their allied regimes all over Europe. They worked across southern France and in collaboration with other humanitarian volunteers and organisations. The Vichy government allowed the USC to operate on its territories as this humanitarian organisation relieved its governmental responsibilities. In a country increasingly impoverished by the war, the French government wanted to focus on its own citizens and welcomed any aid coming from humanitarian agencies, particularly those from the United States. Further, the USC did not pose an existential threat at all to Vichy: neither the rescue of persecuted people nor the medical aid given to refugees appeared to compromise its puppet state.[14]

182    *The long Second World War, 1931–1953*

## The Marseille Clinic during the Second World War: from providing healthcare to European refugees from Nazism to supporting French Resistance fighters

When Noel Field was appointed director of the USC in France to develop its new mission based in Marseille, his wife and life partner since their teenage years in Switzerland, Herta K. Vieser (1904–1980), took over as deputy director. They established 'mutual aid' agreements with other aid organisations, some of which were part of the Nimes Committee, such as the Jewish Children's Aid Society ('Oeuvre de Secours aux Enfants': OSE, hereafter) and others, like the Joint Relief Commission of the International Red Cross (a joint body of the ICRC and the League of Red Cross Societies, created in July 1941 and operational until 1946), the YMCA, the American Quakers, the Jewish organization HICEM, the *Secours Suisse aux Enfants*, and the International Migration Service.[15] To sustain the efforts of the Marseille Clinic, Quakers made a 'generous monthly donation' of food, and the Joint Relief Commission of the International Red Cross sent 'large amounts of vitamins, yeast, calcium, etc.'.[16]

USC's collaboration with the OSE was fostered by the relationship between the Fields and the OSE's director, Joseph Weill (1902–1988).[17] Weill, who had studied and practised medicine in Strasbourg, introduced them to his old friend René Zimmer, a Catholic Alsatian physician, who had become a refugee following the German annexation of Alsace–Lorraine in the spring of 1940. Zimmer was appointed director of the medical programme that the USC promoted from Marseille, not least because his French citizenship seemed to them to facilitate Vichy authorities' approval of the USC's medical and sanitary services based in Marseille.[18] The programme revolved around a medico-social dispensary under the name of *Centre Médico-Social*, of which Zimmer was also the medical director. It was located in a large private apartment shared by the two organisations in a central street –the *rue d'Italie* – in Marseille. In this dispensary, better known as the Marseille Clinic, the USC's activity focused on medical care for refugees (men, women and children), while the OSE developed social work actions oriented towards children based on the extensive experience in the field of this Jewish organisation that had been founded in 1912.[19]

## Unitarian Service Committee's activities     183

Within the Nimes Committee, a health subcommittee was set up, made up of physicians representing their own organisations – René Zimmer for the USC – who were responsible for distributing medical supplies and monitoring their use. After having identified healthcare for foreign refugees without resources as one of the most neglected areas in the humanitarian action deployed, the USC assumed, with the agreement of the other organisations in the Committee, 'the responsibility for centralising relief in medical stores and for supervising the administration of the camps of refugees at Marseilles and in the neighbourhood', without neglecting healthcare for all of them, including French refugees from Alsace–Lorraine and the war zones.[20] The USC had initially focused its work on the various internment camps – *Centres d'Émigration*, according to the terminology then in use by the French authorities – existing in Unoccupied France (e.g. Argelès, Le Barcarès, Gurs, Le Vernet, Les Milles, Noé, Récébédou, Rieucros and Rivesaltes), but its relief activities soon extended to forced foreign workers' camps in both the Hexagon and French colonial Algeria (Colomb-Beschar, Djelfa), on the assumption that their living conditions were similar to those in internment camps.[21]

Though the decision to create the Marseille Clinic had been taken in early April 1941,[22] its opening was delayed until early July because of difficulties in finding premises in a city then so crowded as Marseille. The main purpose of this dispensary was expressly stated in a typewritten pamphlet dated May 1942, which the USC's headquarters produced to publicise the humanitarian activities carried out there: to mobilise solidarity in the United States with the victims of fascism in Europe and, more specifically, to raise funds for its support.[23] Noel Field, the editor of this collective leaflet and the writer of its first part, emphasised in its foreword that the Marseille Clinic provided 'aid and comfort, both material and spiritual, to the foreign refugees in Unoccupied France, especially those forcibly detained in the internment camps'.[24] In practice, relief workers operating in the camps alerted the Marseille Clinic's manager about serious health problems of individual refugees held in the camps, and doctors then went to the camps to determine whether the patients required consultation at the dispensary or even admission to a hospital.

This dispensary provided free medical and nursing care to all refugees in need, whether they were referred directly by the USC or by

184    *The long Second World War, 1931–1953*

other humanitarian organisations operating in the camps (remarkably, Les Milles, but also Rivesaltes, where the USC was developing a child educational project),[25] or sheltered in and around Marseille. Its personnel were made up of health practitioners (physicians and nurses, but also pharmacists and dentists) as well as social workers. All were refugees, many of them Jews. The Marseille Clinic was initially structured around two consultation rooms for adults and children with the support of pharmacy, surgery and dentistry units, but new specialty units like otorhinolaryngology, dermatology, orthopaedics, 'supplementary food' and 'consultations at home' were gradually deployed in addition to sections of X-rays, laboratory, ultraviolet lamps and gymnastics. It carried out between 1,500 and 2,000 consultations every month, approximately one third of them being paediatric.[26] The clinic appears to have done its best to accomplish its mission to help refugees access medical and nursing care. Its contribution to restore patients' good health was perceived as particularly helpful since it was an indispensable consular requirement for obtaining the requested visa for overseas migration.[27]

After November 1942 and the Nazi occupation of the whole of France, it became impossible to continue the operations of the Marseille dispensary in these ways. Not only was the OSE a Jewish organisation, but the USC staff was no longer perceived as 'neutral', the United States having entered the war. The USC's US staff had to flee outside France, which signified the end of US humanitarian aid to the French population. Nevertheless, the USC's activities continued somehow thanks to the complicity of the Marseille city council and a certain indifference of the local prefect of police,[28] under the cover of a supposedly municipal public health centre named *Centre de dépistage et de prophylaxie* led by the chief physician of the municipal hygiene services and making no reference to the USC.[29]

Soon before the Nazis' arrival in Marseille, Noel and Herta Field fled to Geneva where the USC had already transferred its Marseille office in June 1942. Although his name disappeared from the new official organisation chart of the dispensary, Zimmer continued to run the centre and the USC's general administrative and budgetary tasks in the Marseille area in the shadows. After the dissolution of the Nimes Committee, collaboration among the different humanitarian organisations (Joint Relief Commission of the International Red Cross, *Service social d'aide aux émigrants* [SSAE], *Secours*

*Unitarian Service Committee's activities*     185

*Quakers*, and so on) became more and more difficult. The stock of medicines in the USC warehouse was then placed under the management of the Swiss Consulate in Marseille and transferred to the representative of the Joint Relief Commission of the International Red Cross. In the new and increasingly distressing circumstances, this commission had to deal with the supply of medicines – more difficult to procure on the French domestic market – and other basic goods for the refugees.[30] In this crucial task, the USC, Swiss pharmaceutical companies and various relief organisations such as the Quakers, the Swiss Red Cross and the Ecumenical Relief Council cooperated to ensure their distribution and delivery to the camps.[31]

Allegedly, Zimmer then concentrated his efforts on maintaining as much as possible the clinical activities of the dispensary. With the support of its very depleted medical and auxiliary staff, he managed to reinforce the clinical activities by hiring a young and friendly local Christian doctor who was recommended to him by the Medical Order (*L'Ordre des Médecins*) of Marseille.[32] On the other hand, social work with individual cases continued, following Herta Field's instructions from Geneva and now in collaboration with the SSAE – though entirely funded by the USC's own budget. The focus of this work was initially individuals without resources trapped in Marseille, many of them 'intellectuals and people who had relatives in the USA'; and later on, new refugees whom the USC provided material aid of different kinds such as raw materials for their handicraft work, contacts with businesses to sell their products and vouchers for food and meals.[33]

When the consequences of the German occupation of all of France became fully apparent and the Resistance movement against the Nazis grew there, Noel Field and Charles Joy managed, through Dexter, to persuade the USC headquarters in Boston to authorise Zimmer to expand the humanitarian action deployed from the Marseille dispensary beyond refugee relief by assuring 'maintenance to all those "right-thinking people" whose existence was threatened through their activities for the "*bonne cause*"'.[34] Certainly, Zimmer's euphemistic expression concealed clandestine activities, including actions in support of the Resistance such as protecting Spanish Republican refugees from arrest in raids and eventual deportation, assisting Alsatian men who had deserted the German army, providing material and moral support to the families

186     *The long Second World War, 1931–1953*

of imprisoned 'patriots', carrying out intelligence work, and supporting the anti-Nazi propaganda activities of the *Forces Françaises de l'Intérieur* (FFI).[35] Zimmer's own words may reveal a central role of the Marseille dispensary in such activities:

> Our medical work was always a fine cover for all underground activities and the clinic soon became a real center of conspirators. During fictitious consultations, I was often speaking with the patient of everything except of disease. I thought prudent to have secret meetings as less as possible and to meet my agents in the middle of our patients. So, we could not be surprised by an eventual spy insinuating among us to watch our activities.[36]

Regretting the disappearance of the coordinating Nimes Committee, Zimmer deplored the severe difficulties arising from the lack of a common front for joint relief action. Organisational issues were particularly acute when trying to deliver aid to the various local 'Maquis' of the area, since the USC could only provide it in the field of medical work and to a limited extent. However, according to Zimmer, the Marseille Clinic succeeded in developing medico-social activities on such disparate fronts as (1) providing material support to a group of Czech resistance fighters and medical assistance to a children's vacation camp in Vence (Provence); (2) collaborating with a number of external doctors and nurses linked to the municipal and school hygiene departments and the Marseille University Hospital to study the state of health of local schoolchildren (anthropometric studies, X-ray examinations to detect malnutrition, tuberculosis and rickets, dental treatment), with a view to preparing an action plan for immediate relief for those most in urgent need; (3) continuing medical care, in collaboration with the SSAE, for the numerous Spanish refugees left unattended after the dissolution of the Mexican Consulate in Marseille;[37] and (4) giving medical relief to some eight hundred political prisoners through the French Red Cross.[38] This was only possible because the clinic's collaborators continued working for the USC without pay.[39] Their generous and enthusiastic work, Zimmer emphasised, had not ceased even during the six months (from February to August 1944) in which he had been forcibly absent as a result of his arrest by the Gestapo.[40]

With the Liberation of Marseille at the end of August 1944, Zimmer returned to the direction of the Marseille dispensary.

## Unitarian Service Committee's activities

He resumed his collaboration with the OSE and faced a new era of medico-social work with renewed energy and a substantially reinforced budget. In addition to funds coming from private voluntary donations, a very substantial endowment – nearly half a million dollars between October 1944 and September 1945 – was granted by the US federal National War Fund (NWF) for implementing humanitarian programmes in post-war Europe.[41] This new budget allowed the USC to resume their activities in the whole of France and to support more substantially the Marseille dispensary. They started giving aid again to all sorts of European refugees, including Spanish Republicans, and providing medical attention to those just freed from concentration camps who were suffering from severe malnutrition.

### The Hôpital Varsovie at Toulouse and the medical care of Spanish refugees after France's Liberation

In parallel to the development of the Marseille Clinic, the USC contributed to a number of relief projects in southwestern France from 1941. One of them was similar to the Marseille dispensary, though more ambitious in scope. It encountered serious implementation issues. In March 1942, Noel Field reported that the USC was in negotiations with a soon to be retired Toulouse surgeon to take over his surgical clinic of twenty-four beds (which could feasibly be increased to forty to fifty beds), including 'four sisters [of Charity] in charge of ménage, kitchen, etc.'. According to Field's description, this clinic consisted of a complex of buildings round a very attractive courtyard, with 'fully equipped operating, dressing and X-ray rooms, an infirmary and everything that is required for an up-to-date surgical center'. Field conceived it as 'the surgical center for all the camps [that] will thus be Unitarian and our standing in the camps, and with both central and local authorities will be greatly increased'. He nevertheless admitted that it had to be 'reorganized as an inter-denominational enterprise, with the medical direction and services supplied purely by the Unitarians, the Catholics contributing to the rent, the Quakers providing for the kitchen, and the Jewish Children's Aid Society [OSE] taking care of unforeseen expenses'. He hoped that the Toulouse surgical clinic

188     *The long Second World War, 1931–1953*

would work in conjunction with the Récédébou internment camp (Portet-sur-Garonne, Haute-Garonne) and function as both 'a central hospital camp to which sick persons are being transferred from the other camps' and the place for the USC's 'project for fighting starvation'. Finally, Field was very confident that French authorities would approve his plans.[42] In the end, however, the Récédébou hospital camp project, like the nearby camp of Noé (Haute-Garonne), turned out to be an operation of the Vichy regime mostly guided by diplomacy and propaganda purposes instead of by humanitarian relief ones. Récédébou was closed at the beginning of October 1942, after almost all the Jews interned there, who represented half of its population, were deported to Auschwitz. Even though the other half – Spanish Republican refugees – benefited from healthcare in the USC's new surgical centre at Toulouse, this project seems to have been only partially realised.[43]

After the Normandy landings in the summer of 1944, the USC could count on the above-mentioned significant US federal National War Fund grant for implementing its humanitarian programmes in Europe. The USC further joined forces with the Joint Anti-Fascist Refugee Committee (hereafter JAFRC), with whom it had already collaborated since September 1941.[44] Formed by Lincoln Battalion veterans of the Spanish Civil War to provide aid to Spanish Loyalist refugees from Francoist Spain, the JAFRC was led by Edward Barsky (1895–1975), a New Yorker surgeon and political activist who had formerly been the Surgeon General of the International Brigades' medical service.[45] The JAFRC agreed to hand over to the USC the task of channelling all the funds collected in the US to those most in need, not least because it was not licensed to distribute these private funds in Europe.[46] Walter B. Cannon (1871–1945), the prestigious Harvard Medical School professor of physiology who had led in North America the humanitarian medical aid campaign in defence of Spanish democracy during the Civil War, accepted the honorary chairmanship of an appeal fund for the JAFRC's Boston chapter.[47]

The association between the USC and the JAFRC was decisive in setting up and further developing the Unitarian humanitarian activities in France, particularly the organisation and maintenance of the popularly known *Hôpital Varsovie*, based on its location on the *rue Varsovie* in Toulouse, following the failure of the so-called Operation Reconquest of Spain (*Operación Reconquista de*

*Unitarian Service Committee's activities*     189

*España*) in October 1944. This politico-military operation included an armed invasion of the Aran Valley with the aim of provoking in Spain a popular uprising against Franco's dictatorship. The *Operación* had been organised by the communist-oriented *Unión Nacional Española* and carried out by some thousands of exiled Spanish guerrilleros enlisted in the *Agrupación de Guerrilleros Españoles* (AGE) – a part of the FFI, the French resistance fighters in the later stages of the Second World War.[48]

Following the failure of the *Operación*, the FFI and the AGE outfitted an old chateau in a working-class quarter of Toulouse as a hospital to look after wounded and sick Spanish fighters.[49] Eventually, after their demobilisation at the beginning of the spring of 1945, it became a hospital for Spanish civilian refugees in need of healthcare. The Spanish Republican refugee Josep Torrubia (1885–1978), *médecin-commandant* of the French FFI Resistance, was its first director. He became the contact person with the USC in order to achieve support (money, clothes, medicine, medical instruments, and so on) for the new relief institution. Torrubia obtained, in particular, large quantities of penicillin, then a much appreciated 'magic bullet', to perform a series of clinical trials in the wards and its dispensary.[50] In October 1945, just after Cannon's death in Boston, the Hôpital Varsovie added to its name the designation of 'Walter B. Cannon Memorial' as a tribute to his leading role in promoting medical solidarity with the Spanish Republicans during the Civil War and its aftermath, the first years of exile.[51] This posthumous tribute to Cannon reveals a close collaboration between the USC and the JAFRC in this hospital project. This feature was recognised in the 1947 documentary *Spain in Exile*, which devoted two minutes to the Hôpital Varsovie. Both organisations were referred to in the credits of the documentary, and in some sequences devoted to the hospital their names are shown on a banner on the facade of the building.[52] It is interesting to note that the name of the female chief of surgery María Gómez Álvarez (1914–1965) was conveniently invisibilised and surreptitiously replaced by that of Josep Torrubia, the male director of the hospital, in order to reassure its audience.[53]

In February 1948, however, the USC withdrew its support to the hospital. This decision was in part driven by the political climate unleashed by the campaign of the House Committee on Un-American Activities (hereafter HUAC). The USC was in the eye of

190     *The long Second World War, 1931–1953*

the hurricane because of its collaboration with the JAFRC. Unitarian congregations, the American public and government stopped funding it and, as a result, it was forced to cut the number of its programmes in half.[54] Indeed, in the context of McCarthyism and according to the HUAC's demands, the JAFRC had been charged with contempt of US Congress: in June 1947, all the members of the JAFRC's board, including the chairman Edward Barsky, were convicted and, after three years of appeals, sentenced to prison.[55]

In July 1948, five months after the USC had withdrawn its support, the Hôpital Varsovie journal inserted in its first issue and on its first page a JAFRC statement which condemned these prison sentences and vindicated its relief work in favour of the Spanish refugees:

> For many years we have been in charge of providing aid: medical aid, food and clothing to those Spanish Republicans who fought against Franco. We have established a hospital in the south of France, the Varsovie Hospital in Toulouse, and another in Mexico, the Barsky Sanatorium.
>
> Thousands of men, women and children, who otherwise would have died, live today thanks to our work and our effort. Not one of the words uttered in the hundreds of pages of statements and accusations presented before the courts and before the "Anti-American" Committee come to change these facts. Not a single one of the accusations made against us, in the sense that we are not an aid agency for the aforementioned purposes, has been supported by facts.[56]

Despite the USC's insistence that the reference to the Cannon Memorial should be removed from the hospital's name, the JAFRC did not do so until January 1950.[57] By then, the followers of most orthodox Stalinist communism which condemned the independent policy of Yugoslavian communist prime minister Marshal Josip Tito had imposed their line on the leadership of the Varsovie Hospital. This feature implied the purge or discharge from it of a number of members of the Spanish Communist Party (PCE), especially from its Catalan counterpart (*Partit Socialista Unificat de Catalunya*, PSUC), who had been accused of being 'Titoits' and petty-bourgeois nationalists.[58]

Beyond the political tensions unleashed by the Cold War, the USC did not interrupt in 1948 its humanitarian aid to Republican

*Unitarian Service Committee's activities*     191

refugees in southern France, though its financial resources were certainly depleted as a result of McCarthyism. Actually, the USC had opened an office in Toulouse in January 1945. In July 1946, its delegate – the Californian Persis Miller (died 1970) – who had arrived there four months previously, opened in the village of Saint-Goin, near Pau, a shelter for children (*Maison d'Enfants*), which took in 369 Spanish children until its closure in 1952. In most cases, their fathers were dead, disabled or ill, and their destitute mothers were unable to care for and support them; a minority were orphans or abandoned children without families.[59] To run the house, Miller was assisted by Francisco Bosch (1902–1973), a Spanish refugee physician who was overseeing a convalescent home also set up by the USC at Meillon, close to Pau – a centre intended to house former FFI and *Guérilleros Espagnols*, including survivors of Nazi camps, who since 1936 had suffered long years of deprivation and calamity.[60] After 1948, Saint-Goin *Maison d'Enfants* remained open and supported by the USC. It was placed under the direction of the physician Antonio Piñar until its closure in 1952.[61] Providing children's education as well as improving their health, both physical and mental, was the first priority of this *maison d'enfants*. For this purpose, the *Colonia*, as the children used to call it, had a team of caretakers, all of them Spanish refugees, including several teachers, a nurse, two or three cooks, an administrator, a driver and cleaning staff.[62]

While the *Maison d'Enfants* was in operation, the USC office on *rue Homère* in Toulouse centralised applications to admit the children in most need, especially those living with tuberculosis patients, in order to strengthen their health with good nutrition, physical exercise and the fresh air of the Pyrenees. Even after the closure of Saint-Goin in 1952, Persis Miller continued to distribute, from the Toulouse USC office, clothes, food and financial aid to the most destitute Spanish families. When Persis Miller died in January 1970, Dolors Bellido took over the office, which closed its doors two years later.[63]

## Conclusion

Through a detailed study of the USC's humanitarian action in southern France during the Second World War and its aftermath,

192      *The long Second World War, 1931–1953*

this chapter has revealed that the boundary between medical relief activities with refugees fleeing from fascism in many European countries, including Spanish Republican exiles, and active political support to those refugees who chose to stand up to the aggressors became more and more blurred in the course of the war. This became particularly obvious from late 1942, when the Nazis occupied the whole of France and when the repression against the enemy of the regime intensified, leading to a growing number of refugees joining in the Resistance activities against the invader.

Though the UCS's model paralleled that of the American Friends Service Committee, its members did openly support the Allied cause, unlike the Friends who were committed to neutrality and pacifist principles. If the USC's relief activities in France during the Second World War focused on providing medical aid for the most disadvantaged refugees, with particular attention to those held in camps, or in transit to travel abroad, after the Liberation of France, the USC's aid gradually shifted towards Spanish refugees, who were definitely left in a no-man's land as the Allied victory did not impede the survival of Franco's dictatorship until his death in 1975. The ideology of 'religion of the future' held by the hegemonic Radical Unitarian tendency in the United States facilitated during the Second World War years the USC's alliances with socially progressive and left-wing relief organisations, including those linked to the international communist movement as a part of Popular Front coalitions. As a result of the Cold War politico-military confrontation dialectics between the two post-Second World War blocs, anti-communist crusades in the United States eventually found their way into the USC, where Socialist Unitarians and Free Unitarians made a common front against Radical Unitarians, who were sympathetic to the Soviet Union and the cause of international communism, or even members of the Communist Party.[64]

The humanitarian action of different individuals working in relief organisations has always been shaped by their differences from each other in terms of ideology and socio-political agenda. Those differences meant that their humanitarian ethos was guided by diverse values and emotions, as well as contextual circumstances. The cases of a good number of the USC's actors of relief operations in France during the Second World War and its aftermath, and remarkably most of their leaders – for example, Martha and Waitstill Sharp,

# Unitarian Service Committee's activities 193

Robert and Elisabeth Dexter, Noel and Herta Field, René Zimmer, Joseph Weill, Herta 'Jo' Tempi and even Persis Miller – are very illustrative of these changing humanitarian commitments. Their post-Second World War vicissitudes raise fascinating questions about their dilemmas and practical choices, overwhelmed as they were not only by the relentless paranoid 'logic' in the 1940s and 1950s, and the political loyalty conflicts they were compelled to confront, but also by the collaboration of most of them with one or more intelligence services of both blocs at once.[65]

In sum, the case of the USC's humanitarian action in Europe illustrates the extent to which political humanitarianism was transformed from a humanitarianism against fascism in Spain in the late 1930s to one against Nazism in France during Second World War, and finally to a humanitarianism faced with US anti-communism and Soviet Stalinism, either or both, during the early years of the Cold War.

## Notes

1  The research for this article was conducted for the project 'Transnational Humanitarian Medicine and Technological Innovation in Spaces of Confinement, 1870–1950 (TRANSHUMED)', funded by the Spanish State Agency for Research (AEI, PID2019-104581GB-I00).
On the USC's activities in France during the Second World War and the post-war years see, among others, Haim Genizi, 'Christian Charity: The Unitarian Service Committee's Relief Activities on Behalf of Refugees from Nazism, 1940–5', *Holocaust and Genocide Studies*, 2:2 (1987), 261–276; Susan Elisabeth Subak, *Rescue and Flight: American Relief Workers Who Defied the Nazis* (Lincoln, NE: University of Nebraska Press, 2010); Àlvar Martínez Vidal (ed.), *L'Hôpital Varsovie. Exil, médecine et résistance (1944–1950)* (Portet-sur-Garonne: Loubatières, 2011); Aurelio Velázquez-Hernández, 'The Unitarian's Service Committee Marseille Office and the American Networks to Aid Spanish Refugees (1940–1943)', *Culture and History: Digital Journal*, 8:2 (2019), e021, https://doi.org/10.3989/chdj.2019.021; Jon Arrizabalaga, 'La asistencia médica a los refugiados en Francia durante la Segunda Guerra Mundial: la Clínica de Marsella (1941–1945)', *Dynamis*, 40:1 (2020), 67–91, https://raco.cat/index.php/Dynamis/article/view/374648. The USC's archives (USCA) are digitalised and openly accessible online at the Harvard Divinity

194    *The long Second World War, 1931–1953*

School Library. Except for the USCA records most relevant to our purposes, of which a complete reference will be provided, the documents at the USC's archives resorted to in this chapter will be quoted in a simplified form.

2 Although the usual denomination at the time was that of 'concentration camps', French historiography distinguishes between 'internment camps' that were devoted to lodging refugees in better or worse conditions and the 'concentration camps' themselves, which were rather intended for forced labour and annihilation. See Denis Peschanski, *La France des camps. L'internement, 1938–1946* (Paris: Gallimard, 2002).

3 'Saving the Future in Europe: The First-Hand Story of the Unitarian Service Committee's Medical Work in Unoccupied France', Boston, USC, 1942 (Harvard Divinity School Library, USCA, bMS 16035/1 4 [ii]), p. [3].

4 See Isabelle Von Bueltzingsloewen (ed.), *'Morts d'inanition'. Famine et exclusions en France sous l'Occupation* (Rennes: Presses universitaires de Rennes, 2005); and particularly the chapter by Denis Peschanski, 'Morbidité et mortalité dans la France des camps' (pp. 201–212).

5 Subak, *Rescue and Flight*, p. 84. On the inconveniences faced in the migration work, see the 'Confidential Report of Members of the Unitarian Service Committee' signed in about the autumn of 1941 by the Unitarian minister Howard L. Brooks, after having been sent on a mission to France from May to August 1941. See USCA, bMS 16007/10(1), pp. 5–7; Subak, *Rescue and Flight*, pp. 103–107. One year after his mission, Brooks published *Prisoners of Hope: Report on a Mission* (New York: L.B. Fischer, 1942).

6 'Estimated Figures on Unitarian Service Committee Aid, 1943–1946', USCA bMS 16035/2(13).

7 Genizi, 'Christian Charity', p. 265.

8 On Robert Dexter's activities, see Subak, *Rescue and Flight*, pp. xvii, *passim*.

9 Paul Arrighi, *Silvio Trentin. Un Européen en résistance, 1919–1943* (Portet-sur-Garonne: Loubatières, 2007), pp. 182–193, 215–218.

10 Anna Seghers's roman *Transit* (Boston, MA: Little, Brown & Co., 1944) vividly reflects the atmosphere in these circumstances; and Rosemary Sullivan's study *Villa Air-Bel: World War II, Escape, and a House in Marseille* (New York: HarperCollins, 2006) portrays the daily life and vicissitudes of a group of writers and artists who took refuge in this chateau. On the residences and infirmaries (the 'château' of La Reynade and that of Montgrand) that the Mexican consulate in France maintained in the outskirts of Marseille for Spanish refugees, as well as

## Unitarian Service Committee's activities     195

the vicissitudes and setbacks they faced, see the memoirs of Pelai Vilar i Canales, a Catalan Republican doctor, *Memòries d'un metge català a la sanitat republicana* (Barcelona: Permanyer, 2019), p. 231 *et seq.*

11 Subak, *Rescue and Flight*, pp. 28–44.

12 Colin B. Burke, *Red Destinies: From Harvard Square to Stalin's and Mao's Dungeons and the Weathermen, Biographies of American Communists* (preview, 2023: https://userpages.umbc.edu/~burke/titleintro.pdf), Chapter I, pp. 11, *passim.*

13 Subak, *Rescue and Flight*, pp. 33, 84–86. Set up in November 1940, the 'Comité de Nîmes' (Nimes Committee, hereafter), coordinated the efforts of different relief and rescue organisations operating in the internment camps of Unoccupied France (1940–1942) in order to contribute more efficiently to the enormous humanitarian task they had to face. It gathered together about two dozen organisations of very different kinds offering help to refugees, either French or foreign, lay or confessional, ranging from the American Friends Service Committee (Quakers) and the Unitarian Service Committee (Unitarians) to the French Red Cross and the Catholic Church of France, to seven Jewish organisations, and the CIMADE (*Comité Inter Mouvements Auprès des Évacués*), a member of the *Fédération Protestante* of France. For Lowrie's own account of the Nimes Committee, see Donald A. Lowrie, *The Hunted Children* (New York: W.W. Norton & Co., 1963), pp. 82–95.

14 Apparently, by mid-January 1941 Joy was already the USC's 'European director' and Field, the USC's 'director' in France since both of them collaborated with each other under such responsibilities along with someone called 'Madeleine' in a 'Report on the Situation of Spanish Refugees in France' that was signed by a 'Mr Llanos' in Lisbon on 14 January 1941: USCA, bMS 16031/2 (1–2), pp. 5–6. A Spanish refugee with a Cuban passport, since November 1941 Professor Llanos was paid by the JAFRC to work for the Marseille USC office as part of the discreet agreement between both agencies for relief actions concerning the Spanish refugees in France. See Velázquez-Hernández, 'The Unitarian's Service Committee Marseille Office', pp. 6–7.

15 'Saving the Future in Europe', p. [4]. Coordinated actions between the USC and the Joint Commission of the International Red Cross are also reflected in the *Report of the Joint Relief Commission*, pp. 199–200. Examples of coordinated actions between the USC and the American Quakers or, on three sides, with the Joint Relief Commission of the IRC, can be found in American Friends Service Committee, *Records Relating to Humanitarian Work in France, 1933–1950.* Series VIII, Marseille Office, Correspondence Box 52–56, Folders 40 and 41.

196 *The long Second World War, 1931–1953*

16 Noel Field, 'Notes on Visit to Unitarian Dispensary Marseille (May 6th 1942)', USCA bMS 347/49(5), p. 3. For more instances of similar collaborations, see USCA bMS 347/49(1) [September 1941]; and bMS 347/49(4).

17 On Joseph Weill and his concern for diseases associated with hunger in the internment camps in the south of France, see Avi Ohry and Esteban González-López, 'Hunger Disease in Southern France Internment Camps during World War II: The Pioneering Studies of Dr. Joseph Weill', *The Israel Medical Association Journal (IMAJ)*, 24 (2022), 429–432.

18 USCA, bMS 16024/4(11) [5 April 1941], p. 2.

19 Work on the Marseille Clinic has been scarce, and attention to this institution has been limited to forays into studies on the activities of the OSE and the USC in Marseille. See, e.g., Sabine Zeitoun, *Histoire de l'O.S.E. De la Russie tsariste à l'Occupation en France (1912–1944). L'oeuvre de secours aux enfants, du légalisme à la résistance* (Paris: L'Harmattan; 2012), pp. 239–246; Renée Dray-Bensousan, 'Filières juives d'assistance à Marseille: les exemples de l'ORT et de l'OSE', in Jean-Marie Guillon and Robert Mencherini (eds), *La Résistance et les Européens du Sud* (Paris: L'Harmattan; 1999), pp. 143–152. For recent works paying more attention to the topic, see Subak, *Rescue and Flight*, p. 26, *passim*; Velázquez-Hernández, 'The Unitarian's Service Committee Marseille Office', pp. 4–5, *passim*; Arrizabalaga, 'La asistencia médica a los refugiados'.

20 'Saving the Future in Europe', p. [4]; *Report of the Joint Relief Commission*, 1948, pp. 199–200, 204–205, 223–224.

21 A substantial number of the refugees interned in these different spaces were Spanish Republican exiles. The absence in the documentation consulted to date of further specification on the patients treated at the Clinic and its satellite centres between July 1941 and November 1942 prevents us from establishing a percentage distribution of consultations among the different groups of refugees. For the internment camps in France (metropolitan and colonial), see Peschanski, *La France des camps*; Anne Grynberg, *Les camps de la honte. Les internés juifs des camps français, 1939–1944* (Paris: La Découverte; 1999); Anne Boitel, 'Des camps de réfugiés aux centres de rétention administrative: la Cimade, analyse d'une action dans les lieux d'enfermement et de relégation (de la fin des années 1930 au début du XXIème siècle)' (PhD dissertation, Université d'Aix-Marseille, 2016); Andrée Bachoud and Bernard Sicot, *Sables d'exil. Les républicains espagnols dans les camps d'internement au Maghreb (1939–1945)* (Perpignan: Mare Nostrum, 2009); Grégory Tuban, *Camps*

## Unitarian Service Committee's activities 197

*d'étrangers. Le contrôle des réfugiés venus d'Espagne (1939–1944)* (Paris: Nouveau Monde Éditions, 2018).

22 USCA, bMS 16024/4(11) [5 April 1941], pp. 1–2.

23 'Saving the Future in Europe'. Noel Field's initials ('N.H.F.') and date of production ('May 1942') are listed at the end of the part written by him (pp. [3–19]), while the names of the remaining authors, all of whom were staff of the Marseille Clinic, are listed in the preface by Robert C. Dexter as the executive director of the USC (p. [2]).

24 'Saving the Future in Europe', p. [3].

25 USCA, bMS 16024/4(11) [5 April 1941], p. 2.

26 Arrizabalaga, 'La asistencia médica a los refugiados', pp. 72–86.

27 *Ibid.*, pp. 76–77.

28 'Report of Our Activities during the German Occupation of Marseilles (1942–1944)', Centre Médico-Social – Unitarian Service Committee, Marseille, *c.* November 1944 (Harvard Divinity School Library, USCA, bMS 16035/1 4 [i]), pp. 3–4. Since the devastating fire in a department store in Marseille in 1938, and throughout the Second World War, there were no mayors in Marseille, but 'administrators' under trusteeship. Louis Barraud was presumably the municipal 'administrateur' when the UCS's activities had to go underground.

29 'Report of Our Activities', pp. 3–5. This report, apparently sent from Lisbon to the USC headquarters in Boston, describes the forcedly clandestine activities of the Marseille Clinic during the nearly two years of German occupation (November 1942 to August 1944) and the first four months after liberation. Although unsigned, its writing is attributed to René Zimmer and is dated towards the end of 1944.

30 To know more precisely how Red Cross actors viewed the USC's partisan humanitarianism would require systematic research in the ICRC and the League archives, which is beyond the scope of this chapter. Yet, the ICRC and the League apparently continued to cooperate with the USC. We tend to think that the USC's collaboration with other relief agencies and the power of persuasion developed by Noel Field from Geneva itself, along with the increasingly dramatic circumstances, could have helped to maintain this cooperation even after the Nazi occupation of the whole of France.

31 *Report of the Joint Relief Commission*, 1948, p. 204. American Friends Service Committee Archives, 1933–1950, folder 40, pp. 3–4, 6, 7, 8, 9, 10; folder 41, pp. 46–47, 51.

32 'Report of Our Activities', p. 8. It should be stressed that the *Ordre des Médecins* was in general very pro-Vichy. Thus, their recommending a physician for this underground dispensary on an unspecified date soon after the Nazis had occupied Marseille might have meant a change

198 *The long Second World War, 1931–1953*

of attitude at the local level, though he was a 'French and Christian physician of Marseilles', as Zimmer pointed out in his report of November 1944. On this issue, see Julie Fette, *Exclusions: Practicing Prejudice in French Law and Medicine, 1920–1945* (Ithaca, NY and London: Cornell University Press, 2012), pp. 162–202.

33 'Report of Our Activities', pp. 8–10.

34 'Report of Our Activities', p. 10.

35 'Report of Our Activities', p. 11.

36 'Report of Our Activities', p. 11.

37 On the relevant humanitarian relief work of the Mexican Consulate in Marseille between 1939 and 1944, see Gérard Malgat, *Gilberto Bosques. La diplomatie au service de la liberté. Paris-Marseille (1939–1942)* (Marseille: L'Atinoir; 2013). Leaning on new sources so far unknown, the role of Gilberto Bosques and the Mexican consulate at Marseille has been revisited by Daniela Gleizer, 'Gilberto Bosques y el consulado de México en Marsella (1940–1942). La burocracia en tiempos de guerra', *Estudios en Historia Moderna y Contemporánea de México*, 49 (2015), 54–76.

38 'Report of Our Activities', pp. 12–13.

39 'Report of Our Activities', p. 13.

40 'Report of Our Activities', p. 14.

41 Genizi, 'Christian Charity', pp. 271–273. Significantly, the USC devoted 2,500 dollars to the University of Minnesota Starvation Project, a clinical trial in which states of malnutrition then suffered by many people in Europe were experimentally reproduced in voluntary healthy individuals.

42 Noel Field, 'Report ... on work in France' (6 March 1942): USCA bMS 347/49 (4), pp. 5–6.

43 The Noé camp was first opened for two years (1941–1943) as a pseudo-hospital camp, then as a conventional internment camp until its Liberation on 19 August 1944, and finally as the antechamber of courts charged with judging collaborationist acts until its definitive closure in 1947. Éric Malo, 'De Vichy à la Quatrième République: le camp de Noé (1943–1945)', *Annales du Midi: revue archéologique, historique et philologique de la France méridionale*, 104:199–200 (1992), 441–458; Peschanski, *La France des camps*, pp. 104, 119, 238–240, 366–367. See also USCA bMS 16181/2 (4), Toulouse Clinic pictures: W454951, W454955, W454956.

44 Velázquez-Hernández, 'The Unitarian's Service Committee Marseille Office', pp. 5–7.

45 On the JAFRC, see Sebastiaan Faber, 'Image Politics: U.S. Aid to the Spanish Republic and Its Refugees', *Revista Forma*, 14 (2016),

## Unitarian Service Committee's activities 199

21–34. On Edward Barsky, see SIDBRINT (https://sidbrint.ub.edu/ca/content/barsky-edward-k).

46 Faber, 'Image Politics'.

47 Elin L. Wolfe, A. Clifford Barger and Saul Benison, *Walter B. Cannon: Science and Society* (Cambridge, MA: Harvard University Press, 2000), pp. 516–517; Jon Arrizabalaga and Àlvar Martínez-Vidal, 'Medicine, Religion, and the Humanitarian Ethos: Walter B. Cannon, Unitarianism, and the Care of Spanish Republican Refugees in France Cannon', *Journal of the History of Medicine and Allied Sciences*, 77:2 (2022), 158–185, https://doi.org/10.1093/jhmas/jrac002.

48 Jordi Guixé i Coromines, 'Solidarité humaine et résistance politique sous contrôle policier: l'Hospital Varsovia dans le cadre de la Guerre Froide (1944–1950)', in Àlvar Martínez Vidal (ed.), *L'Hôpital Varsovie. Exil, médecine et résistance (1944–1950)* (Portet-sur-Garonne: Loubatières, 2011), pp. 57–79.

49 We know that this was not the only convalescence centre for Spanish resistance fighters after Operation Reconquista. There were others, founded and supported by the USC, in various locations of southern France, but they were soon closed; one of them was in Lourdes. See Rosa Toran and Àlvar Martínez-Vidal, *El metge Josep Torrubia Zea. Lliurepensador, maçó i socialista* (València: Afers, 2021), pp. 251–252.

50 Àlvar Martínez-Vidal and Xavier García-Ferrandis, 'Las secuelas patológicas de los campos de concentración entre los refugiados españoles en Francia', *Dynamis*, 40:1 (2020), 93–123, https://raco.cat/index.php/Dynamis/article/view/374652.

51 Arrizabalaga and Martínez-Vidal, 'Medicine, Religion, and the Humanitarian Ethos'.

52 Àlvar Martínez-Vidal and Antoni Adam-Donat, '*Spain in Exile*: l'Hospital Varsovia mis en scène', in *L'Hôpital Varsovie. Exil, médecine et résistance*, pp. 91–98. See also Carolina Fenoll Espinosa, *Spain in Exile (Guillermo Zúñiga, 1947): una película recuperada del cine de propaganda antifascista* (Madrid: Universidad Complutense de Madrid, Trabajo Fin de Máster, 2014).

53 Àlvar Martínez-Vidal, 'The Powers of Masculinization in Humanitarian Storytelling: The Case of the Surgeon María Gómez Álvarez in the Varsovia Hospital (Toulouse, 1944–1950)', *Medicine, Conflict and Survival*, 36 (2020), 103–121, https://doi.org/10.1080/13623699.2019.1710902.

54 Faber, 'Image Politics'.

55 On the imprisonment of Barsky and other members of the JAFRC board in 1950, see Faber, 'Image Politics'. On political repression

## 200 *The long Second World War, 1931–1953*

against physicians during the Cold War Era, see Merlin Chowkwanyun, ' "The Neurosis That Has Possessed Us": Political Repression in the Cold War Medical Profession', *Journal of the History of Medicine and Allied Sciences*, 73:3 (2018), 255–273.

56 'Nuestra protesta', *Anales del Hospital Varsovia – Walter B. Cannon Memorial*, 1, 1948, p. 1 (my translation from Spanish).

57 The *Anales del Hospital Varsovia*, its quarterly hospital journal, only failed to include 'Walter B. Cannon Memorial' in its title from its seventh issue (first term 1950). Arthur Schlesinger, Cannon's son-in-law since 1940, claimed –without hiding his antipathy towards communists– that the name of Cannon had been instrumentalised 'purely to raise funds in the United States'. Moreover, he stated that 'Socialist and trade union sources among Toulouse refugees [had] testified that the Varsovie Hospital was Communist-controlled and discriminated against non-Communists as both doctors and patients.' See Arthur Meier Schlesinger, *A Life in the Twentieth Century: Innocent Beginnings, 1917–1950* (Boston, MA: Houghton Mifflin, 2000), p. 403.

58 Jordi Guixé Coromines, *La República perseguida. Exilio y represión en la Francia de Franco, 1937–1951* (Valencia: Publicacions de la Universitat de València, 2012), pp. 403–405. Toran and Martínez-Vidal, *El metge Josep Torrubia Zea*, pp. 233–238 (the so-called 'Afer Comorera'). For the evidence of the expulsion from the PCE of the Varsovie Hospital doctor Josep Torrubia and pharmacist Pau Cirera, accused of being Titoists, see Archives Départementales de la Haute-Garonne (ADHG, Toulouse), 2042W 292, dossier nº 1, chemise 5. The headings of the confidential report (*Renseignements*), dated 4 February 1950 and numbered 955, are as follows: 'OBJET: A/S de la mission officielle qu'avait confié le Comité Central du P.C.E. du Colonel Fernando Claudin: Constater les effets du "Titisme" dans la région toulousaine et prendre les mesures nécessaires pour les combattre. SOURCE: Correspondant du service. VALEUR: sérieuse'.

59 Annette Mülberger, ' "Ells necessiten ser tractats psicoterapèuticament": l'impacte psicològic de la guerra entre els infants espanyols acollits a França', in Roger Barrié, Martine Camiade and Jordi Font (eds), *Actes du 2d Séminaire Transfrontalier. Déplacements forcés et exils au XXe siècle – Le corps et l'esprit* (Perpignan: Talaia, 2013); Annette Mülberger, 'Ciencia y política en tiempos de guerra fría: un examen psicológico de niños españoles en el exilio', *Universitas Psycologica*, 13:5 (2014), 1941–1953. See also Pierre Ferrer, *La colonia de l'Unitarian Service Committee à Saint Goin* (Toulouse: Messages SAS, 2021).

# Unitarian Service Committee's activities    201

60 Guixé i Coromines, 'Solidarité humaine', pp. 57–79, in the context of the huge population movements that took place on European soil after the end of hostilities in 1945, the French Ministry of Prisoners, Deportees and Refugees took a series of measures between mid-May and mid-June 1945 regarding the humanitarian treatment to be given to the Spanish Republican deportees who had survived the Nazi camps. The main measure was the creation of the *Villa Don Quichotte*, in the former Récébédou Camp (Portet-sur-Garonne) near Toulouse, to house those deportees who had no family or friends to take them into their homes. The French authorities were aware that their return to Spain was impossible due to the reprisals awaiting them from Franco's regime. See Joan M. Calvo Gascón and Rosa Toran Belver, 'Quan s'obriren les portes dels camps. La nova odissea dels republicans deportats. Una història singular', *Mayurqa*, 5 (2023), https://doi.org/10.22307/2386.7124.2023.01.004

61 Mülberger, 'Ciencia y política en tiempos de guerra fría', pp. 1945–1946.

62 Ferrer, *La colonia de l'Unitarian Service Committee*, pp. 25–28.

63 *Ibid.*, p. 37. Dolors Bellido, Persis Miller's assistant, was a daughter of the exiled Catalan physician Jesús M. Bellido, former professor of pharmacology at the University of Barcelona and close friend of Walter Cannon. Just before the end of the Civil War, Bellido has been designed the Minister of [religious] Cults by the Republican prime minister Negrín. For a contextualisation of the aid to Spanish refugees in Toulouse during the middle decades of the twentieth century, see Alicia Alted, 'La ayuda asistencial española y franco-española a los refugiados', in Alicia Alted and Lucienne Domergue (eds), *El exilio republicano español en Toulouse, 1939–1999* (Madrid: UNED Ediciones – Presses Universitaires du Mirail, 1999), pp. 73–90.

64 Burke, *Red Destinies*, Chapter 3, p. 39; and Chapter 18, p. 22.

65 On this issue, see Subak, *Rescue and Flight*, pp. 217–238; and Burke, *Red Destinies, passim.*

# 8

# Cultural actors in rehabilitation: Second World War craft therapy and white, ableist, heteronormative masculinity

*Jennifer Way*

When the US entered the Second World War in December 1941, the American Red Cross (ARC) expanded its purview from attending to refugees and the war wounded in Europe to include caring for American and Allied troops, too. Concurrently, the ARC led efforts to alert civilians in the US to the needs of American troops.[1] As part of their work to reduce ill and wounded troops' suffering and aid in their healing and wellness, in military hospitals abroad and at home the ARC facilitated what doctors prescribed as craft therapy—"healing by directed activity," for which ARC nurses and volunteers guided patients in making craft objects.[2]

The practice of craft therapy diverted the attention of the convalescing war wounded so that instead of dwelling on their pain, they turned their minds to enjoyable tasks such as bookbinding, leather work, metal work, needlecraft, pottery, puppetry, reed work, textiles, weaving, woodwork, and minor crafts—braiding and weaving mats, crocheting, finger painting, hooking rugs, knitting, knotting, and more.[3] Importantly, in addition to providing diversion, crafting served as a curative therapy. As they handled and shaped leather, metal, fiber, clay, wood, and paper, these troops and veterans became accustomed to their new amputation stumps and in some cases their new prosthetic limbs, finetuned the coordination of their minds and bodies, and built mental and physical stamina.[4] Craft therapy accommodated a wide range of abilities as well as diversity in locations of care ranging from mobile tent hospitals and hospitals in repurposed and more permanent facilities abroad to fixed hospitals and medical campuses in the US.

## Cultural actors in rehabilitation 203

Although widespread during the war, craft therapy remains understudied in its historical frameworks of war and caregiving.[5] This chapter contributes to a better understanding of craft therapy by highlighting its expansion from its primary deployment in military medical settings to civilian medical and especially non-medical places, a development that occurred in the US during the Second World War and the years immediately following, and that the ARC originated. As they had done during the First World War, ARC nurses and aids continued to teach rehabilitating patients how to make craft objects while observing their mastery of fabrication techniques as a sign of their progress in healing. New, however, was that the ARC oversaw a craft-focused program that brought civilian craftsmen into craft therapy to work with patients and train nurses along with new ARC volunteer craft aids who would also work with patients directly. In 1942, renowned American textile artist Dorothy Liebes originated the ARC's new Arts and Skills program and, serving as its National Art Director, she launched its first efforts in New York, Chicago, and San Francisco.[6] 1943 saw the Arts and Skills program develop as a unit of the Hospital and Recreation Corps in army, navy, and air force hospitals and gradually expand into private hospitals and the homes of invalids.[7] Little known is that in addition to individual craftsmen, the Arts and Skills program was working with cultural actors, and some quickly developed their own programs. To get a sense of these developments, this chapter samples craft therapy-related activity and materials from the American Craftsmen's Cooperative Council (ACCC), a non-governmental, national affiliation of craftsmen and their advocates,[8] American art world journals such as *Design* and the ACCC's *Craft Horizons*, the Metropolitan Museum of Art (Met), the ACCC's Education Council's School for the American Craftsmen (SAC), and the Museum of Modern Art (MoMA) and its War Veterans Art Center (WAC).

Previously, these organizations, media platforms, institutions, and programs in the visual and material arts were not involved with caregiving. Yet, during and after the war they brought to troops and veterans who were recuperating in the US new opportunities to participate in craft therapy. Despite their different approaches, collectively, they aimed to reduce troops' and veterans' suffering,

204    *The long Second World War, 1931–1953*

improve their mental and physical abilities, and enhance the quality of their lives. To this end, they practiced humanitarian agency, that is, an ability to think and act with authority and legitimacy on behalf of rehabilitating patients and civilians, for the good of "broad collective purposes."[9] For example, the leaders of museums that hosted craft therapy programs contemplated the role of the museum as a contemporary social institution that must address broad civilian needs for wellness during and after the war. Frances Henry Taylor, Director of the Met, claimed the world was "tottering on the brink of a new 'world order'" and he held up museums as one of the "arsenals for intellectual and moral rearmament" from which "spiritual regeneration" would spring from "the hard thinking of carefully cultivated minds."[10] Psychologist Dr. Edward Liss, advising MoMA, wrote in that museum's bulletin: "We are now faced with the problem of a sick world and increased responsibilities to our armed forces and civilians who are striving to bring about a betterment in man's lot."[11] Liss recommended that art museums "prepare ... the sick and ailing for the art of living when they become well again."[12]

Although cultural actors professed a concern for "spiritual regeneration" and spoke about bettering "man's lot," as they facilitated the flow of information about and the practice of craft therapy from military hospitals into civilian American life via art magazines, museums, and educational programs, they represented and played a part in privileging white, ableist, heterosexual masculinity, as the military did, along with its tendency to discriminate against Black troops and veterans. The situation alerts us to notice that while cultural actors promoted craft therapy and the visual arts to heal military and civilian Americans, nevertheless, their humanitarian efforts also participated in the "construction of identities [that were] central to the creation and perpetuation of divisions of difference and inequality in society."[13]

Until recently, research on craft therapy mainly emerged from the social sciences, tended to be published in medical and therapy journals, and addressed the professional concerns of craft and other types of therapy providers.[14] However, a growing number of humanities scholars are exploring craft therapy's historical contexts and cultural and social significance. This chapter builds on the work of Tara Tappert, whose broad chronology of American troops

*Cultural actors in rehabilitation* 205

and veterans working with craft for purposes of healing across the twentieth and twenty-first centuries provides a crucial touchstone for researching developments that emerged during a more limited set of years, such as the Second World War era.[15] Equally foundational are the many publications of Ana Carden-Coyne. Along with studying the cultural and social significance of war wounds,[16] Carden-Coyne has examined the somatic element of injured troops and veterans responding to craft therapy with creativity and resilience at MoMA's WVAC during the Second World War.[17] This chapter applies her approach to studying craft therapy discursively by being mindful of its interconnecting military, medical, social, and cultural contexts as it analyzes the messages and meanings of cultural actors' engagements with craft therapy.

The discussion here is guided also by the work of Sebastien Farré, Jean-François Fayet, and Bertrand Taithe on humanitarian exhibitions, in particular, their examinations of the ways in which "images, photographs, semiotics, [and] narratives" reflect the social values and priorities of modern humanitarian organisations.[18] Building from their work on cultural representations of humanitarian ideas and aspirations,[19] this chapter examines American Second World War–era craft therapy photographs, texts, and programs. It shows that, beginning with the ARC Arts and Skills program, cultural actors extended craft therapy from the military into civilian places and populations. Importantly, an analysis of this material suggests that through craft therapy, cultural actors troubled if not contradicted their humanitarian intentions to serve the needs of the war wounded and improve conditions for human thriving by promoting concern and support for humankind while maintaining anti-Black racism and privileging the needs of white men.

As Katherine Ott notes, "human relationships are established and mediated through ... objects" and images.[20] Interestingly, relevant images of making craft objects for this chapter depart from an iconic trope of wartime humanitarian outreach—"the suffering victim and the heroic aid worker"—that Wendy Asquith notes has persisted in the propaganda of humanitarianism since the First World War.[21] Instead, what comes to the fore are images of white convalescing men demonstrating their ableness by making something without appearing to suffer from their illnesses and impairments. What is more, rather than victim status, the visual prominence

## 206 The long Second World War, 1931–1953

that cultural actors and craft therapy gave these men reaffirmed their white privilege—"the series of advantages that come to white Americans in their daily lives because, typically, they have been free of the labeling, stereotyping, and discrimination, past and present, that people of color experience"[22]—and iterated anti-Black racism by absenting Black men and marginalizing their presence in inter-racial scenes of care. This visual practice associated convalescing white male troops and veterans with power and prominence over white female nurses and craft therapy aids and Black servicemen. At the same time, a pattern of depicting pairs of white men and women promoted heteronormativity.

Scholarship on gender, race, and the military undergirds this chapter's analysis of the mid-twentieth-century material, in particular, Stephanie Szitanyi's work on the American military as a "gendered and gendering institution."[23] According to Szitanyi, the American military "favor[s] men of the dominant race, ethnicity, and sexuality" and privileges "male dominance, a masculinist culture, and homosociality," or bonds between men that enhance their collective power yet constitute not homosexuality but heterosexuality as a set of "social and cultural norms associated with gender."[24] The scholarship of Donna B. Knaff, Sara Perry Myers, Christina Jarvis and others respectively shows that during the Second World War— as servicemen were injured and unable to continue in their military roles, and women took on jobs that during peacetime had been the reserve of men, entered the armed forces, albeit in female-segregated branches of service, and even wore uniforms to serve as craft therapy aids—images published in U.S. government and military authored posters and pamphlets and in business advertisements helped to "restore masculine power and normalcy within society" and per-petuate it.[25] Importantly, cultural actors participated in this devel-opment by conveying the predominance of white masculine power and heteronormativity to American civilians through craft therapy images and activities.[26] Intersecting this research is scholarship that excavates race-based social inequities in Second World War–era healthcare and anti-Black racism in the military.[27] It corroborates this chapter's understanding that cultural actors' craft therapy rein-forced the lion's "share of power and prestige [for] those who could claim status as white"[28] and male while at the same time it neglected, if not failed, to depict caregiving for Black troops and veterans.

# Cultural actors in rehabilitation

207

## Ward work: American Red Cross Arts and Skills and *Design* and *Craft Horizons*

By early 1943, the ARC's Arts and Skills program had launched in the New York City area. MoMA and the Brooklyn Museum of Art selected "head craftsmen" or highly qualified craftsmen from the region, who then interviewed and selected volunteer craftsmen, overseeing their work at specific hospitals. They worked with patients and they trained nurses as aids to work with patients, too.[29] To support the new program, *Design* magazine and *Craft Horizons* magazine urged craftsmen to turn their skills from "the arts of peace to those of war"[30] and aid the Surgeon General by augmenting the work of occupational therapists.[31] To expedite the volunteer process, *Craft Horizons* published a questionnaire asking craftsmen to identify the crafts they could teach to troops and veterans who were recuperating in military hospitals.[32]

In these magazines as well as military publications, occupational therapy textbooks, and sociology literature, image and text representations of craft therapy emphasized not the craft therapy aids but their support of, if not subservience to, their white convalescing male patients located on wards, in hospital workshops, and outside, on hospital grounds. Pictorially, these publications treated the patients as "the dominant race, ethnicity, and sexuality"[33] by pairing them with white female craft aids and nurses in ways that allude to heterosexual relationships. This occurred, for example, through the spatial proximity, the physical nearness, of the women to the male patients, the often attractive youthfulness of the women and, despite their status as recuperative, the men, too, along with intimations of conviviality if not intimacy. Women's hands appear near to or touching the men's, or their heads bend together (see Figure 8.1). Group pictures show young women paired with a young man. The heterosexual tone of these images is heightened by the absence of all-male groups or much older aids and nurses with younger or middle-aged male patients or female patients. Additionally, the dominance of the men comes to the fore in these heterosexual contexts. Visually, pictorially, men predominate by appearing in the center of compositions with women placed to the side, and the men take up more pictorial space than the women or they appear larger, or they may act or interact as a female nurse or aid stands or sits still. These

# CRAFTSMEN and THE WAR

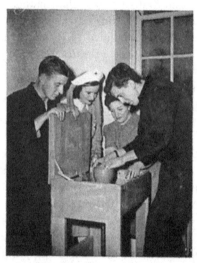

actual work being done by the craftsmen in pitals is under Miss LeMaire's committee. ticle is written work is only being done in h three areas. New York (at the Brooklyn N St. Albans, Halloran, and Fort Jay Hospi cago, and San Francisco. An Advisory C under the Chairmanship of Mr. James Sc Museum of Modern Art, acts as a clearing all applicants in the New York area. In ad Committee advises on matters of policy, d organization. In Chicago the work is bein close collaboration with the Art Institute a lieve this is also the case in San Francisco such advisory committees it is hoped that ard of the work done will be high and add tural education of the men as well as recreation.

All teachers are volunteers, donating thei and already skilled craftsmen. Materials plied by the Red Cross. Each craft being t a head craftsman in each hospital who is r for the technical excellence of their wo who sees they are prompt and regular in tendance. These head craftsmen are in tur responsible to Miss LeMaire's Committ craft is taught at least three days a week probably be taught five days a week sh volunteers give at least a full day a we work. Textiles, which includes rugs, woo weaving, embroidery; ceramics; woodworki working, and leather work are the crafts ta other specialties, such as fly-tying or c

A member of the volunteer potters groups supervises the throwing of a bowl by one of the patients at Halloran Hospital, while a Red Cross Gray Lady and another wounded man look on.

Figure 8.1 "Craftsmen and the War," *Craft Horizons* 2:2 (May 1943), p. 12 (American Craft Council)

visual strategies of organizing subjects in photographs connote male emphasis and importance supported by female assistance.

Rather than zero in on the men's distress and need for help with sitting, eating, and walking, pictures of craft therapy focused attention on their ability to learn and practice new ways to make something with materials and tools while they rehabilitated from broken limbs and mental injuries. Their ability to rise above their pain to make craft objects suggested strength, if not stoicism, and helped to counteract anxieties about craft's associations with femininity and the feminine as the weaker sex and the possibility that working with craft would effeminize men.[34]

Visual references to heterosexuality buttressed these inferences. In *Craft Horizons*, putting aside the two male patients' bedclothes

## Cultural actors in rehabilitation 209

and the two women's aid uniforms, the lighthearted interaction between tall young white men and smaller white women, with all of their heads bent close to examine something of interest, suggests a group of young people enjoying a double date.[35] It signifies servicemen not lost to their injuries or effeminized by craft but demonstrating a mastery of pottery and enjoying the moment with attractive female caregivers, an act that dovetailed with wartime messaging to male troops that women were worth fighting for and coming home to.[36] Thus, besides contributing to "the task of restoring injured servicemen to their 'proper place' in society through work" by way of showing a convalescing war patient making pottery,[37] the image in *Craft Horizons* augurs a return to normality in social relationships as an element of the men's progress in their rehabilitation. It does so through a display of their virility, based on having the strength to stand and work at a potter's wheel and the energy for socializing with the opposite sex. This display may have put to rest fears that residual impairments would prevent rehabilitating men from performing sexually, a topic of great concern to servicemen.[38] Furthermore, it would have allayed what Jarvis explains is the male wounded body's potential to pose threats "to America's post-war strength and return to normalcy."[39]

At the same time, women's visibility in the war economy and armed forces troubled the American military and citizens on matters of their femininity—was civilian work and military service masculinizing women?[40] If yes, would their masculinization lead women to lesbianism and correspondingly destabilize the heterosexually based family as the bedrock of American society?[41] Adding to these challenges to masculine and feminine social roles, scholars tell us that the identity of the military as uniformly heterosexual was a fiction, as the gender identity of its troops and personnel was "never stable and always relational."[42] The realization brings into view "the ever-present possibility of military transformations and the inherent instability within militaries' gendered cultures and structures"[43] that could tip into civilian life.[44] Consequently, a military wanting to maintain the profile of its rank and file as strong, capable, and combat-ready likely would need to reassert this idea of masculinity, perhaps all the more in situations where men were not physiologically, psychologically, or emotionally strong.

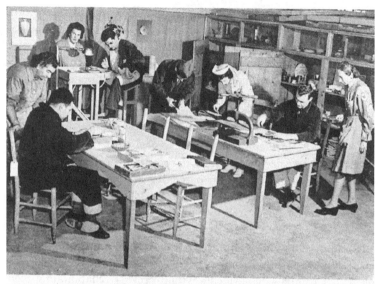

**Figure 8.2** Mildred G. Burrage, "Craftsmen Can Help: An Account of the Arts and Skills Unit of the New York Chapter of the American Red Cross at Halloran Hospital," *Craft Horizons*, 3:6 (August 1944), p. 18 (American Craft Council)

Published images of craft therapy accommodated these needs by pairing white male patients and white female craft aids as dominant and supporting, respectively (Figures 8.1, 8.2). Male–female pairs appear in the War Department's publications, too. In its *Technical Manual for Occupational Therapy*, 1944 (Figure 8.3) a young white female craft aid stands at the bedside of a young white male veteran recuperating from a severe leg injury. It's not simply their youthfulness or good looks or that they both gaze at his craft work that connects them. The center of the picture features one of her well-manicured fingers touching one of his fingers as she helps him securely hold the belt he is knotting. This gesture subtly suggests a heterosexual connection, accentuated by the ring on his left hand, which may underscore a marital commitment and signal his faithfulness even as he interacts closely with a female aid. This goes beyond the dry tone of a manual providing technical information

Cultural actors in rehabilitation 211

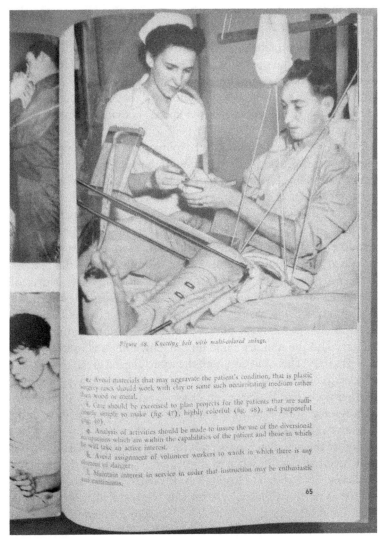

Figure 8.3 War Department, *Technical Manual for Occupational Therapy*, TM-8291 (Washington, DC: U.S. Government Printing Office, 1944), p. 65 (U.S. Government)

212     *The long Second World War, 1931–1953*

about therapy. In the same publication, another example shows a young female aid smiling as she stands close behind and watches a man with a prosthetic leg working with a floor loom.[45] As a reminder of the hierarchy of gender in heterosexual relationships, in these and other examples women stand close to the side of or behind men. They watch and sometimes they help, but they do not obscure visual access to the men's activity or monopolize their space.

Still, *Craft Horizons* cautioned potential craft volunteers that many of the war wounded struggled: "If the opportunity arises, consider the teaching of crafts to a wounded man as the rope thrown to help him climb out of the pit, a pit which will often be full of mental as well as physical pain."[46] The metaphor of a veteran "climbing out of his pit" of pain and injury mystified the multiple staff and resources that in actuality his rehabilitation required, as did mainstream rehabilitation literature. Despite urging that "the veteran problem is one of the most important—if not the most critical of our time," in *The Veteran Comes Back*, 1944, sociologist Willard Waller omitted discussing how veterans' service experiences differed in significant ways due to race-based discrimination in the military and the military's inability or unwillingness to keep Black troops safe.[47] This omission is all the more glaring given that Waller alluded to unresolved racial conflict in the US but did not elaborate. Furthermore, like Waller, often other social scientists studying veteran reintegration remained silent about the impact of racism on veterans' rehabilitation.[48]

Before the war, Black-only craft therapy appeared in a context of pride and racial uplift when examples from patients at the all-Black Tuskegee US Veterans Hospital in Tuskegee, Alabama, were displayed as part of Chicago's 'American Negro Exposition' of 1940, and the Black press, such as *The Chicago Defender*, published some of the photographs (Figure 8.4).[49] Yet, scholars recognize that historically, the character of the US military was a "most foundational, ubiquitous, institutionalized, and consequential racist division split [of] 'colored' from white—or, in today's terms, black from white."[50] During the Second World War, Black men comprised around 11 percent of troops,[51] and all branches of the military remained segregated until President Harry S. Truman signed Executive Order 9981 in 1948. Military healthcare was segregated,

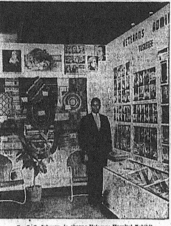

Figure 8.4 "Tuskegee Veteran Hospital Exhibit at Exposition Shows How Patients Are Cured," *The Chicago Defender*, August 24, 1940, p. 4

too. Correspondingly, rare interracial scenes of craft therapy used a variety of pictorial techniques to separate Black men from white men and white female aids and give visual prominence to white men over white women and Black men.

A good example from *Design* magazine featured the new Forest Glen Annex, a convalescent section of Walter Reed Hospital, the Army's leading military medical institution in the US. The photograph of craft therapy outdoors focuses on a white male patient sculpting a voluptuous white female figure as a white female craft aid stands adjacent to him and bends towards the sculpture (Figure 8.5). Of importance here is that the white soldier and white aid stand above a seated Black soldier from whom they are separated physically by a table. Moreover, everyone looks at the white man's clay figure and ignores the Black man's project and, in contrast to the white man, no one tends to the Black man.[52] These pictorial dynamics put into question the quality and inclusiveness of

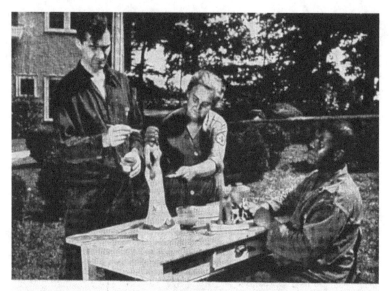

C. N. Beck of Buffalo is touching up his "Pink Lady" sculpture with the help of Mrs. George Thompson, instructor. Eddie Fuller looks up from his work on a sculpture of a cat. Forest Glen Hospital, Maryland.

**Figure 8.5** "Creative Work for Veterans," *Design Magazine* (March 1945), p. 14

the craft therapy program summarized in *Design*: "Excellent results as to rehabilitation and recreation prevail. The project proves art to be emotional and spiritual balance."[53]

Additional techniques of separation spatially organized pictures to message the importance of white men and women over Black men. Examples from the War Department (Figure 8.7) and Lawson General Hospital in Atlanta, Georgia (Figure 8.6) represent Black troops and veterans in fewer numbers than white men and women, placing them on the margins of spaces where craft therapy was practiced (Figures 8.5, 8.6, 8.7). Additionally, they depict Black convalescent men working with very different materials than white men active in the same space (Figure 8.7); they position Black men in profile or looking away from the viewer, in contrast to white men and women who appear more forward-facing (Figures 8.5, 8.6, 8.7); and they reproduce images of Black men on pages separate from groups of white men and women (Figure 8.8).

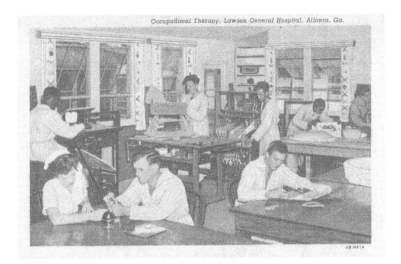

Figure 8.6 Occupational therapy, Lawson General Hospital, Atlanta, Georgia, 1944 (Newberry Library)

These techniques constituting white male dominance pictorially reflected racism sanctioned by the Second World War–era military, including diminished access to resources, fewer resources, and overall challenges of care for Black servicemen.[54] Wounded Black veterans faced difficulty in obtaining the entitlements they had earned,[55] and their injuries were disregarded due to racist assumptions about their health and abilities.[56] Physicians misdiagnosed Black injured soldiers by presuming they were "somehow naturally predisposed to physical and mental illness," discounted their injuries and suffering,[57] and failed to consider that their injuries resulted from "the prevalence of racial terrorism within the armed forces—murders, beatings, extreme and cruel forms of punishment [that] produced its own racially specific traumas."[58] At the beginning of the war, although less by the end, general hospitals and station hospitals segregated Black medical staff and troops.[59] Segregated environments widespread across the South lacked necessary staff and resources.[60] There were problems with Black nurses being able to enlist in the Army Nurse Corps, and once they could, the numbers remained low because of a military-imposed quota,[61] while only two Black

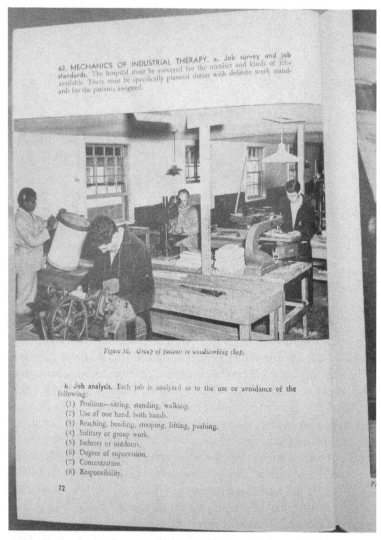

**Figure 8.7** War Department, *Technical Manual for Occupational Therapy*, TM-8291 (Washington, DC: U.S. Government Printing Office, 1944), p. 72

medical schools graduated students and white medical schools graduated very few Black men.[62] These inequities in medical care caused Black troops and veterans to suffer, and "many black veterans experienced severe bouts of acute depression, helplessness, and dependence."[63]

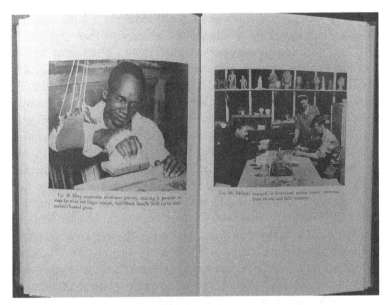

Figure 8.8 Helen S. Willard and Clare S. Spackman, *Principles of Occupational Therapy* (Philadelphia, PA: J. B. Lippincott Company, 1947) (Wolters, Kluwe Health Inc.)

### White privilege in promoting ability: the Army Handicrafts Contest Exhibition and School for American Craftsmen

Meanwhile, publicity about achievements by veterans making craft objects privileged white perspectives and bodies, and an important opportunity for professional training in craft ignored Black veterans.

In New York City, the Met's support of veterans' craft led the museum to help organize and present the Army Handicrafts Contest Exhibition, which took place from December 21, 1945, to January 10, 1946. The exhibition displayed over two hundred handicraft objects that hospitalized enlisted men from the Second Services Command of New York, New Jersey, and Delaware made using salvage materials and then submitted for a juried competition. A panel of white civilian reviewers renowned in the American craft and art worlds evaluated the entries,[64] and the museum exhibited those selected with the name of each maker and his hospital affiliation.[65]

218     *The long Second World War, 1931–1953*

A New Jersey newspaper's photograph and caption depicting local enlistee Pfc. Harold B. Whiting—who as part of the competition won first prize for his near-perfect small replica of an army jeep—and Ann Friga, a "civilian employe [sic] of the Special Service section of the Indiantown Gap, Pa., Military Reservation,"[66] bristled with racial distinctions and hierarchies that socially elevated Friga, a white woman, above Whiting, a Black serviceman. Although the newspaper identified Whiting as "a musician, mechanic, photographer and hobbyist,"[67] it also explained that he served in "the all-Negro Army Service Forces Band" and it identified him as "Negro,"[68] whereas it said nothing about Friga's racial identity. Other evidence of her white privilege involved Friga's and Whiting's locations and interaction in a photograph that showed them both with the jeep Whiting created. In what appears as a cramped space, the jeep is nevertheless positioned lengthwise and used to physically separate Whiting, who crouches behind the jeep, and Friga, who kneels in the foreground right corner where she takes up more vertical space than Whiting and puts her hand on the jeep's front tire. Although both appear to look at the jeep, the newspaper remarked only on Friga's looking and coded it as an authoritative, racially dominating gaze. The paper tells readers that she "looks on with approval"[69] at the object Whiting crafted, while it ignores Whiting's actions and thoughts.

Three years earlier, a program to train veterans in craft skills and help them launch their own businesses had developed in the Northeast and might have interested Whiting. Yet, there is no indication that it recruited Black veterans. During February 1943, the ACCC's Division for Group Education received a charter from the Regents of the State of New York to develop a Rehabilitation Training Program.[70] Initially, the program aimed to give returning disabled veterans the skills to make "an independent living through craftsmanship" by producing high-quality hand-crafted objects[71] that would "raise the level of our [American] own cultural life."[72] The program launched in 1945 in collaboration with the Student Workshop that was established at Dartmouth College in 1941.[73] Under the direction of Virgil Poling, students honed their skills in woodworking, ceramics, metal work, weaving, and decorative work using designs sourced from the program's Design Committee.[74] 1945 also saw the program's name change to the School for American Craftsmen (SAC).

*Cultural actors in rehabilitation*          219

In the early years, as the program sought to attract applicants, *Craft Horizons* publicized SAC as "ideally suited to many returning men who may be so disabled, either physically or nervously that they cannot cope with industry or return to their former occupations."[75] Further, the ACCC "believed that craftsmanship may become a way and means of life both for the disabled man and the one suffering from psychoneurosis,"[76] although to participate, students had to be ambulatory, able to care for themselves, and sighted.[77] The program claimed that barring its training, these men would be left to depend for support on the government, charity, or their own resources."[78]

*Craft Horizons* listed the School's merits, such as contributing to a post-war society "geared towards finding employment for all," which it said amounted to a basic national need,[79] and the magazine shared that the first students were a former Marine and a former Seabee, although it did not mention that both were white.[80] In a photograph of ex-Marine Claire Moore published in the *Dartmouth Alumni Magazine* (Figure 8.9), Moore fills the left half of the photograph and his white male mentor teacher the right. Appearing in profile, Moore's face expresses concentration. Leaning into his work, his bodily strength and agility are evident and appear unencumbered by any impairments. The image also promotes Moore's status as a budding professional artisan. His mentor wears a shop coat, which indicates his role as Moore's teacher and the seriousness of the work-oriented setting of the studio. The image confirms that this white male veteran is intellectually and physical abled in his pursuit of a career for which he was selected to receive educational guidance and support.

Despite linking the program to a national agenda of "finding employment for all," SAC's early selections and corresponding press favored white veterans. In part, the exclusion of Black veterans probably resulted from the program filling at least some of its enrollment through referrals from the Veterans Administration,[81] while the G. I. Bill helped to offset training costs.[82] Neither government program was particularly amenable to giving Black veterans the entitlements they had earned.[83] Moreover, for Black veterans who left military service with a blue military discharge resulting from responding to unsolicited threats and acts of violence from white troops, they were ineligible for their G. I. benefits, and this

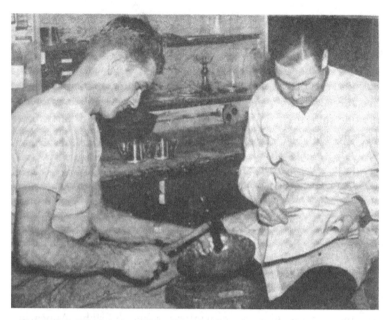

**Figure 8.9** "Ex-Marine Claire Moore, the school's first trainee, shapes a bowl in the metal class, under direction of Aiden Wood," *Dartmouth Alumni Magazine* (March 1945), p. 12

disqualified them from SAC.[84] Additionally, there was the question of whether Black veterans would want to participate in a program that initially was associated with Dartmouth College, which prior to 1967 matriculated only one or two Black students annually.[85]

On top of this, SAC required its students to live in the community to demonstrate they could establish a financially viable livelihood.[86] However, it was not exactly clear what the program meant by "community"—was this code for "white society"? If yes, would Black veterans be welcomed to establish craft practices in the larger New England region? Maybe, although following demobilization everywhere, Black veterans faced disenfranchisement and vulnerability to harassment and police brutality, including on all manner of public transportation.[87] At the same time, white anxiety intensified from a fear that Black veterans would become militant as they sought the civil rights and access to resources denied to them in military service.[88] These inequities, discriminations, omissions, and

*Cultural actors in rehabilitation*        221

anxieties together likely made participating in the program difficult if not unappealing to disabled Black veterans. Consequently, while it claimed a national purview, SAC reiterated the nation's tendency to reserve "American" as a descriptor for white men.[89]

## Post-hospitalization and post-war: the Museum of Modern Art's War Veterans Art Center

Overseen by Victor D'Amico, MoMA's Director of Education, the War Veteran's Art Center (WVAC) opened on October 30, 1944 "as an activity of the Museum's Armed Services Program."[90] Before closing on June 30, 1948, twenty-four instructors would teach nearly fifteen hundred troops and veterans in classes that treated the making of craft and art objects as a practice blending craft therapy's diversion and healing with pre-vocational training.[91] D'Amico interviewed veterans who enrolled and then placed them in design and foundational courses. Following these, the veteran students enrolled in courses for clay, metal, wood, and paint, where they pursued self-paced projects.[92] Instructors worked with them individually and laddered their challenges to gradually master materials and techniques.[93] These instructors also taught volunteers working with veterans in hospitals for the New York State Association for Occupational Therapists and for the ARC Arts and Skills program.[94]

The WVAC reported that more than 50 percent of the men who enrolled bore physical disabilities,[95] while "emotional disturbance[s] were still common to most,"[96] and it promoted its courses to help veterans "find their way back through art into civilian pursuits and pleasures"[97] while recuperating psychologically and physically. In late 1945, D'Amico stated that he found the first enrollees uprooted, lost, and "obviously emotionally upset."[98] Kendall Bassett, who taught *Advanced Woodworking*, reported that his classes accommodated "occasional cases of men whose physical co-ordination was temporarily lost or atrophied because of wounds received in action. Special exercises in hand and machine work were devised for them, often on their doctor's recommendation." Bassett recalled that many students "were non-combat discharges—the so-called 'psycho' cases. As a result much of the work was therapeutic."[99]

222    *The long Second World War, 1931–1953*

Regarding "emotional disturbance" and "non-combat discharges," D'Amico noted that "most veterans use art as a means of getting rid of disturbing experiences which they try to project onto paper or canvas."[100] In this way, "veterans adjust themselves through the creative process."[101] D'Amico expected that in making craft and art objects, veterans turned inward, looking inside themselves to reflect on and come to terms with their personal struggles from war. The process hinged on ideas about one's authentic self as a private, individual, and unique inner self. In making craft and art objects, ostensibly, veterans got in touch with their innermost self and used materials to express if not resolve their war-related psychological wounds, and this process helped "adjust" them to post-war life.[102]

There is no archival evidence that Black veterans enrolled at the WVAC. Like SAC, the WVAC recruited students by writing to "veterans agencies, the American Red Cross and hospitals,"[103] and if these organizations typically ignored Black veterans, their names would not have surfaced as potential enrollees recommended to the WVAC. Had the WVAC welcomed their enrollment, Black veterans may have found several circumstances off-putting, such as D'Amico's paradigm for veterans self-reflexively coming to terms with their individual war traumas as a key part of their "reconversion to civilian life."[104] To be sure, like all war survivors who had served in the military, certainly Black veterans bore personal trauma that could benefit from a supportive veterans aid program. However, in addition to dealing with their individual injuries, many Black men experienced "racial terrorism within the armed forces,"[105] and there is no evidence that courses addressed this more systemic dimension of racism. On top of this, for some Black veterans a "reconversion" to civilian life may have looked more like activism to eradicate social injustice and inequality and achieve civil rights, and less like a corporate office space for creatives, which is the image a WVAC poster distributed (Figure 8.10).[106]

The image depicted white male veterans as independent, abled, and white-collar, career-aspirational men.[107] Gone were the military uniforms for service, and pajamas and robes for recuperating in a hospital ward, with female Arts and Skills aids in attendance nearby. Instead, wearing dress shirts and ties, some in blazers,

*Cultural actors in rehabilitation* 223

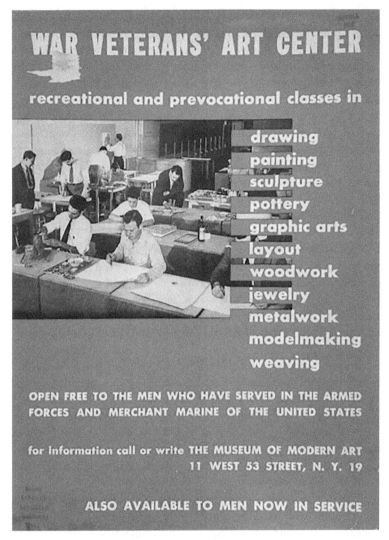

**Figure 8.10** Poster, War Veterans' Art Center, 1942, Early Museum History: Administrative Records, I.3.o. (The Museum of Modern Art Archives, New York). © The Museum of Modern Art/Licensed by SCALA/Art Resource, NY.

## 224 *The long Second World War, 1931–1953*

each man worked at his own table. Together, the veteran art and craft students resembled a group of young corporate professionals working individually yet with some group interaction in a modern space outfitted with modular geometric tables and stools, with at least one wall serving as a common critique board.[108] That WVAC classes were held at night to accommodate veterans who worked during the day suggests, along with their dress, that the veterans who enrolled worked daytime white-collar jobs. Their aspirations for middle-class life were also reflected in *Art for War Veterans*, September 26 to November 25, 1945, an exhibition MoMA held to mark the WVAC's first year of operation. The exhibition included a series of photographs depicting a white male veteran making something.[109] Words and phrases appearing above their images—including the personal pronoun "I" as part of self-reflexive statements—invested the men with agency. Below the photographs, additional words and phrases stressed characteristics of their courses, such as "prevocational training" and "individual instruction," along with takeaways like "creativeness" and "personal satisfaction." The men's appearance in the WVAC's poster epitomized their transition from the unit focus of military life to an I-centered, agentic post-war self.[110]

Other photographs from *Art for War Veterans* pointed to additional types of good outcomes for white veterans enrolled at the WVAC. One features a young white male veteran demonstrating his skills on a pottery wheel to an older white male on the left—Kenneth Chorley, Chairman of the WVAC, and an older white male on the right—Admiral Monroe Kelly (Figure 8.11). Together, Chorley and Kelly signified the interests of military leadership and civilian cultural leadership merging in support of the WVAC helping to reintegrate this young man. Crucially, with the addition of the veteran explaining his pottery, this small group portrayed a genealogy of white patriarchy: the two older white male leaders represented the white male descendants from which the young white male veteran emerged. Now experienced and recuperated from his service, perhaps one day he would support the rehabilitation of yet another generation of white men returning from war to eventually assume positions of productivity and perhaps even leadership in civilian society.

*Cultural actors in rehabilitation* 225

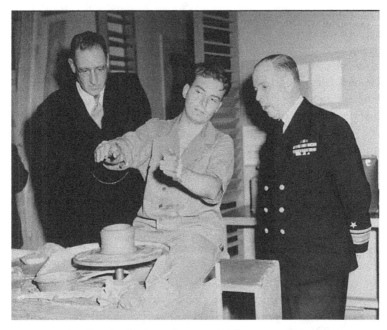

Figure 8.11 Kenneth Chorley, Chairman of the War Veterans' Art Center, and Admiral Monroe Kelly (right) watch veteran at potter's wheel at the opening of the exhibition Art for War Veterans, September 26, 1945 to November 25, 1945 (Photographic Archive, The Museum of Modern Art Archives, New York. Photograph by Henry Mallon). © The Museum of Modern Art/Licensed by SCALA/Art Resource, NY.

## Conclusion

Humanitarian-led efforts to care for wounded troops and rehabilitate them for civilian life through craft therapy and pre-vocational craft activity did not necessarily deliver inclusion. Despite organizations like the American Red Cross and museum leaders professing concern for humankind, during and following the war, as care flowed from military hospitals into civilian care facilities and cultural institutions, programs in the latter venues reiterated segregation and racism associated with the armed forces that privileged white men in an abled capacity over Black troops and women

226    *The long Second World War, 1931–1953*

and underscored their heterosexual orientation. Image and text representations in art and craft journals and mass print media, along with features of education programs, exhibitions, and pre-vocational training conveyed this privilege, as did the military and civilian cultural and business worlds. While there may be additional stories that are not part of these records of craft therapy that offer divergent points of view and experiences, those examined here indicate that craft participated in shoring up these social dominances during wartime as well as in the post-war period.

To this last point, after the war, MoMA published a series of how-to-make books beginning with *How to Make Pottery and Ceramic Sculpture*, 1947, followed by *How to Make Modern Jewelry*, 1949, and *How to Make Objects of Wood*, 1951. The series maintained elements of occupational therapy textbooks of the period by referring to patients with male pronouns and reproducing photographs of white men busy in "the production of something," which *Practical Occupational Therapy for the Mentally and Nervously Ill* implied was a standard activity for men.[111]

An example of producing something appeared in MoMA's *How to Make Objects of Wood* (Figure 8.12). A photograph near the end of the book portrayed a white man working with wood in a home garage amply outfitted with a workbench and tools. Perhaps he was a veteran. MoMA's book series maintained links to veterans by reproducing photographs and course content from the WVAC. In this book, the photograph contributed a positive ending. Near the end of the book, it offered an image of suburban home ownership following other photographs of veteran students working with wood at the WVAC. As a narrative ending, it suggested success for the veteran who had rehabilitated from his war injuries and reconverted to civilian life.

The photograph also reiterated privileges that MoMA was helping to pass on to suburbia. The WVAC and other cultural actors had worked on behalf of white male veterans, beginning with their support of the ARC's Arts and Skills program. Their efforts left out Black veterans—in visual representations and records of access, recruitment, and participation. As they took up a general humanitarian ethic of supporting veterans by facilitating, organizing, and delivering craft therapy and craft therapy-informed programs, they reiterated the military's mixture of racial and gender privileges and

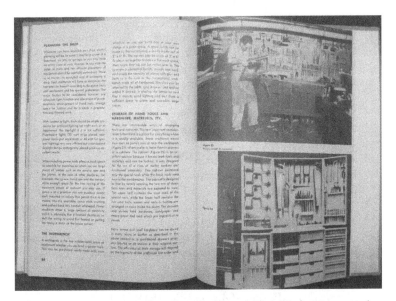

Figure 8.12 *How to Make Objects of Wood* (New York: Museum of Modern Art with Simon & Schuster, 1951) (Simon & Schuster)

oppressions. Soon, many Americans would challenge this status quo by advocating for more inclusive civil rights, including in the cultural sector.[112]

## Notes

1 Julia Irwin, *Making the World Safe, The American Red Cross and a Nation's Humanitarian Awakening* (New York: Yale University Press, 2013), pp. 199–207. See also Allan M. Winkler, *Homefront USA: American during WWII*, 3rd ed. (Wheeling, IL: Harlan Davidson, Inc., 2012); Emily Yellin, *Our Mothers' War: American Women at Home and at the Front during World War II* (New York: Free Press, A Division of Simon & Schuster, Inc., 2004).
2 Marjorie B. Greene and Dorothea Cooke Lythgoe, *Occupational Therapy* (Boston, MA: Bellman Publishing Company, Inc., 1941), pp. 5, 7.
3 Greene and Lythgoe, *Occupational Therapy*, pp. 14–15.

228     *The long Second World War, 1931–1953*

4 *Ibid.*

5 See the notes and bibliography in Jennifer Way, "Prolegomena for Craft Therapy during World War 1," in Chandan Bose and Mira Mohsini (eds), *Encountering Craft: Methodological Approaches from Anthropology, Art History, and Design* (Abingdon and New York: Routledge, 2023), pp. 93–113.

6 Mrs. Cass Canfield [Jane Sage White], "Report of First Year," April 1, 1944, American Red Cross, Arts and Skills Corps. From Library, Gallery of Ontario, p. 1.

7 Arts and Skills Service [pamphlet], *Volunteer Services: The American National Red Cross* (Washington, DC). Dorothy Liebes Papers Art, Archives of American Art.

8 "Our History," American Craft Council, www.craftcouncil.org/about/our-history (accessed April 1, 2024).

9 John W. Meyer and Ronald L. Jepperson, "The 'Actors' of Modern Society: The Cultural Construction of Social Agency," *Sociological Theory*, 18:1 (2000), 102.

10 Francis Henry Taylor, "Humanism and Human Responsibility," *The Metropolitan Museum of Art Bulletin* (1941), 2–4.

11 Edward Liss, "Creative Therapy," *The Bulletin of the Museum of Modern Art* (1943), 13–16.

12 Liss, "Creative Therapy," pp. 14–15.

13 Stephanie Taylor, "Identity Construction," in Karen Tracy (ed.), *International Encyclopedia of Language and Social Interaction* (Hoboken, NJ: John Wiley, 2015), p. 11.

14 Way, "Prolegomena for Craft Therapy."

15 Tara Tappert, "In Service to the Nation: Military Arts and Crafts," LaSalle University, 2012.

16 Ana Carden-Coyne, *Reconstructing the Body: Classicism, Modernism, and the First World War* (New York: Oxford University Press, 2009); *The Politics of Wounds: Military Patients and Medical Power in the First World War* (Oxford: Oxford University Press, 2014).

17 Ana Carden-Coyne, "Butterfly Touch: Rehabilitation, Nature, and the Haptic Arts in the First World War," *Critical Military Studies* 6:2 (2019), 176–203 and "The Art of Resilience: Veteran Therapy from the Occupational to the Creative, 1914–1945," in Leo Van Bergen and Eric Vermetten (eds), *The First World War and Health: Rethinking Resilience* (Leiden: Brill, 2020), pp. 39–70.

18 Sebastien Farré, Jean-Francois Fayet, and Bertrand Taithe, "Exhibiting Humanitarian Identities: The Role of Exhibitions in the Modern Humanitarian Project, An Introduction," in Sebastien Farre, Jean-Francois Fayet, and Bertrand Taithe (eds), *The Humanitarian*

Cultural actors in rehabilitation 229

*Exhibition (1867–2016)*, (Geneva: Georg Editeur, 2022), pp. 14–27, at pp. 18, 20, 22.

19 Farré, Fayet, and Taithe, "Exhibiting Humanitarian Identities," p. 18.

20 Katherine Ott, "Disability Things: Material Culture and American Disability History, 1700–2010," in Susan Burch and Michael Rembis (eds), *Disability Histories* (Urbana, Chicago, and Springfield, IL: University of Illinois Press, 2014), pp. 119–135, at p. 126.

21 Wendy Asquith, "Constituting Communities of Humanitarian Feeling: The League of Nations, The United Nations, and World Expos," in Farre, Fayet, and Taithe (eds), *The Humanitarian Exhibition (1867–2016)*, pp. 82–115, at p. 88.

22 Kathleen. J. Fitzgerald, "White Privilege," in Richard T. Schaefer (ed.), *Encyclopedia of Race, Ethnicity, and Society* (Thousand Oaks, CA: Sage Publications, 2008), pp. 1403–1405.

23 Stephanie Szitanyi, *Gender Trouble in the U.S. Military: Challenges to Regimes of Male Privilege* (Cham: Springer Nature, 2020), pp. 4, 5.

24 *Ibid.*

25 The quotation is from Christina Jarvis, *The Male Body at War: American Masculinity during World War II* (DeKalb, IL: Northern Illinois University Press, 2004), p. 102. See also Chapter 2 in Donna B. Knaff, *Beyond Rosie the Riveter: Women of World War II in Graphic Art* (Lawrence, KS: University of Kansas Press, 2012); Sarah Parry Myers, "'The Women Behind the Men Behind the Gun': Gendered Identities and Militarization in the Second World War," in Kara Dixon Vuic (ed.), *Routledge Histories: The Routledge History of Gender, War, and the U.S. Military* (London: Routledge, 2018); and Donna B. Knaff, "Homos, Whores, Rapists, and the Clap: American Military Sexuality since the Revolutionary War," in Vuic (ed.), *Routledge Histories: The Routledge History of Gender, War, and the U.S. Military*, pp. 269–285.

26 Szitanyi, *Gender Trouble in the U.S. Military*, p. 5.

27 On race and health see Keisha Ray, *Black Health: The Social, Political, and Cultural Determinants of Black People's Health* (New York: Oxford University Press, 2023); Robert F. Jefferson, "'Enabled Courage': Race, Disability, and Black World War II Veterans in Postwar America," *The Historian*, 65:5 (2003), 1102–24; Todd L. Savitt, *Race and Medicine in Nineteenth- and Early-Twentieth Century America* (Kent, OH: The Kent State University Press, 2007); and Robert J. Parks, "The Development of Segregation in U.S. Army Hospitals, 1940–1942," *Military Affairs*, 37 (1973), 145–150. On anti-Black racism and the military see Phillip McGuire (ed.), *Taps for a Jim Crow Army: Letters from Black Soldiers in World War II* (Lexington, KS: University Press of Kentucky, 2014); Kimberley L. Phillips, *War! What Is It Good For?*

230    *The long Second World War, 1931–1953*

*Black Freedom Struggles and the U.S. Military from World War II to Iraq*, The John Hope Franklin Series in African American History and Culture (Chapel Hill, NC: University of North Carolina Press, 2012); Robert E. Jefferson, *Fighting for Hope: African American Troops of the 93rd Infantry Division in World War II and Postwar America* (Baltimore. MD: Johns Hopkins University Press, 2008).

28  Thomas A. Guglielmo, *Divisions: A New History of Racism and Resistance in America's World War II Military* (New York: Oxford University Press, 2021; online ed, Oxford Academic, 2021), p. 7. https://doi.org/10.1093/oso/9780195342659.001.0001.

29  Mrs. Cass Canfield [Jane Sage White], "Report of First Year," April 1, 1944, American Red Cross, Arts and Skills Corps, p. 1; "Arts and Skills Program," *Design*, 46:4 (December 1944), p. 24; Minutes, Arts and Skills Meeting, Museum of Modern Art, December 31, 1942, American Occupational Therapy Association Archives.

30  "Craftsmen and the War, A Symposium," *Craft Horizons*, 1:2 (May 1942), p. 3. See also "Craftsmen and the War: A Continuation," 2:1, *Craft Horizons* (November 1942), p. 4.

31  Mildred G. Burrage, "Craftsmen Can Help: An Account of the Arts and Skills Unit of the New York Chapter of the American Red Cross at Halloran Hospital," *Craft Horizons*, 3:6 (August 1944), p. 18; "Craftsmen and the War: A Continuation," p. 5.

32  "Craftsmen and the War: A Continuation," p. 5.

33  Szitanyi, *Gender Trouble in the U.S. Military*, pp. 4, 5.

34  Roszika Parker, *The Subversive Stitch: Embroidery and the Making of the Feminine* (London: Women's Press, 1984); Eileen Boris, "The Subversive Stitch: Embroidery and the Making of the Feminine Rozsika Parker," *The Journal of Modern Craft*, 5:1 (2012), 119–121; Clive Edwards, "'Home Is Where the Art is': *Women, Handicrafts and Home Improvements 1750–1900*,"*Journal of Design History*, 19:1 (2006), 11–21.

35  There are similar examples in Margery Hoffman Smith, "Arts and Skills Workshop," *Design*, 46 (October 1944), p. 16, and Kay Peterson Parker, "Calling all Artists," *Design* (February 1945), p. 13.

36  Myers, "'The Women Behind the Men Behind the Gun.'"

37  Jarvis, *The Male Body at War*, p. 115.

38  Jarvis, *The Male Body at War*. See Chapter 3, "Representing Wounded Bodies: Personal, Popular, and Medical Narratives."

39  Jarvis, *The Male Body at War*, p. 89.

40  Charissa Threat, "'Patriotism Is Neither Masculine nor Feminine': Gender and the Work of War," in Vuic (ed.), *Routledge Histories: The Routledge History of Gender, War, and the U.S. Military*, pp. 233–245.

## Cultural actors in rehabilitation  231

41  Knaff, *Beyond Rosie the Riveter*, pp. 59–71; Knaff, "Homos, Whores, Rapists, and the Clap."
42  Szitanyi, *Gender Trouble in the U.S. Military*, p. 4.
43  *Ibid.*, p. 8.
44  *Ibid.*, pp. 4, 5.
45  War Department, *Technical Manual for Occupational Therapy*, TM 8-291 (December 1944), Figure 43, page 48.
46  "Craftsmen and the War," *Craft Horizons*, 2:2 (May 1943), p. 13.
47  Willard W. Waller, *The Veteran Comes Back* (New York: The Dryden Press, 1944), 86–87; Douglas Walter Bristol, Jr., "Terror, Anger, and Patriotism: Understanding the Resistance of Black Soldiers during World War II," in Douglas Walter Bristol and Heather Marie Stur (eds), *Integrating the US Military: Race, Gender, and Sexual Orientation since World War II* (Baltimore. MD: Johns Hopkins University Press, 2017), pp. 10–25).
48  See, for instance, Frank T. Hines, "The Medical Care Program of the Veterans Administration," *The Annals of the American Academy of Political and Social Science*, 239 (1945), 73–79; Wilbur B. Brookover, "The Adjustment of Veterans to Civilian Life," *American Sociological Review*, 10:5 (1945), 579–586; Leo P. Crespi and G. Schofield Shapleigh, "'The' Veteran—A Myth," *The Public Opinion Quarterly*, 10:3 (1946), 361–371.
49  Rebecca Stiles Taylor, "Tuskegee Veteran Hospital Exhibit at Exposition Shows How Patients are Cured," *The Chicago Defender* (August 24, 1940), p. 4. See also Starr Smith, "The Road Back Leads to Tuskegee, from There the Road Leads Home: Vets Rest at Huge Hospital," *The Chicago Defender* national edition, November 22, 1947, p. 13, which includes a photograph captioned, "Cabinet Making, Instructor shows patient the fine points of cabinet making. Course is part of hospital's rehabilitation program."
50  Guglielmo, *Divisions*, p. 3.
51  "Minority Service in World War II," U.S. Army Center of Military History, https://history.army.mil/documents/wwii/minst.htm (accessed April 1, 2024).
52  *Arts and Skills Corps Newsletter*, National Headquarters, Washington, DC, no. 3 (February 1946), Dorothy Liebes Papers, Archives of American Art.
53  Calvin O. Stanton, "Arts and Skills, A Program Sponsored by the Red Cross, My Art Experience," *Design*, 46 (November 1944), p. 15.
54  Jefferson, "'Enabled Courage,'" p. 1103.
55  Jefferson, "'Enabled Courage,'" p. 1109.
56  Jefferson, "'Enabled Courage,'" p. 1103.

232 *The long Second World War, 1931–1953*

57 Jennifer C. James, *African American War Literature from the Civil War to World War II* (Chapel Hill, NC: University of North Carolina, 2007), p. 243.

58 James, *African American War Literature*, p. 243.

59 Parks, "The Development of Segregation in U.S. Army Hospitals, 1940–1942."

60 Jefferson, " 'Enabled Courage,' " p. 1111.

61 "African American Nurses in World War II," National Women's History Museum, July 8, 2019, www.womenshistory.org/articles/african-american-nurses-world-war-ii (accessed February 2024).

62 Savitt, *Race and Medicine in Nineteenth- and Early-Twentieth Century America*, pp. 265–266.

63 Jefferson, " 'Enabled Courage,' " p. 1114.

64 Loan exhibitions held 1945, Army Handicrafts, 1945 – L7806, Metropolitan Museum of Art Archives, Metropolitan Museum of Art.

65 Press Clippings, Army Handicrafts Contest Exhibition, Metropolitan Museum of Art Archives.

66 "Plainfielder's Jeep Shown at Museum," *Courier-News*, Plainfield, New Jersey, January 28, 1946. Press clippings from Handicraft Exhibition 1945. Metropolitan Museum of Art Archives.

67 *Ibid.*

68 June Ying Yee, "Whiteness," in Richard T. Schaefer (ed.), *Encyclopedia of Race, Ethnicity, and Society* (Thousand IOaks, CA: Sage Publications, 2008), pp. 1398–1399.

69 "Plainfielder's Jeep Shown at Museum."

70 Aileen Webb to Mrs. Dorothy Liebes, letter, February 11, 1943. Dorothy Liebes Papers, Archives of American Art.

71 "What's New Under the Sun," *Craft Horizons*, 3:6 (August 1944), p. 1.

72 Aileen Webb to Mrs. Dorothy Liebes, "Memorandum on Design Committee, from Mrs. Webb to Mrs. Draper," Dorothy Liebes Papers, Archives of American Art.

73 C.[harles]E.[dward]W.[idmayer], "School for Craftsmen, Dartmouth Cooperates in a New Educational Approach," *Dartmouth Alumni Magazine* (March 1945), pp. 13–15. https://archive.dartmouthalumnimagazine.com/article/1945/3/1/school-for-craftsmen (accessed April 5, 2024).

74 Rehabilitation through Craftsmanship, The American Craftsmen's Educational Council, Minutes of Special Meeting of Board of Directors, 1943. Dorothy Liebes Papers, Archives of American Art.

75 "The School for American Craftsmen," *Craft Horizons*, 4:10 (August 1945), p. 8.

76 Rehabilitation through Craftsmanship.

*Cultural actors in rehabilitation* 233

77 "The School for American Craftsmen," p. 8.
78 Rehabilitation through Craftsmanship.
79 "The Editor Speaks: The Professional Attitude," p. 3.
80 "American Craftsmen's Educational Council Notes," *Craft Horizons*, 6:14 (August 1946), p. 35.
81 "The School for American Craftsmen," p. 8.
82 Widmayer, "School for Craftsmen, Dartmouth Cooperates in a New Educational Approach," pp. 13–15.
83 Jefferson, " 'Enabled Courage,' " p. 1109.
84 Matthew F. Delmont, *Half American: The Epic Story of African Americans Fighting World War II at Home and Abroad* (New York: Viking, 2022), p. 270.
85 Bill Platt, "Forty Years On: The Changing Face of Dartmouth," *Dartmouth News*, June 17, 2013, (accessed November 2023).
86 Bulletin No. 1, *The War Veteran's Art Center, An Experiment in Rehabilitation in Art, 1944–1948*, EMH, I.3.p., The Museum of Modern Art Archives, New York (hereafter MoMA Archives).
87 Margaret Burnham, "Soldiers and Buses: All Aboard," *Race and Justice*, 5:2 (2015), 91–113.
88 Jefferson, " 'Enabled Courage,' " pp. 1104–1105.
89 Gary Gerstle, *American Crucible: Race and Nation in the Twentieth Century* (Princeton, NJ: Princeton University Press, 2017); Ian Haney Lopez, *White by Law: The Legal Construction of Race* (New York: New York University Press, 1996).
90 *The War Veteran's Art Center.*
91 Laurel Humble, "Response and Responsibility: The War Veterans' Art Center at the Museum of Modern Art (1944–1948)" (MA Art History thesis, City University of New York, 2016), pp. 17, 27–28.
92 Humble, "Response and Responsibility," p. 19.
93 *The War Veteran's Art Center*, p. 7.
94 *Ibid.*, p. 8.
95 Press release, *Art for War Veterans.*
96 "Museum of Modern Art Establishes Art Center for War Veterans," Press release, *Art for War Veterans*, September 21, 1945, p. 9, www.moma.org/momaorg/shared/pdfs/docs/press_archives/1003/releases/MOMA_1945_0037_1945-09-21_45921-30.pdf (accessed October 2024).
97 *Ibid.*
98 Minutes of the meeting of the Advisory Committee of the War Veteran's Art Center, December 11, 1945, JTS N.C.4. MoMA Archives.
99 Kendall Bassett, *Advanced Woodworking Design*, pp. 29–30. VDA, III.A.13. MoMA Archives.

234 *The long Second World War, 1931–1953*

100 *The War Veteran's Art Center*, p. 5.

101 *Ibid.*, p. 8.

102 Jorden Pitt, "American Masculinity after World War II," July 23, 2021, The National WWII Museum, www.nationalww2museum.org/war/articles/american-masculinity-after-world-war-ii (accessed November 2024).

103 Humble, "Response and Responsibility," p. 17.

104 Press release, *Art for War Veterans*.

105 James, *African American War Literature*, p. 243.

106 Bristol, "Terror, Anger, and Patriotism."

107 Poster for the War Veterans' Art Center, 1942. APF, War Veterans Art Center, MoMA Archives.

108 See a reproduction of the photograph in *The War Veteran's Art Center*, p. 9.

109 Installation view, *Art for War Veterans*, www.moma.org/calendar/exhibitions/3180?installation_image_index=0 (accessed November 2024).

110 Press release, *Art for War Veterans*.

111 Louis J. Haas, *Practical Occupational Therapy for the Mentally and Nervously Ill* (Milwaukee, WI: The Bruce Publishing Company, 1944), p. 15.

112 Bristol, "Terror, Anger, and Patriotism."

# 9

# Trauma of warfare: maxillofacial surgery and medical relief in wartime China, 1948–1956

*Jinghong Zhang*

In May 2009, the 19th International Conference on Oral and Maxillofacial Surgery (ICOMS) was held in Shanghai. At the conference, Qiu Weiliu, one of the leading maxillofacial surgeons in China, was elected the "Distinguished Fellow of 2009" by the International Association of Oral and Maxillofacial Surgeons (IAOMS). Being the first Asian oral and maxillofacial surgeon to receive the award, Qiu emerged as the iconic figure representing the global recognition of China's oral and maxillofacial surgery field.[1] Whereas maxillofacial surgery is an important component of Chinese stomatology (*kouqiang yixue*) – a system based on the Soviet model that combined dentistry with oral and maxillofacial surgery, it only emerged as a medical specialty in China during the early People's Republic of China (PRC). This chapter argues that while it was initially part of the circulation of transnational medical knowledge and practice from the United States to China in the late 1940s, its development in China was provoked by warfare and later enhanced by the Learning-from-the-Soviet-Union Campaign in the early 1950s. The substantial role played by maxillofacial surgeons during the Korean War (1950–1953) earned them a distinct and significant recognition within the new system of stomatology established by the PRC regime.

Maxillofacial surgery played a significant role in managing and repairing facial injuries of wounded soldiers during and after both the First and Second World Wars. The war, as acknowledged by oral and maxillofacial surgeons, facilitated the creation of medical services "dedicated to the recovery and reconstruction of the

236     *The long Second World War, 1931–1953*

wounded."[2] In particular, the treatment of facial injuries during and after the First World War (1914–1918) led to the birth of plastic and reconstructive surgery and later the disciplinary formation of oral and maxillofacial surgery. Throughout the duration of the Second World War (1939–1945), maxillofacial surgery remained a pivotal component in the treatment of facial injuries sustained by wounded soldiers. Even though the Second World War officially concluded in 1945, the mission of maxillofacial surgery to restore functionality to the disabled and reintegrate them into society continued.[3] This also led to the further exchange of surgical expertise, practices, and medical professionals across different spaces as well as between military and "civilian" medicines.

In contrast to its evolution in the European and American regions, the development of maxillofacial surgery in China and the other East Asian regions occurred significantly later. This specialty only reached China in the late 1940s, following the end of the Second World War, and saw extensive implementation for the first time during the Korean War (1950–1953). Shortly after the Korean War, the Learning-from-the-Soviet-Union Campaign in the 1950s introduced the Soviet system of stomatology to China, which facilitated the institutionalization of oral and maxillofacial surgery as well as its incorporation into the new system of Chinese stomatology.

Tracing the development of maxillofacial surgery in China from the late 1940s to the early 1950s, this chapter explores the underexamined transfer of medical knowledge and practices between China and the United States and later the Soviet Union. Recent studies have demonstrated the transnational influence on the formation of science in socialist China, be it from the former Soviet Union or the United States.[4] In her recent monograph on medicinal animals in the PRC, for instance, Liz P. Y. Chee has demonstrated the importance of the Soviet influence on China's formation of socialist medicine in the 1950s.[5] Combining and localizing both the US and Soviet impacts, the development of maxillofacial surgery in China thus offers a concrete case study of the transnational making of medical knowledge and practices across spaces and wars in the twentieth century.

The transnational circulation of maxillofacial surgical knowledge and practices transcended the conventional Second World

*Trauma of warfare* 237

War chronology of 1939 to 1945 and enables us to think about the "long" Second World War from the vantage point of the wounded soldiers and medical practitioners. As historian Ana Carden-Coyne argues, reconstruction indicated the aftermath of the war, aligning with broader humanitarian and cultural objectives aimed at advancing civilized societies.[6] During and after the war, medical and welfare organizations and actors were primarily concerned with the rehabilitation of wounded soldiers. By emphasizing the restoration of both mental and physical wellbeing, rehabilitation became demilitarized after the war as "men transformed from warriors to citizens."[7] Hence, the wartime obligations of medical practitioners and the suffering of the wounded soldiers did not cease with the war coming to an end. Instead, they extended into the post-war phase of rehabilitation and reconstruction. The ability of maxillofacial surgery to *reconstruct* was thus significant in the newly established PRC. By reconstructing the facial structure of the wounded soldiers, maxillofacial surgery managed to restore the function and appearance of their faces, which also helped to reconstruct their social identity after the war. The reconstruction held significance in both the social recovery from the war and the construction of a new People's Republic of China during the early 1950s.

In the rest of the chapter, I will first give a brief introduction of the historical development and disciplinary formation of plastic and reconstructive surgery as well as maxillofacial surgery in the Euromerican world over the two world wars. Next, I will examine how the Chinese physicians dispatched by the Nationalist government following the Second World War introduced maxillofacial surgical practices from the United States to China. Subsequently, I delve into the account of surgical teams sent to assist North Korea during the Korean War (1950–1953) and their wartime encounters. These experiences and practices played a pivotal role in establishing maxillofacial surgery as a formal medical specialty in the early PRC. Finally, I switch the gaze from the surgeons and the medical specialty to the experience of the injured, theorizing how maxillofacial surgery mattered to the reconstruction of their facial structure and later their affective experience and social identity, which was crucial to reintegrating them into the newly established socialist society.

238        *The long Second World War, 1931–1953*

## The rise of maxillofacial surgery on the battlefield

The recognition of maxillofacial surgery as a medical specialty is a relatively recent event. Originally a branch of general medicine, maxillofacial surgery became a specialty that combined dentistry and surgery in the early twentieth century, establishing its identity from its important role in managing and repairing neck, head, and particularly facial injuries during the First World War.[8] During the First World War, facial injuries were frequently inflicted by the conditions of trench warfare and the deployment of grenades, machine guns, and shrapnel, while soldiers had limited protection against these dangers.[9] War injuries of the jaw, which were common among the wounded soldiers at the time, refer to "severe injuries of the maxilla which are caused by projectiles such as bullets, pieces of shell, or bombs striking the bone at high velocity."[10] Given that the lower jaw is the least securely anchored bone in the human body, its comminution easily disrupts the muscle equilibrium on the remaining part of the jaw. This disruption leads to compromised jaw functions, tooth loss, and facial deformity.[11] The task of the maxillofacial surgeons, therefore, is to restore the remaining portions of the jaw to the proper positions as well as to retain and repair them.[12]

At the beginning of the First World War, there was significant neglect of plastic surgery in the army in both Europe and the United States.[13] As the American surgeon John Staige Davis recalled, when England first witnessed a surge in maxillofacial wounds among soldiers in 1914, there were no trained physicians to deal with these cases.[14] When the United States later joined the war in 1917, a few physicians served the US army to help treat soldiers who were suffering from battlefield wounds, burns, and facial injuries. Harold H. Gilles, an otolaryngologist without any precedent experience in plastic surgery, was assigned to do the work.[15] Among these surgeons, some of them were volunteer dental surgeons who collaborated with their medical colleagues in treating facial injuries caused by the war.[16] Although most of the early treatment work was done "by trial and error," the knowledge gained in the process soon began to be applied to plastic reconstruction of the maxillofacial region for the wounded.[17] By the end of the First World War, the realm of military medicine had witnessed evident progress in "the treatment of fractures of the jaw, and in the repair of destructive

*Trauma of warfare* 239

wounds of the maxillae, by bone grafting and by adequate and ingenious prostheses."[18] These methods "stood the test of time" and soon came into use and were greatly improved later during the Second World War.

Over the First World War, the significant contributions of these American surgeons in effectively treating facial and jaw injuries among soldiers garnered newfound recognition for plastic surgery as a distinct medical specialty for the very first time. After the war, the American plastic surgeons returned home and continued with the post-operative care of patients at the Veterans Hospitals.[19] J. Howard Crum, an American surgeon who was advocating facelifts, noted that plastic surgery was crucial to the reconstruction of the post-war society in 1928: "the world felt that horrible disfigurement of face was too great a pride for one to pay for his patriotism ... The modern man and woman are more sensitive to facial beauty, and, unlike their ancients, cannot stoically look at faces disfigured by war and other causes. The prospect of a considerable number of war-mutilated men being let loose upon the streets seemed appalling."[20] In Europe, photography played a vital role in disseminating images of patients going through reconstructive surgeries during and after the First World War, which evoked the horror of war among the public.[21] For instance, in the Weimar Republic, images of war-wounded individuals exploded as symbols of the meaninglessness of the war, and the missing or mutilated faces were interpreted as the visual emblematic of the "loss of humanity."[22] Amid the horror and the public presence of reconstructed faces of veterans, plastic surgery began to claim a more important role in the society in the 1920s. The post-war era's increased focus on the significance of reconstructive surgery in enhancing aesthetic sensibility, fostering social stability, and contributing to the rebuilding of civilization led to an elevated social standing for plastic surgery.

The challenges posed by wartime facial reconstruction cases, especially those involving previously uncharted injuries, necessitated a tight partnership between dentistry and surgery. The repair process demanded a fusion of expertise and knowledge from both dentists and surgeons. In a meeting held at the Royal Society of Medicine in London in 1916, for instance, it was noted that "the details of the making and adjusting of the necessary splints were obviously outside the sphere of the general surgeon, and could only be dealt with by the trained dental surgeon."[23] Surgeons and dentists thus

240    *The long Second World War, 1931–1953*

worked in groups to exchange their expertise and knowledge as well as collaboratively analyzed cases during the First World War. In 1921, the American Association of Oral and Plastic Surgeons was officially established to facilitate the exchange of experiences and skills between dentists and surgeons.[24] Based on their collaboration with plastic surgeons in their wartime experience, oral surgeons also extended their interests and expertise beyond the mouth to the adjacent facial regions afterwards.[25]

While the treatment of jaws and the repair of destructive wounds of the maxillae were advanced in the First World War, regular medical corps of the armed services still paid little attention to it, and nor was there much official recognition of the necessity of plastic surgery either in the army or navy until the Second World War.[26] At the onset of the Second World War, facilities for plastic and maxillofacial surgeries were notably lacking, as officials had not foreseen the substantial number of plastic surgery cases that would arise. Commencing in 1943, a total of nine centers within the newly established Army General Hospitals in the United States were designated specifically for plastic surgery procedures.[27] John Staige Davis, an American pioneer plastic surgeon, acknowledged the splendid work of the Dental Corps in their domain of expertise. He emphasized the crucial collaboration between the plastic and dental services in most of the Plastic Centers, allowing for joint problem-solving in the realm of maxillofacial reconstruction. In particular, the dental service played a pivotal role in crafting prostheses, plates, and assorted splints. By the end of the Second World War, plastic and reconstructive surgery assumed an unprecedentedly significant role within the military services. Concurrently, oral and maxillofacial surgery, which focused on restoring the disfigured oral and facial regions and served as a bridge between dentistry and surgery, reached a level of maturity as a distinct medical discipline.

### Maxillofacial surgery: from the United States to China in the 1940s

While oral and maxillofacial surgeons in Europe and America made great contributions over the two world wars, it was during the Second World War that the Chinese Nationalist government

*Trauma of warfare* 241

realised the lack of oral and maxillofacial surgeons.[28] During the Second Sino-Japanese War (1937–1945), China witnessed substantial development in both military and civilian health services.[29] As historian Nicole Barnes observes, the catastrophic war spurred the expansion of public health sectors, both in quantity and scope: many Chinese people "had their first encounter with state-directed public health during the war."[30] In addition to the efforts of state public health services and physicians, Barnes also notes that "unorthodox actors" such as women and foreigners participated in the wartime medical care, as citizens were also caring for each other.[31] In the domain of plastic surgery, however, China faced a lack of specialists capable of treating maxillofacial injuries. As Song Ruyao, the widely acknowledged "Father of Plastic Surgery in China," recollected:

> In 1942, a few wounded soldiers with mandibular trauma and a pilot with facial and hand burns were sent to the Huaxi (West China) Dental Hospital for treatment.[32] Lacking maxillofacial and plastic surgeons, we could do nothing but stare blankly at these soldiers with disformed faces, unable to speak or eat, suffering psychological and biological pain. In the end, the pilot was sent to the US and stayed for more than a year there receiving treatment. As a result, the government decided to send me to the US to study plastic surgery.[33]

Song Ruyao graduated from the dental school of West China Union University in 1939. In 1942, Song was sent to study plastic and reconstructive surgery in the US by Generalissimo Chiang Kai-shek. Song arrived in New York in 1943 and worked as a resident at Rochester University Hospital for a year. In 1944, he travelled to Pennsylvania to study with Dr. Robert H. Ivy, a leading American plastic surgeon who served as a commissioned captain in the US army during the First World War and was also highly involved in creating the disciplinary framework of maxillofacial surgery as a specialty afterwards.[34] Ivy also had ties to China as he spent some of his childhood and two years of adulthood in Shanghai.[35] During his time at Penn, Song learned a series of surgical techniques from Ivy as well as from other surgeons there.

After the end of the Second Sino-Japanese War in 1945, the Nationalist government decided to send more Chinese physicians to study in the United States in 1946. Zhang Disheng, a Chinese

242    *The long Second World War, 1931–1953*

surgeon who served the Chinese Expeditionary Force (CEF) during the Burma Campaign in 1944, was among the physicians that went to study in the US in 1946.[36] In Burma, each division of the Chinese army was equipped with a US surgical team, which often consisted of ten American military personnel, including physicians and nurses.[37] During Zhang's time in Burma, he worked closely with the American surgical team and performed a number of trauma surgeries for the CEF soldiers. Zhang's wartime experience as a military surgeon in Burma laid the foundation for his later specialized study in plastic surgery. Funded by the American Bureau of Medical Aids to China (ABMAC), Zhang went to the Medical School at the University of Pennsylvania to study plastic and reconstructive surgery with Dr. Robert Ivy from 1946 to 1948.[38]

In 1948, both Song and Zhang completed their study in the US and decided to return to China. Song took up a job offer from his alma mater, Huaxi (West China) University in Chengdu, the widely acknowledged birthplace of modern Chinese dentistry. Because of his experience working as a medical resident as well as a teaching assistant of anatomy in the US, Huaxi directly hired him as a tenured professor to jointly teach plastic surgery at the medical school and maxillofacial surgery at the dental school.[39] Similarly, Zhang also commenced his teaching career at the medical school of Tongji University in Shanghai. Song saw this as a significant historical moment because "it marked that China was the first country in Asia to be able to offer courses on plastic surgery. Even Japan could not at the time."[40] In 1948, Dr. Richard Webster, a prominent American plastic surgeon, organized a plastic and reconstructive surgery workshop in Shanghai. Both Zhang and Song participated in this event to further enhance their training and knowledge in the field.[41]

Even though both Song and Zhang introduced plastic surgery to China in the late 1940s, the Nationalist government was in the process of retreating to Taiwan during that period and was unable to devote attention to the advancement of plastic and reconstructive surgery. As a result, while Song was instructing medical and dental students in both plastic and maxillofacial surgery, the actual execution of these surgical procedures on patients was relatively infrequent until the Korean War.[42]

*Trauma of warfare*   243

## Surgical teams to aid North Korea, 1950–1952

Maxillofacial surgery was practiced on a large scale for the first time in China during the Korean War (1950–1953). In June 1950, the Korean War between South Korea (backed by the US) and North Korea (supplied by the Soviet Union) broke out. In October, China made the pivotal decision and decided to send a People's Volunteer Army (PVA) to resist the US-led United Nations coalition and aid North Korea (*kangmei yuanchao*). Without enough helmets, most of the PVA soldiers had to fight on the battlefield with their faces and heads exposed. The UN forces used napalm weapons in the Korean War, which could lead to severe wounds on the head and face as well as untreatable burns on the skin.[43]

In 1951, when medical schools all over China organized medical teams to go to the battlefield, the Shanghai municipal government decided to send a medical team to the Korean War front line, which consisted of over four hundred physicians and nurses.[44] Zhang Disheng was in the surgical team and served as the leader of the maxillofacial surgical section.[45] Zhang left Shanghai with the medical team in January 1951 and worked in a hospital in Changchun city, Jilin province of northeast China. As many soldiers at the time suffered from chemical burns and cold injuries, Zhang's team managed to establish a Center for Burn and Cold Injury Treatment (*dong shaoshang zhiliao zhongxin*), which was the first plastic surgery center since the establishment of the PRC.[46]

With the increasing demand for plastic and reconstructive surgeries on the northeast battlefield, the Southwest Military Area Command ordered Huaxi to form a plastic surgery team to help treat the wounded PVA soldiers in 1951. Being a foremost authority on plastic and maxillofacial surgeries in China during that period, Song Ruyao was chosen as the team leader. Song subsequently handpicked a team consisting of three young dentists from Huaxi, a resident surgeon from the affiliated hospital of Huaxi, an orthopedist, a technician, two head nurses, and a secretary.[47] The ten-person surgery team was officially named "the southwest plastic surgery team to aid Korea" (*Xinan zhengxing waike yuanchao shoushudui*).

In April 1951, the Huaxi surgery team left Chengdu for Chongqing and joined another thoracic and abdominal surgery

244 *The long Second World War, 1931–1953*

team. Together they formed a "southwest surgical team to aid Korea" (*xinan yuanchao shoushudui*), which was the first medical team sent from Sichuan to the Korean War.[48] In early July, the southwest surgical team finally arrived in Changchun. As the Shanghai medical team had completed their service and would head back in late July, Song's team took over the plastic and reconstructive surgery task from Zhang Disheng. By the time Song's team arrived, the entire city had been severely bombed. The only intact buildings were the eight departments of the Manchurian government building that had been constructed by the Japanese administration to house the government from 1931 to 1945, so the surgical team decided to set up a field hospital there. After the hospital was prepared, the team immediately started to treat the wounded soldiers that were sent from Korea, most of whom had been bombed or burned by the napalm weapons.

In the spring of 1952, the Huaxi surgery team (see Figure 9.1) returned to Chengdu from the front line and continued to treat the wounded soldiers. As one of the rear treatment bases for the PVA, Chengdu was full of wounded soldiers waiting to receive treatment. The team brought back useful experience in the treatment of war wounds, particularly related to maxillofacial surgery and facial reconstruction. In 1953, Huaxi officially established the very first maxillofacial surgery ward in China, which was expanded from the maxillofacial inpatient department that had been set up earlier in 1951.[49] Other hospitals in Beijing and Shanghai also established maxillofacial surgery wards in the early 1950s to continue with the treatment of the wounded PVA soldiers. The Korean War, for the first time, provided a practical opportunity for the further development of maxillofacial surgery in China. As Song Ruyao summarised it:

> The Korean War marked China's inaugural foray into conducting extensive plastic surgery and facial reconstruction efforts on a large scale. This endeavor heightened the awareness of both the Party-state and the masses about the pivotal role of plastic and reconstructive surgery. It became evident that without plastic surgery, the survival of wounded soldiers would have been uncertain, impeding their transition from military service to civilian life, productive work, and the ability to lead fulfilling social lives.[50]

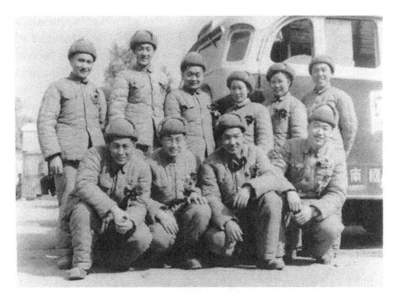

Figure 9.1 The Huaxi plastic surgery team, 1952, Chengdu. Photograph reproduced with kind permission of Mr. Deng Changchun, the son of Deng Xianzhao.

## Institutionalizing maxillofacial surgery: the Soviet impact in the 1950s

While the Korean War provided a practical opportunity for the development of maxillofacial surgery, the Soviet experts in China during the 1950s offered substantial help in the theoretical and academic training of Chinese maxillofacial experts.[51] From 1949 to 1956, the newly established PRC intensively emulated the Soviet model in various fields including the economy, medicine, industry, and agriculture.[52] Against the background of the Learning-from-the-Soviet-Union Campaign, dentistry in the early PRC was claimed to have drawn from the Soviet model, which merged maxillofacial surgery with dentistry and together constituted the new field of stomatology. Denoting the study of the mouth and its disorders and diseases, the name stomatology was thus translated as *kouqiang yixue*.[53]

246    *The long Second World War, 1931–1953*

Wang Hanzhang, a disciple of Song Ruyao and subsequently a prominent maxillofacial surgeon in China, was also a member of the Huaxi surgical team during the Korean War. Following the end of the Korean War, in the winter of 1953, Wang Hanzhang was selected to participate in the Medical Russian Language Training Class held by Harbin Medical University. More than thirty young physicians from all over the country attended the Russian-language training workshop. "Most tutors are Russian, with an additional four Chinese assistants helping us with the language training," Wang recalled.[54] Wang spent six months studying there, mastering this entirely new language. He returned to Huaxi in the summer of 1954 after receiving a completion certificate. Upon his homecoming to Huaxi, he took on the role of a part-time language tutor for the Intensive Russian Language Training class, a mandatory three-month program attended by over 98 percent of the physicians and professors. At that time, all English classes were suspended and replaced by Russian language training.[55]

In the 1950s, there was an increased exchange of maxillofacial surgical knowledge and practices between China and the Soviet Union. In 1955, Wang Hanzhang, who had already been promoted to director of the teaching-research group of maxillofacial surgery at Huaxi, was sent to Beijing to participate in a national advanced class of oral and maxillofacial surgery held at Beijing Medical College from fall 1955 to spring 1956.[56] The instructor was Dr. C. F. Kosykh, a Soviet stomatologist hired by the Ministry of Health to teach maxillofacial surgery at Beijing Medical College for two years.[57] In the class, Dr. Kosykh systematically introduced the development of maxillofacial surgery and stomatological education in the Soviet Union. Similar to the situation in China, the development of maxillofacial surgery in the Soviet Union had been stimulated by the need to treat soldiers on the Eastern Front during the Second World War. Many leading maxillofacial experts in China at this time attended the class, including Wang Hanzhang and Song Ruyao.[58] Leveraging their extensive practical experience in conducting maxillofacial surgeries during the Korean War and receiving comprehensive training from Soviet stomatologists, these individuals emerged as the driving force behind the advancement of maxillofacial surgery and the broader stomatological discipline in the PRC.

*Trauma of warfare*    247

In 1956, the CCP government sent Song Ruyao to visit and study in the Soviet Union. Song visited hospitals and plastic and reconstructive surgery centers in Moscow and Leningrad and returned to China in early 1957.[59] In August 1957, Song officially established China's first plastic and reconstructive surgery specialized hospital. This hospital extended its services to civilians dealing with burns, injuries, and congenital malformations, broadening the application of plastic and reconstructive surgery from the military sphere to the civilian domain.

Initially transferred from the US, maxillofacial surgery became localized through the practices in the Korean War and was enhanced by the Soviet training. In July 1956, the Ministry of Health issued higher education guidelines for all medical subjects.[60] In the guidelines for stomatology, the name of oral surgery (*kouqiang waikexue*) was officially changed to maxillofacial surgery (*kouqiang hemian waike xue*), marking the official recognition of maxillofacial surgery as a subfield under stomatology. In 1959, after years of work and editing by the top maxillofacial experts in China, the first maxillofacial surgery textbook in Chinese was published by the People's Medical Publishing House, along with textbooks on oral medicine and oral orthopedics. The publishing of the first set of domestic textbooks for higher education in stomatology in 1959 also became the landmark of the successful establishment of a new system of stomatology in the first decade of the PRC, in which maxillofacial surgery played a key role.

## Reconstructing the face: between function and appearance

For the soldiers suffering from oral and maxillofacial injuries, the wounds were not only life-threatening, physically painful, and dysfunctional, but also emotionally devastating and even provoking disgust once they caused deformation to the face. As sociologist Bill Hughes vividly puts it, "disability is a life lived before a looking glass that is cracked and distorted by the vandalism of normality."[61] Even if a soldier recovered from maxillofacial injuries, persistent facial malformations would prevent them from being perceived as normal, as the constant sensational corporeal moments would serve as continual reminders of their abnormality.

248        *The long Second World War, 1931–1953*

Many years later, when being interviewed by a journalist about the Korean War, Wang Hanzhang recalled his experience with a twenty-year-old PVA soldier named Jin Hankui, who was sent to the field hospital on the day of its operation during the Korean War. Wang said that his heart still ached whenever he thought of Jin.[62] Jin was severely burned by a napalm bomb. "He was awake and could still talk to me. But his nose and ears were gone; hands and feet were left with palms and soles only; lower eyelids were inside out, and the eyeballs were completely exposed; lips were distorted in the shape of the fish mouth. The only intact part was the skin on his abdomen," Wang recalled. Wang spent half a year trying to treat him and performed four surgeries on him, each time taking part of the skin on his abdomen to graft on his face. As he was gradually recovering, Jin felt hopeful and was looking forward to going home and marrying his fiancée once he fully recovered. One day, he accidentally saw his malformed face in the mirror of the bathroom. Desperate and unable to accept his distorted look, Jin lost control of his emotions on the spot, smashing the window and jumping off the building. Wang recalled sobbing as he asked himself, "Why couldn't he hold on for longer?"[63]

Jin's tragic story is a vivid example of how negative emotions associated with facial abnormalities can lead to catastrophe. As a recent medical journal points out, maxillofacial injuries may cause sensory impairment, aesthetic compromises, and dysfunction, yet the importance of the facial region in influencing social and emotional behavior is hardly considered when assessing the disability and eligibility for compensation.[64] In particular, the psychological impact of facial disfigurement, as shown in Jin's case, is difficult to measure and can be long-lasting. It can also be closely linked with the so-called "direct psycho-emotional disablism," which refers to the "disavowal of disability" in everyday experiences. This includes situations where individuals are excluded or invalidated, such as being stared at by strangers, becoming the subject of jokes about their impairment or disfigurement, or being commented on by others.[65] Hard to classify as a specific type of disability, maxillofacial injuries create a dilemma for the wounded, as they are suffering physically, psychologically, and financially without proper compensation.

Following the unique features of maxillofacial injuries, maxillofacial surgery thus has two significant goals – to treat injuries of the

*Trauma of warfare* 249

oral and maxillofacial region, and to reconstruct the deformed face. In fact, the war was a pivotal moment for surgeons to reconsider the meaning of their care and aftercare for patients. The responsibilities of maxillofacial surgeons extended beyond the immediate objectives of preserving lives and reinstating facial functions. Their role encompassed a more profound mission – the intricate task of reconstructing not only the physical attributes of a patient's appearance but also the very essence of their self-identity and their reintegration into society after the war. In a Chinese textbook of oral and maxillofacial surgery, the author also explicitly introduces the two-fold meaning of maxillofacial surgery:

> The injury of the oral and maxillofacial region has great impact on both the physiological function and appearance of the patient. It creates great obstacles to eating, chewing, and speaking. If the injury affects respiratory tract and blood vessels, the patient can die of airway obstruction and massive hemorrhage. The handling of oral and maxillofacial injuries also matters to their personal look afterwards, which has great impact on their mental health and life quality.[66]

In socialist China, maxillofacial surgery and the facial reconstruction of the wounded PVA soldiers, later extended to treating civilians, aligned with the following value held by the communist state: to "relieve the suffering of the working people," as Song Ruyao noted.[67] The military body, as Suzanne Bierroff puts it, is more than "flesh and blood" but is "a symbolic site invested with political as well as personal meaning."[68] In the aftermath of the war, the process of post-war reconstruction for the wounded soldiers carried profound implications, not only in clinical terms but also on a political front. This period held a dual significance as the CCP-led state transitioned from the exigencies of war to the larger imperatives of national reconstruction and the implementation of socialist initiatives. The medical practitioners' commitment to post-war reconstruction was a testament to their dedication not only to their patients but also to the broader welfare of socialist China.

On the political front, this phase of post-war reconstruction served as a bridge, channelling the transformative energy that had fueled the war effort into constructive nation-building endeavors. As the guns fell silent, the focus shifted from the battlefield to rebuilding the nation's infrastructure, economy, and social relations. As plastic

250    *The long Second World War, 1931–1953*

and reconstructive surgery continued to establish its vital role in the post-war care of wounded soldiers, it also began to extend its reach to the broader population as a significant component of socialist medicine. When *People's Daily*, the official newspaper of the CCP state, covered Song Ruyao's practice of maxillofacial surgeries during the socialist era, the showcased cases were strategically chosen to carry significant political implications:

> A rural girl in her teens suffered from a congenital cleft lip. Professor Song performed surgery for her, and the cleft lip vanished. She could confidently smile at herself in the mirror. An outstanding caretaker, who had sustained facial burns while rescuing a child, experienced profound dismay. Following facial reconstructive surgery, she re-engaged with the children and was even recognized as an exemplary worker.[69]

Both narratives exemplify the broader significance of plastic and constructive surgery within the socialist framework. Beyond the realm of aesthetics, reconstructive surgery became a tool for inclusion, empowerment, and social mobility. It enabled individuals to overcome physical barriers and fully participate in the collective progress of society, aligning with socialism's emphasis on collective welfare and individual development. The CCP's transition from war to post-war reconstruction was emblematic of its ability to harness the nation's collective determination and redirect it towards rebuilding a new and rejuvenated society. The transition of maxillofacial surgery from its wartime role on the front line to its application among civilians within the socialist society underscored its enduring success in establishing a sustainable presence within socialist China.

## Conclusion

The political and cultural meanings of plastic and reconstructive surgery turned out to be very slippery later in the Mao years. Song Ruyao recalled that "emphasizing the recovery of function was legitimate for a proletariat. The aesthetic concern, however, was deemed a capitalist concept of treatment."[70] In 1969, at the height of the Cultural Revolution (1966–1976), Song's plastic surgery hospital was condemned as a "bourgeois beauty salon" and shut down.[71] Song himself was also purged and convicted of crimes. It was only later in the reform period (1978–present), when the concept of "medical aesthetics" began to emerge in the socialist market economy, that the aesthetic function of maxillofacial surgery was re-emphasized in a very different commercial setting.

In the contemporary global medical world, maxillofacial surgery remains a unique dentally based specialty that "continues to bridge medicine and dentistry in its education and training."[72] The progression of maxillofacial surgery in modern China encapsulates not only the transfer of medical knowledge and practices between China, the US, and the Soviet Union, but also provides insight into wartime medical care and post-war aftercare. The transnational dissemination of maxillofacial surgical knowledge and practices went beyond the conventional Second World War timeline of 1939 to 1945. It thus prompts us to contemplate the extended duration of the Second World War from the perspective of both wounded soldiers and medical professionals.

Aiming at the recovery of both function and appearance, maxillofacial surgery represents a kind of bodily reconstruction crucial to wounded soldiers' physical and mental health as well as their reintegration into society. In the late twentieth century, with the wide range of maxillofacial injuries beyond the war setting (such as those from sports and car accidents), Chinese maxillofacial surgeons were able to take advantage of the large number of patients and surgical opportunities, leading to a few breakthroughs in the 1980s and 1990s. When China resumed international cooperation and medical knowledge exchange in the 1980s, this young and burgeoning field that stemmed from wartime medical care soon asserted its place in the international oral and maxillofacial surgery community and became a source of national pride, being referred to as "maxillofacial surgery with Chinese characteristics."

## Notes

1 Yan Weimin, *Jiandan qinxin, shangxia qiusuo: Qiu Weiliu* [Searching High and Low: The Biography of Qiu Weiliu] (Shanghai: Shanghai Jiaotong University Press, 2015), p. 23.

252 *The long Second World War, 1931–1953*

2 Daniel Lew, "A Historical Overview of the AAOMS," published by the American Association of Oral and Maxillofacial Surgeons, p. 2.

3 *Ibid.*

4 Zuoyue Wang, "Transnational Science during the Cold War: The Case of Chinese/American Scientists," *Isis*, 101:2 (2010), 367–377; Sigrid Schmalzer, *Red Revolution, Green Revolution: Scientific Farming in Socialist China* (Chicago, IL: University of Chicago Press, 2016); Lijing Jiang, "Crafting Socialist Embryology: Dialectics, Aquaculture and the Diverging Discipline in Maoist China, 1950–1965," *History and Philosophy of the Life Sciences*, 40:3 (2018).

5 Liz P. Y. Chee, *Mao's Bestiary: Medicinal Animals and Modern China* (Durham, NC: Duke University Press, 2021).

6 Ana Carden-Coyne, *Reconstructing the Body: Classicism, Modernism, and the First World War* (Oxford and New York: Oxford University Press, 2009), p. 22.

7 Carden-Coyne, *Reconstructing the Body*, p. 23.

8 Kevin C. Lee and Sung-Kiang Chuang, "History of Innovations in Oral and Maxillofacial Surgery," *Frontiers of Oral and Maxillofacial Medicine*, 4 (2022).

9 Jason Bate, "Facilitating Exchanges: Photography as a Link between Dentistry and Surgery in the First World War," *History and Technology*, 32:1 (2016), 91–103, at p. 92.

10 H. Baldwin, "Discussion on War Injuries of the Jaw and Face," *Proceedings of the Royal Society of Medicine 9*, Odontol. Sect. (1916), 63–67, at p. 63.

11 *Ibid.*

12 *Ibid.*

13 John Staige Davis, "Plastic Surgery in World War I and in World War II," *Annals of Surgery*, 123:4 (1946), 610–621, at p. 610.

14 *Ibid.*

15 *Ibid.*

16 Lew, "A Historical Overview of the AAOMS," p. 2.

17 Davis, "Plastic Surgery in World War I and in World War II," p. 610.

18 *Ibid.*, p. 611.

19 Frank McDowell, "Plastic Surgery in the Twentieth Century," *Annals of Plastic Surgery*, 1:2 (1978), 217–224, at p. 220.

20 J. Howard Crum, *The Making of a Beautiful Face or Face Lifting Unveiled* (New York: Walton Book Company, 1928), p. 17.

21 Sander L. Gilman, *Making the Body Beautiful: A Cultural History of Aesthetic Surgery* (Princeton, NJ: Princeton University Press, 1999), p. 159.

22 Gilman, *Making the Body Beautiful*, p. 162.

## Trauma of warfare 253

23 Anon., "Reports of Societies. Discussion on War Injuries of Jaws and Face," *The British Medical Journal*, 1 (1916), 375–376, at p. 375.
24 *Ibid.*
25 *Ibid.*
26 Davis, "Plastic Surgery in World War I and in World War II," p. 612.
27 *Ibid.*, p. 613.
28 Roger A. Meyer, "Historical Milestones in Oral and Maxillofacial Surgery," *Journal of Oral and Maxillofacial Surgery*, 74:12 (2016), 2336–2337.
29 Nicole Elizabeth Barnes, "Health and State Making: The Expansion of State Health Services during the War of Resistance Against Japan (1937–1945)," *Twentieth-Century China*, 47:1 (2022), 60–70.
30 Barnes, "Health and State Making," p. 61; for more on the spread of public health organizations during the war, see Barnes' map illustrations on pp. 62–63.
31 *Ibid.*, p. 69.
32 The Huaxi (West China) Dental Hospital is the widely acknowledged birthplace of modern Chinese dentistry.
33 Song Ruyao, "Woguo zhengxing waike fazhan de lishi huigu" [A Historical Retrospect of Plastic Surgery in China], *Chinese Journal of Plastic and Burn Surgery*, 3:4 (1987), 241.
34 Meyer, "Historical Milestones in Oral and Maxillofacial Surgery," p. 2.
35 S. I. Rosenbaum, "The Name of Song Ruyao," *Penn Medicine*, 29:3 (2018), 30–35; Ivy's father was a British dental practitioner in Shanghai.
36 Zhang Disheng, Wang Wenhu, and Fang Mengmei, *Shenzai xing wai: Zhang Disheng zhuan* [Spirit Exists Beyond the Physical Form: The Biography of Zhang Disheng] (Shanghai: Shanghai jiaotong chuban she, 2006), p. 36.
37 Zhang Disheng et al., *Shenzai xing wai*, p. 38.
38 Jia Shurong, Zhang Zhengzhi, Ma Rong, and Li Shirong, "Dui zhongguo zhengxing meirong waike fazhan zuochu tuchu gongxian de zhuanjia xuezhe – Zhongguo zhengxing waike de dianjiren" [Prominent Experts and Scholars Who Have Made Significant Contributions to the Development of Plastic and Cosmetic Surgery in China—the Pioneers of Chinese Plastic Surgery], *Zhongguo meirong zhengxing zazhi* [Chinese Journal of Aesthetic and Plastic Surgery], 10 (2018).
39 Song Ruyao, "Woguo zhengxing waike fazhan de lishi huigu," p. 241.
40 *Ibid.*
41 Song Ruyao (ed.), *Meirong zhengxing waike xue* [Plastic and Reconstructive Surgery] (Beijing: Beijing chuban she, 1990), p. 10; Song's account mentions that a renowned American plastic surgeon

254  *The long Second World War, 1931–1953*

named Webster conducted a workshop in China, potentially referring to Dr. Richard Webster. However, further evidence is required to definitively establish this connection.

42 *Ibid.*

43 S. I. Rosenbaum, "The Name of Song Ruyao," p. 34.

44 Zhang Disheng et al., *Shenzai xing wai*, p. 63.

45 *Ibid.*, p. 63.

46 *Ibid.*, p. 64.

47 Wu Hua, Zhang Honghui, and Wang Yunbao, *Chisheng wuhui: Wang Hanzhang zhuan* [No Regret of This "Tooth" Life: The Biography of Wang Hanzhang] (Beijing: zhongguo kexue jishu chuban she, 2017), pp. 112–113.

48 Wu Hua et al., *Chisheng wuhui*, p. 116; from 1950 to 1952, there were also other medical teams, including two surgery teams from Shanghai and Nanjing that went to northeast China to treat wounded soldiers.

49 Zheng Linfan, ed., *Zhongguo kouqiangyixue fazhan shi*, p. 106; Huaxi was officially renamed Sichuan Medical College in 1953 until 1985 when it was named Huaxi Medical University again. To maintain consistency and avoid confusion, I continue to use the name Huaxi while being aware of the name shifts.

50 Song Ruyao, "Woguo zhengxing waike fazhan de lishi huigu," p. 242.

51 Wu Hua et al., *Chisheng wuhui*, p. 136.

52 For more, see Hua-Yu Li and Bernstein, Thomas P. (eds), *China Learns from the Soviet Union, 1949–Present* (New York: Rowman & Littlefield, 2010).

53 According to the online etymology dictionary, the prefix – stoma – originates from Greek and means "mouth, mouthpiece." The English word "stomatology" is derived from the French word "stomatologie."

54 Wu Hua et al., *Chisheng wuhui*, p. 131.

55 *Ibid.*

56 Wu Hua et al., *Chisheng wuhui*, p. 133.

57 In the Chinese source, his name is translated as Kesuihe (柯绥赫).

58 Zhang Yi, "Jianguo yilai wo guo kouqiang hemian chuangshang zhuanye fazhan de huigu" [A Review of the Development of Maxillofacial Surgery Since the Establishment of the PRC], *Chinese Journal of Stomatology*, 52:7 (2017), 393–399.

59 Song Ruyao (ed.), *Meirong zhengxing waike xue*, p. 10.

60 Wu Hua, *Chisheng wuhui*, p. 137.

61 Bill Hughes, "Invalidating Emotions and the Non-Disabled Imaginary: Fear, Pity, and Disgust," in Nick Watson, Alan Roulstone, and Carol Thomas (eds), *Routledge Handbook of Disability Studies* (New York: Routledge, 2019), p. 91.

# Trauma of warfare 255

62 Yang Dan, "Kangmei yuanchao zhengxing yisheng yi: zhanshi shaoshang juewang zisha" [The Memory of a "Resist the US Aid Korea" Doctor: A Desperate Burn Soldier Committed Suicide by Jumping Off the Building], *Tianfu Zaobao*, October 25, 2010.

63 *Ibid.*

64 Navin Shah, Soniya Palan, Amit Mahajan, Parshwa Shah, Rakesh Shah, and Prachur Kumar, "Why and How Maxillofacial Disability and Impairment Due to Trauma Should Be Quantified for Compensation: A Need for Nationwide Guidelines," *Journal of Maxillofacial & Oral Surgery*, 13:4 (2014), 425–430.

65 Donna Reeve, "Psycho-Emotional Disablism: The Missing Link?" in Watson, Roulstone, and Thomas (eds), *Routledge Handbook of Disability Studies*, p. 103.

66 Li Zubin (ed.), *Kouqiang hemian chuangshang zhiliao xue* [The Study of Oral and Maxillofacial Injury Treatment] (Wuhan: Hubei kexue jishu chunban she, 2002), p. 1.

67 S. I. Rosenbaum, "The Name of Song Ruyao," p. 34.

68 Suzannah Biernoff, *Portraits of Violence: War and the Aesthetics of Disfigurement* (Ann Arbor, MI: University of Michigan Press, 2017), p. 4.

69 Ding Fan and Fu Xu, "Yiliao zhengrong, miaoshou huichun: fang zhuming zhengxing waike zhuanjia, zhengxing waike yiyuan yuanzhang, Song Ruyao jiaoshou" [Medical Aesthetics: Skilled Hands Revitalizing Youth: Interview with Professor Song Ruyao, Renowned Plastic Surgeon and Director of a Plastic Surgery Hospital], *People's Daily*, June 28, 1984, A05.

70 *Ibid.*

71 S. I. Rosenbaum, "The Name of Song Ruyao."

72 Daniel M. Laskin, "Oral and Maxillofacial Surgery: The Mystery Behind the History," *Journal of Oral and Maxillofacial Surgery, Medicine, and Pathology*, 28 (2016), 101–104, at p. 104.

# 10

# Dying on enemy ground: the ICRC and the German soldiers killed in France during the Second World War

*Taline Garibian*

In 1940, as the war intensified, the question of bodies emerged.[1] Surprisingly, this did not concern the dead of the current conflict but those of the previous world war and the people taking care of their graves. Indeed, at that time, the Imperial War Grave Commission wrote to the International Committee of the Red Cross (ICRC) to enquire about the fate of the gardeners of the numerous British cemeteries – who, as foreigners, in France were interned by the Germans – and the state of those cemeteries, since their maintenance could no longer be carried out.[2] The ICRC, which carried out several visits, noted that even if in some places the graves had been damaged by shell pieces, the cemeteries were in good condition, despite the high grass.[3] This episode reflects a particular sensitivity in relation to the dead and their burial which, since the First World War, have been the subject of formalised state grave policies in many Western countries.[4]

During the interwar period, the management of war deaths was further codified by international laws. The belligerents were required to communicate to one other all the names of the dead and any information that could help in their identification. Death certificates were to be provided, burials or cremations were to be preceded by identification and a report was to be produced.[5] However, despite this legislation, managing bodies often turned out to be more complicated than expected. Post-conflict, the large number of corpses, the weaknesses of state structures and the symbolism related to human remains were all obstacles to the scrupulous application of the precepts.[6]

The emotion aroused by the poor maintenance of First World War graves underlined the gap between policies pursued in times of peace and those difficult to implement in times of war. It also demonstrates the interest of states in war cemeteries as a signifier of the collective war effort. As Paul Betts, Alon Confino and Dirk Schumann wrote about Germany, 'mass death was related to private life as much as it was to the nation and to ideology'.[7] Bodies were highly symbolic objects, and while international law required that they be treated in a dignified manner, identified and buried, these operations were complicated, both materially and politically. While historians have studied state policies regarding First and Second World War military graves and cemeteries,[8] few have investigated the treatment of enemy bodies. If 'in reality, the end of the war is fundamentally a violent time, when the hateful representations forged during the conflict are at work, either underground or openly', as stated by Bruno Cabanes and Guillaume Piketty,[9] one can imagine that the fate of the bodies of the enemies was an important stake at the end of the war, materially and symbolically.

In this chapter, I examine the work of the ICRC and its delegation in France after the war to stimulate the efforts of the French authorities in the handling of German corpses located on their soil, and to supplement them where possible. I show that the policy of the French state reveals a modest interest in the enemy corps and a temptation to delegate their handling to private or, possibly, communal entities. For its part, the ICRC's initiative seems to extend both the work already begun with the dead bodies of the First World War and its activities to help prisoners of war, particularly in terms of tracing. While religion usually plays an important role in funeral treatments, the sources consulted here are relatively silent on the subject. This might be interpreted as a proof of the determination of state and humanitarian actors to place their actions within a secular framework. Overall, I argue that the failures of France and the willingness of the ICRC in this matter reflect different views of the corpses, what purpose they should serve and, above all, in what time frame. On the one hand, a dominant vision within state structures was that the bodies must serve the national narrative of the sacrifice of the victors. On the other hand, a more common approach in non-governmental organisations was to be more attentive to the individual value of the bodies, viewing them

258     *The long Second World War, 1931–1953*

as exempt from political significance and focusing on the mourning of loved ones, which required action to be taken as quickly as possible.

## Who cares for the enemies' corpses?

In the aftermath of the war, it was the duty of France to locate the bodies or graves of the soldiers who died on its soil, including those of the Germans, care for the graves and provide Germany with all the necessary information on this subject. Early on, French authorities anticipated this issue and took measures concerning the management of soldiers' bodies and their burials, some of which also concerned enemy corpses.[10] After the war, the country adopted further regulations to deal with this matter. The United States and the United Kingdom for their part were responsible for bodies in their area. An agreement between the President of the Provisional Government of the French Republic and the Allied authorities stipulated that the British and the Americans would proceed with the burial of German soldiers, killed by their armies, according to their zones of operation.[11] These regulations, which required the authorities to treat the bodies of the enemy army the same as those of the national army, would have been difficult to apply, given that distinguishing the bodies was one of the concerns of the Resistance fighters when they reclaimed control of the ground.[12] As early as July 1945, the ICRC was concerned about the arrangements made by the French regarding this issue. Already experienced in the tracing of prisoners of war during the First World War, the ICRC was probably also prompted to act by the demands it received from Germany. Moreover, in the absence of a sovereign German state, it assumed the role of protective power for German prisoners of war (PoWs).[13]

An ICRC report dated 13 September 1945 detailed the procedure followed by the French authorities. The tombs, which were often scattered, were being located and listed and the exhumation was planned for November. In the case of identified bodies, a death certificate would be issued and sent to the registry office. For those who remained unidentified, a report of exhumation would be made.[14] According to Bonnet, the Director of the *Service Central de l'Etat civil, des successions et des sépultures militaires*, around

50 per cent of the bodies were unidentifiable. The identification procedure relied partially on the work of the municipalities in charge of locating and gathering the scattered tombs located on their territories. As much as it responded to international standards, this policy was a form of territory as well as mourning management. After the war, French authorities took measures to avoid communal cemeteries being used for German bodies, although exceptions were possible for a small number of bodies, that is, five at most. In 1946, they also specified that no German cemetery resulting from the fighting could remain on private or communal property unless it was already integrated into a communal cemetery.[15]

While the procedures seemed to be clearly planned, there appears to have been some delay, since in the summer of 1946, the ICRC expressed its concerns on this subject to its Delegation in Paris. This delay was particularly unfortunate in the eyes of the ICRC because the more time that passed, the more difficult it was to locate the tombs and identify the soldiers. It was also pointed out that in Italy, a specialized team of German PoWs had been working for several months to identify the graves of German soldiers, in order to group them together and maintain the cemeteries.[16] Obviously, the corpses of German soldiers were not the first concern of the French authorities. Pierre Boissier, a legal expert and delegate attached to the Paris Delegation, had little doubt in this regard. 'He has seen that the service that deals with this issue shows ill will and slowness.'[17] The goodwill of the French official responsible for the task was clearly in doubt. 'It seems that Mr [Pierre-Cyrille] Lavaud is doing just enough to ensure that it cannot be said that he is not dealing with this problem.'[18] In addition to the bodies, the service dealt with successions, and here too, there was a significant delay, since the service was still dealing with the cases of French people who died during the First World War. The successions of the fifty-five thousand Germans who died in action or in captivity in France were therefore not ready to be settled, and Boissier estimated that this task would not commence for another two years.[19]

The ICRC, therefore, sent a note to its delegates in France recommending that they monitor the process and, as far as possible, pass on information to the countries requesting it. The task was complicated since many tombs had been hastily dug, were often not very deep and were located along the roads. They were marked

260    *The long Second World War, 1931–1953*

with wood with a helmet on top, to which was attached an identity plate. However, this layout probably did not last very long. 'Given the state of mind that prevailed during the first months after the liberation, it is certain that in most cases these graves could not be maintained, it was dangerous for a civilian to want to take care of the thing. Little by little the helmets were removed, as well as the objects, which were considered by the civilians to be collectors' items.'[20] By May 1947, the Geneva Committee seemed a little more optimistic about the work of the French than its Delegation based in Paris. It noted: 'This French government agency [the *Service de l'Etat civil et des recherches du Ministère des Anciens Combattants et Victimes de la Guerre*], is engaged in issuing death notices of German servicemen who fell during the fighting in the French campaign.'[21] This goodwill did not appear to be shared by all bodies, as the civil authorities, who were responsible for grouping the graves, still seemed uncooperative. According to the Paris delegation they were 'totally uninterested in this question', partly for financial reasons, but also because of the 'still very marked antipathy of the population towards the Germans'.[22]

In fact, the ICRC very soon took on a task that it had never undertaken previously. Faced with the number of requests for information that it received from next of kin at the end of the war, it took the decision to send information on the deaths of soldiers directly to German families.[23] Besides this work, it lobbied France to put in place a clear policy for the transmission of death notices and, if necessary, for the search for bodies and identification. However, the scope of its intervention was subject to debate within the organisation itself. During a meeting of ICRC delegates in France, held in September 1947, several positions were expressed, revealing the different sensibilities coexisting within the organization. As William Michel explained: 'If the French authorities fail to act, the ICRC cannot take their place. It does not have the material and financial means to do so, and if it did, it would have to set them aside to relieve the living PoW.'[24] A lengthy discussion, which was not recorded in the minutes, took place to establish whether the ICRC should be more actively involved in this work. Finally, while the delegates noted that something urgently needed to be done, they, except for R. Roth and Emile Filliettaz who favoured a more substantive intervention, agreed that this was not a role for the ICRC.

# Dying on enemy ground    261

The ICRC used the example of Italy, where a German commission, the *Deutsche Gräberfürsorge*,[25] looked after the graves of German nationals, to persuade France to allow a similar initiative. Of course, the situation in Italy was very different from that in France; as a former ally of Germany, it was far less reluctant to have a German organisation working on its soil. The committee was in contact with the unit based in Italy and could send a delegate to set up a similar team in France, who would have knowledge of how such a unit should be implemented in this country.[26] But the Paris Delegation was also faced with the difficulties caused by a lack of clarity within the French administration regarding who should take on this role. These difficulties were compounded by the lack of financial resources devoted to this type of work.[27] This last point prompted the ICRC to request a contribution from the German PoWs themselves. Moreover, the ICRC pointed out that the sooner the work began in France, the easier it would be to mobilize the German PoWs still present on the territory.

> We assume that there must be among the POWs held under French control, elements having belonged in the German Army, to the units [taking care] of the graves and who would be able to accomplish with full knowledge of the facts, the work which would be required of them. Regardless of the technical nature of this question, we are of the opinion that it would be preferable to ask German soldiers to take a census and group together the graves of their comrades, because, for reasons that are easy to understand, they would bring more interest and precision to this task than the French authorities.[28]

After several meetings requested by the ICRC Delegation in Paris with the various competent French authorities to fulfil these obligations, a global exhumation plan emerged. With a budget of almost 1 billion francs, the plan was primarily devised to exhume the bodies of the French; however, the costs for the research and maintenance of German graves were also taken from this budget. The *Ministère des Anciens Combattants* intended to create German military cemeteries, either adjacent to certain municipal cemeteries or created from the outset. In any case, these would be large cemeteries, able to group together bodies scattered over several departments.[29]

If this plan were to be positively received in Geneva, the international committee would not fail to remind its Parisian delegation

262 *The long Second World War, 1931–1953*

that the identification and processing of successions were also essential. The gathering of bodies and the maintenance of cemeteries were tasks that the French could hardly avoid, as the presence of graves scattered over the territory was likely to make it difficult to return to normal daily life. On the other hand, the identification of bodies could appear to be a secondary task, even a luxury offered to former enemies. Moreover, German soldiers were equipped with identification plates on which only a number appeared and not their full name, making the tracing of identities more complex. The committee was well aware of the difficulties that could arise for the identification of bodies and the issuing of death certificates.

> We are also ready to receive lists of such numbers, which we could forward to the WAST [Wehrmachtsauskunftstelle] to provide us in return with the nominal indications that could be used later to indicate on the grave who is buried there, and to establish by the same a complete report or death certificate that could be used by the family. In fact, it seems to us that it is not enough to gather graves, it is also necessary that this work brings a practical result, that of knowing who was exhumed.[30]

Although in the eyes of the ICRC the French work on the German bodies was too slow, Paul Thomas, an ICRC delegate, acknowledged that the situation was no better regarding the French corpses.[31] In a report produced in March 1948, he admitted that many French bodies remained to be exhumed and reburied. 'In short, the problem of regrouping German graves is more advanced than the problem of French graves, especially since a recent law grants perpetual concessions to French soldiers and civilians killed during the Liberation battles, which brings the total number of French graves to be regrouped from 150,000 to 300,000.'[32] Ironically, France also depended on the Germans to find the bodies of certain soldiers, such as those from Alsace–Lorraine, forcibly enrolled in the Wehrmacht and who died in France in German uniforms. In a letter dated June 1948, the *Ministère des Anciens Combattants et Victimes de la Guerre*, addressed the German authorities to request that the lists of dead German soldiers that he sent them be processed quickly and that the names of any Alsatians appearing on them be communicated to him as soon as possible.[33]

In the first years following the conflict, the management of the bodies was thus deficient. The absence of a German sovereign state undoubtedly favoured the intervention of the ICRC, including in the field, even if the relevance of this action was debated even within the organisation. This evolution reflects the growing intervention of private actors as well as municipalities in the management of the bodies and the memorialisation of the conflict to the detriment of the state. This shift was also visible in the field of the politics of remembrance and commemorative plaques in France. It can partially be explained by the lack of resource of the central state.[34] The slowness with which the French authorities acted was in fact more the result of a shortage of means. This approach, which was more bureaucratic than humanitarian, did not reflect a real aversion to the idea of offering a burial for former enemies. Indeed, as early as 1945, the communist newspaper *L'Humanité* denounced the presence of swastikas on the graves of certain German soldiers who had died during the occupation and were buried by their compatriots. The newspaper reported that the Ministry of Veterans Affairs was reluctant to have these symbols removed in the name of respect for military graves.[35]

## Scattered corpses and differing practices

This absence of a central policy led to a diversity of practices. Faced with what it considered the apathy of the French authorities, the ICRC urged the chaplains and trusted men in the PoW camps to gather as much information as possible on the location of the graves and the identity of the deceased, and to pass this on to the Geneva agency, hoping that this kind of initiative would put pressure on the French. In the Drôme and Ardèche departments, for example, the PoWs from the Montélimar camp carried out searches and maintained some tombs. They were able to locate 679 tombs, where lay identified bodies and 700 unidentified corpses, some of whom remained in mass graves.[36] During a visit, the delegate of the ICRC in Lyon acknowledged the work that had been done and asked that copies of the lists of PoWs or soldiers buried, as well as the sketches of isolated graves, be sent to Geneva.[37]

264     *The long Second World War, 1931–1953*

A meeting held in Annecy on the work done in Haute-Savoie in August 1947 revealed that the French authorities had not yet implemented a clear policy and procedure in the search for German corpses and tombs. Several administrative military entities worked in parallel, and their results were not always consistent. The work was complicated by the circumstances in which many German soldiers died, as in Vieugy, where forty executed German soldiers lay in a mass grave. The *Forces Frances de l'Intérieur* (FFI) refused to allow them to be buried in coffins. The bodies were probably no longer identifiable and only the combatants who carried out the execution could have given information regarding their identities, but these combatants used pseudonyms and were themselves unidentified.[38] In some regions, the French Red Cross was also involved in the exhumations. This was, for example, the case regarding the exhumation of four German soldiers killed in the maquis at Haute-Rivoire in the Rhone department. Frère Benoît, head of the exhumation team of the Red Cross, was accompanied by the German chaplains from depot 141 of Saint-Fons.[39]

The exhumations and transfers of corpses in the *Département de l'Orne* were described in a detailed report produced by Paul Thomas in October 1947;[40] Thomas was the ICRC delegate for the 3rd military region, which covered the northwest area of France.[41] He rapidly became a respected interlocutor of the committee in relation to the graves, particularly because the region in which he was located had been the scene of many battles.

According to Thomas, the *Ministère des Anciens Combattants et Victimes de la Guerre* (Ministry of Veteran's Affairs and War Victims) was behind the operation which aimed to group together the graves of German soldiers. At the time of writing, some one thousand bodies had already been exhumed and transferred to a cemetery in Gorron, created by the Americans, and Paul Thomas estimated that a further four thousand were still to be exhumed. Thomas noted that, in some cases, only bones remained, while in others the decomposition of the bodies was not yet complete. Identification was made by the inscriptions on the cross if they were readable, the identity plate if there was one or by the presence of documents kept in a bottle in the immediate vicinity of the body. Several years after the end of hostilities, few indicators remained,

*Dying on enemy ground* 265

and many bodies were no longer identifiable. The commando in charge of proceeding to the exhumation was divided into three teams. The first exhumed the cadaver or human remains; the second put the bodies in coffins that were divided in two by a partition, each coffin containing the remains of two people for transport purposes. Finally, the secretarial team registered all the information available regarding the identity of the dead bodies. Once transferred to the cemetery, the bodies were placed in individual coffins, except for the unidentified corpses found in a common grave, which were also reburied together. According to Thomas, the commando was able to undertake forty to sixty exhumations per day. In another communication regarding the efforts made in the department of La Manche, Thomas informed the ICRC that in this department, more than half of the German graves located outside the cemeteries had been registered. In addition, the delegate estimated that 70 per cent of the bodies were still identifiable.[42]

In another report on the situation in the north and west of France, dated only a couple of weeks later, Thomas noted that the Americans had essentially finished their task of burying the German soldiers. ' "The American Graves Registration Command", created in the departments of the Manche, of Finistère, of the Mayenne and of the Eure, registered several German cemeteries containing around 25,000 tombs.'[43] The maintenance of these cemeteries was then transferred to the French authorities. The same report noted that the British had just resumed this work after the French had reminded them of the agreement made. It is worth pointing out that the bodies were subject to different policies within the Allied armies. The Americans put considerable effort into identifying their own. 'We were able to see the extreme care taken by the American authorities in identifying the remains of their soldiers. After exhumation of the bodies or what was left of them, the bones were cleaned, embalmed and scientifically measured. The identification research continues down to the smallest details: dentition, body features, etc. are scrupulously noted.'[44] By contrast, the British army seemed less meticulous: 'Isolated British graves – in accordance with the English law that British servicemen who have fallen on foreign soil are not exhumed but remain in situ – will remain in the communal cemeteries.'[45]

266    *The long Second World War, 1931–1953*

Regarding the German corpses, Thomas was concerned about the following up of indicators which could reveal the identity of the deceased.

> For the time being, PoWs are busy with the exhumation work itself and can therefore accurately and unmistakably record the indications on a cross or an identity plate found on the remains. However, once this information is passed from the commando of PoWs who carry out the exhumation work to the higher level who centralise the information for one or more departments, there are no longer PoWs but French people whose qualifications for this kind of work are not always certain.[46]

These kinds of difficulties were also prevalent in Italy, where Italian workers, unable to read the German gothic script often used in funerary inscriptions, made errors. Moreover, from December 1948 onwards, no more German PoWs were held on French soil. As the French now had to deal with the regrouping and maintenance of the graves and sometimes even the exhumations, one of the prisoners' representatives of the Douai depot wrote to the ICRC to ask them to take over.[47]

The work of the ICRC is at the intersection of several issues and encroaches on sensitive areas, such as the execution of Germans during the liberation, who were buried in mass graves. 'We have been approached by several families and even the German Red Cross with cases such as the 16 German soldiers in a mass grave in St Julien [near] Bergerac, Dordogne. In such cases, we believe that sending an enquiry to the city hall, to a Depot, or directly to the DGPG, would not lead to any result.'[48] The organisation's policy remains very cautious with regard to such cases. 'It is not our role in investigating matters to justify the reasons why executions were carried out at the time of the liberation of France. All we want is to be able to answer questions about such cases.'[49] The ICRC, anxious not to get involved in a more political field, is careful to limit itself to the search for bodies, their identification and the transmission of information to German authorities.

Although a legal obligation and a state mission, the management of bodies was therefore characterised by a multitude of actors with varying practices. Like in the aftermath of the First World War, this gave rise to obvious abuses, such as when a French contractor

# Dying on enemy ground

267

maltreated bodies in order to split them up to artificially increase the number of cases treated.[50]

## The mission of Paul Thomas

By September 1948, Paul Thomas had located more than fifteen thousand tombs or common graves on French territory, focusing on those situated on private grounds, as well as those situated in military or communal cemeteries that had already been identified.[51] By the end of 1948, the ICRC confirmed the identity of nearly seventy thousand bodies and this information was passed on to the German *Gräberfürsorge*. At the beginning of 1949, the committee decided to support the efforts of Paul Thomas by commissioning him to produce a report on the exhumation and reburial of German soldiers' bodies throughout France, the number of which was estimated to be two hundred thousand.[52] Obviously, this was not only a question of collecting information and monitoring the work carried out by the French; more importantly, it was a matter of exerting a certain pressure so that this work was not neglected. As Eugène de Weck explained at a meeting held in Geneva in the presence of Thomas and the representatives of the *Gräberfürsorge*: 'The role of the ICRC delegate is not only to collect lists himself, but by his activity and presence to draw the attention of the French authorities to the problem of German graves in France and thereby to activate the solution.'[53]

The mission's tasks included locating the cemeteries where German combatants or PoWs were buried, contacting the local authorities responsible for the conservation of these cemeteries, assessing the progress of the work and forwarding the information to the *Gräberfürsorge*.[54] Finally, instead of a six-month mandate, the model of one-month specific missions was finally adopted. By 14 June, two reports had been produced covering the situation in more than fifteen departments. However, the mission was not pursued, and it was claimed to be mainly on account of financial reasons. Nevertheless, the ICRC did not fail to put pressure on Germany to contribute to the costs of such work. During a meeting held in Geneva, it was indeed agreed that Thomas would not go, as planned, to the southeast and would first visit the headquarters

268 *The long Second World War, 1931–1953*

of the *Gräberfürsorge*, to let the German administration know that the mission could not continue without additional funding.[55] This strategy worked, since during the meeting between the committee and the German entities, held in Geneva in September 1949, the Germans agreed to cover the costs of Thomas's mission.

However, Thomas seemed to face the same problems as before, as the French authorities still proved to be overwhelmed. In November 1949, he explained: 'In some departments in the Paris region, in response to my request, I was given some documents in the form of notebooks for consultation. These notebooks contained lists of German graves from the 1914–1918 war (!). It was then explained to me that for the 1939–1945 lists, the town halls would be notified, we would see, we would be written to, etc.'[56] Nevertheless, in some cases, Thomas praised the efforts made, especially in the Lyon region, where Frère Benoît and volunteers from the Red Cross were active.[57]

By February 1950, Thomas's mission had made it possible to communicate the identity of 150,000 Germans to the *Gräberfürsorge*.[58] However, the fact remains that this mission, which essentially consisted of collecting information on the graves, their location and the identity of the Germans buried there, was largely dependent on the French services that carried out the exhumations. In this respect, the situation was not much better in the early 1950s. In addition to a general lack of resources, Thomas complained of a lack of communication between the different administrations and levels. Moreover, the officials of the *Ministère des Anciens Combattants et Victimes de la Guerre* were overwhelmed. Charged with grouping together the 400,000 bodies of Frenchmen who died during the liberation, minimal efforts were made to recover the enemy dead – a situation which, according to Thomas, could be explained by the anti-German tendencies that persisted in France, as had already been noticed a few years earlier. 'There is still in some quarters a feeling of mute, invisible, sometimes malevolent resistance to anything that has to do with the German label.'[59]

The extent of the work to be done in terms of the handling of the French bodies, as well as the tensions between France and Germany, also explained the reluctance of the French to repatriate to Germany the remains of soldiers claimed by their families. When the question arose in 1949, the French were far from having completed the repatriation of the bodies of their compatriots who had died in Germany; nor had they carried out all the internal transfers of those who had died in France or North Africa. Furthermore, by 1950 they also had to deal with the return of the bodies of their soldiers who died in Indochina.[60] Thomas therefore considered it 'doubtful' that they would accept the repatriation of Germans.[61] Faced with these difficulties, the ICRC, which regularly acted as an intermediary between German families and the French authorities, was entrusted with funeral tasks, such as when a German father, through the help of a Swiss acquaintance, sent the ICRC plates to be affixed to the graves of his son and three of his comrades, who died in France.[62]

In fact, it was not until 1954 that France and Germany signed an agreement on the burial of German soldiers.[63] It ratified the fact that the German government delegated to the *Gräberfürsorge* the responsibility of managing the German cemeteries in France and therefore formalised their maintenance by assigning this responsibility to the German organisation. In 1966, a second convention on the burial of the soldiers of 1914–1918 and those of 1939–1945 was signed by Charles de Gaulle at the ceremony marking the fiftieth anniversary of the battle of Verdun. While many of its principles had already been formulated in the 1954 agreement, this convention reflected a desire to make the graves an element of remembrance. The text provided for a 50 per cent discount on train tickets in France for relatives of the German deceased who wished to visit their graves in France. This offer was limited to one thousand people per year.[64] This agreement thus indicated a new stage in the Franco-German reconciliation and gave the enemy's graves and cemetery an importance that they had never known before. It also corresponded well to the desire expressed by de Gaulle at the end of the conflict to associate the two world wars and to combine their remembrance.[65]

## Corpses: between national and international borders

In contrast to its role of intermediary in the matter of graves during the First World War, the ICRC clearly stepped into the field following the Second World War. Its delegate travelled the country

270  *The long Second World War, 1931–1953*

to assess the progress of its work, draft reports and meet state agencies. The corpses of the conflict were thus quickly caught up in two different logics with their own temporalities. Faced with the demands of German families, the ICRC engaged in lobbying French authorities, who were already struggling to manage their own dead. This humanitarian approach, oriented towards the relatives and the grieving processes, did not fit in well with the logic of the French state, constrained by financial and logistical imperatives. For the French state, German bodies were certainly not a priority, and their management was more a matter of territorial management than of mourning. This changed when the graves served the Franco-German reconciliation narrative.

In the late 1940s, the drafting of an international convention regarding the issue of missing persons and death certificates began. More specific than the existing regulations, this aimed to establish a framework for the transmission of declarations of death between the parties involved in the conflict, thus providing an administrative solution for missing persons whose bodies would probably never be found or identified. This can certainly be explained by the difficulties encountered in identifying dead soldiers, sometimes exhumed several years after their death, despite the measures taken since the First World War, such as the generalisation of detachable double identity plates. As the question of bodies became a humanitarian issue, the ICRC did not fail to promote its competences. While a first version of the text proposed the creation of an international death notification office, the ICRC was concerned that its acclaimed offices would not be called upon, since the Central Prisoners of War Agency had already taken on part of this work. When consulted, the ICRC reiterated its willingness to take on this role. It also proposed amendments to broaden – or to make less political – several points in the text; for example, it proposed to replace the wording 'Whereas military events and racial, political or religious persecutions during the Second World War caused the disappearance of persons whose deaths cannot be ascertained with certainty' with 'Whereas events and persecutions caused the disappearance of persons whose deaths cannot be ascertained with certainty.'[66] The ICRC justified this approach by pointing out that the first phrasing drafted by the Preparatory Commission for the International Refugee Organization – probably on the basis of the cases with

Dying on enemy ground 271

which it had dealt – could result in the omission of a number of missing persons.

Clearly, the ICRC advocated a broad understanding of the issue that went beyond the strict confines of the military sphere of responsibility, and this approach made it a key stakeholder in the process. But it also had the effect of promoting a depoliticised view of bodies as mere objects to be handed over to families, rather than a political vehicle for state communication. Notably, the ICRC suggested the implementation of scientific or medical tools – such as the Bertillon method or the recording of soldiers' skull X-rays – to facilitate soldiers' identification.[67] However, the conference considered that it was the responsibility of each country to make its own arrangements in this matter, indicating the limits of the humanitarian organisation's approach. The corpses' management and handling were still to remain a prerogative of the state and its military organisation.

## Notes

1 The research for this chapter was generously funded by the Swiss National Science Foundation (n. 100011_220032).
2 Archives of the ICRC (hereafter ACICR), B G 035_007, Letter from Fabien Ware to the ICRC, 9 April 1941. According to Ware, there were more than 400,000 British soldiers' graves in France at that time, most of them being in the occupied part of France.
3 ACICR, B G 035_007, Note entitled: Cimetières anglais et canadiens de la Guerre 14–18 en France occupée, visités au début de juin 1941 par les délégués du CICR, Paris, 8 June 1941.
4 See, for example, Philip Longworth, *The Unending Vigil: A History of the Commonwealth War Graves Commission, 1917–1969* (London: Constable, 1967), Laura Tradii, '"Their Dear Remains Belong to Us Alone": Soldiers' Bodies, Commemoration, and Cultural Responses to Exhumations After the Great War', *First World War Studies*, 10:2–3 (2019), 245–261; Antoine Prost, 'Les cimetières militaires de la Grande Guerre, 1914–1940', *Le Mouvement social*, 237:4 (2011), 135–151; Annette Becker and Stéphane Tison (eds), *Un siècle de sites funéraires de la Grande Guerre* (Nanterre: Presses universitaires de Paris Nanterre, 2018). Of course, many human remains could never be identified and the killed in action were never found, which motivated the development of a new burial practice: the creation of graves to honour the unknown soldier.

272  *The long Second World War, 1931–1953*

5 Convention for the Amelioration of the Condition of the Wounded and Sick in Armies in the Field, signed in Geneva in July 1929, article 4.

6 See, for example, Jean-Marc Dreyfus, 'Remettre les corps en place à la Libération: exhumations, identifications et transferts après 1944', *Guerres mondiales et conflits contemporains*, 285:1 (2022), 129–147.

7 Paul Betts, Alon Confino and Dirk Schumann, 'Introduction: Death and Twentieth-Century Germany', in Paul Betts, Alon Confino and Dirk Schumann (eds), *Between Mass Death and Individual Loss: The Place of the Dead in Twentieth-Century Germany* (New York and Oxford: Berghahn Books, 2008), p. 4.

8 See, for example, Serge Barcellini and AnnetteWierviorka, *Passant, souviens-toi! Les lieux de souvenir de la Seconde Guerre mondiale en France* (Paris: Editions Graphein, 1999); Serge Barcellini, 'La gestion du deuil par l'État français au lendemain de la Seconde Guerre mondiale', in Francine-Dominique Liechtenhan (ed.), *Europe 1946. Entre le deuil et l'espoir* (Brussels: Éditions Complexe, 1996); Luc Capdevila and Danièle Voldman, 'Rituels funéraires de société en guerre (1914–1945)', in Stéphane Audoin-Rouzeau, Annette Becker, Christian Ingrao and Henry Rousso (eds), *La Violence de guerre 1914–1945* (Brussels: Editions Complexe, 2002).

9 Bruno Cabanes and Guillaume Piketty, 'Sortir de la guerre: jalons pour une histoire en chantier', *Histoire@politique*, 3:3 (2007), 1.

10 Décret concernant les lieux de sépulture à établir pour les soldats des armées françaises et alliées "morts pour la France" au cours d'opérations de guerre, JORF, 25 February 1940, pp. 1390–1391.

11 ACICR, B G 035_014, Report on the graves of German soldiers, written by Paul Thomas, 27 February 1948.

12 See Dreyfus, 'Remettre les corps'.

13 Fabien Théofilakis, *Les prisonniers de guerre Allemands. France, 1944–1949. Une captivité de guerre en temps de paix* (Paris: Fayard, 2014), p. 68.

14 ACICR, B G 035_011, Rapport. Visite du 13 septembre 1945 au Service Centre de l'État civil des successions et des sépultures militaires.

15 'Regroupement des tombes des militaires américains et des militaires allemands tués au cours des combats livrés par les troupes américaines', 30 April 1946, in *Bulletin officiel de la ville de Paris*, 4 May 1946, p. 833.

16 ACICR, B G 035_01, Letter from Barbey to M. Michel, 7 August 1946.

17 ACICR, B G 035_011, Minutes of the meeting between P. Boissier and E. de Weck, 9 September 1946. All quotations are translated from French by the author.

# Dying on enemy ground 273

18 ACICR, B G 035_011, Minutes of the meeting between P. Boissier and E. de Weck, 9 September 1946.

19 ACICR, B G 035_011, Minutes of the meeting between P. Boissier and E. de Weck, 9 September 1946. It is difficult to say what this figure of fifty-five thousand mentioned by P. Boissier corresponds to, as it may only be the cases currently identified and processed by the French administration. In fact, according to Fabien Théofilakis, the number of Germans who died in French captivity is about forty thousand, to which must be added those who died during the liberation. See Théofilakis, *Les prisonniers*, p. 96.

20 ACICR, B G 035_011, Letter from the Paris Delegation to the ICRC, 1 October 1946.

21 ACICR, G 8/51 XIX, Letter from E. de Weck to the Paris Delegation, 29 May 1947.

22 ACICR, G 8/51 XX, Note from the Paris Delegation to the ICRC, 27 August 1947.

23 ACICR, G 8/51 XX, Note to the ICRC Delegation in Paris, 18 July 1947.

24 ACICR, G 8/51 XXI, Minutes of the meeting of the ICRC delegates in France, 22, 23 and 24 September 1947.

25 The *Volksbund Deutsche Kriegsgräberfürsorge* or People's Association for the Maintenance of German War Graves was a private organisation, close to right-wing groups, created in 1919 to care for the graves of German soldiers. For more information about its history during the interwar period, see Johann Zilien, 'Der "Volksbund Deutsche Kriegsgraeberfuersorge e. V." in der Weimarer Republik', *Archiv für Kulturgeschichte*, 75:2 (1993), 445–478.

26 ACICR, B G 035_011, Letter from E. de Weck to the Paris Delegation, 7 July 1947.

27 ACICR, B G 035_011, Letter from the Paris Delegation (R. Roth) to the ICRC, 11 July 1947.

28 ACICR, B G 035_011, Letter from E. de Weck to the Paris Delegation, 19 November 1947.

29 ACICR, B G 035_012, Document from the Delegation of the ICRC in France to the ICRC, 9 February 1948.

30 ACICR, B G 035_012, Note à la Délégation du CICR à Paris, 19 February 1948. The Wehrmachtsauskunftstelle was a German agency created in 1939, whose task was to keep records of German soldiers.

31 On the exhumation of French soldiers and Resistance fighters see: Dreyfus, 'Remettre les corps'.

32 ACICR, B G 035_016, '*Gräberfürsorge*' Rapport concernant les tombes des combattants allemands inhumés en France, Guerre

274 *The long Second World War, 1931–1953*

1939–1945, Paul Thomas, 18 March 1949, pp. 10–11. Later estimations put the number of French bodies to be exhumed at 400,000.

33 ACICR, B G 035_016, Letter from the Ministry of Veteran's Affairs and War Victims, 16 June 1948.

34 Olivier Wieviorka, *La mémoire désunie. Le souvenir politique des années sombres, de la Libération à nos jours* (Paris: Editions du Seuil, 2010), p. 111.

35 'Tout le monde le pense, L'Huma le dit!', *L'Humanité*, 17 November 1945, p. 1. On German cemeteries created in France during the occupation, see Nina Janz, 'From Battleground to Burial Grounds – The Cemetery Landscapes of the German Army during the Second World War', in Sarah K. Danielsson and Frank Jacob (eds), *War and Geography. The Spatiality of Organized Mass Violence* (Paderborn: Ferdinand Schöningh, 2017), pp. 147–162.

36 ACICR, B G 035_011, Translation of an article published in the journal of the camp of the DPG 147 in Montélimar, probably in August or September 1947.

37 ACICR, B G 035_011, Letter from Emile Fillietaz to the ICRC, 18 November 1947.

38 ACICR, B G 035_011, Rapport pour la direction de l'Agence, dated 1 September 1947.

39 ACICR, B G 035_012, Letter from the ICRC to E. Fillietaz, 24 July 1948.

40 ACICR, B G 035_011, Rapport concernant l'exhumation et le transfert des dépouilles des combattant allemands tombés dans le département de l'Orne, établi par P. Thomas, délégué CICR, 25 October 1947.

41 These military regions were established by decree on 18 February 1946. The 3rd region, with its headquarters in Rennes, included the following departments: Ille-et-Vilaine, Côtes-du-Nord, Calvados, Manche, Sarthe, Mayenne, Orne, Morbihan, Finistère, Loire inférieure, Maine-et-Loire, Vendée.

42 ACICR, B G 035_012, Note to the ICRC Delegation in Paris, 19 February 1948.

43 ACICR, B G 035_014, Report on the graves of German Soldiers written by Paul Thomas, 27 February 1949.

44 *Ibid.*

45 *Ibid.*

46 ACICR, B G 035_014, Minutes of meeting between P. Thomas and E. de Weck, 8 March 1948.

47 ACICR, B G 035_012, Letter from Bayerer to the ICRC, 19 November 1948.

*Dying on enemy ground* 275

48 ACICR, G 8/51 XXI, Note to the ICRC Delegation in Paris, 12 December 1947.

49 *Ibid.*

50 'L'entrepreneur d'inhumation menait la grande vie en multipliant à coup de pelle le nombre de ses clients', *Libration. Le Quotidien républicain de Paris*, 5 March 1951, p. 5. On the misdeeds of the management of the bodies of the First World War, see Béatrix Pau, *Le Ballet des morts État, armée, familles: s'occuper des corps de la Grande Guerre* (Paris: La librarie Vuibert, 2016).

51 ACICR, G 8/51 XXV, Minutes of the meeting between the ICRC delegates in France, held in Paris on 27 and 28 September 1948.

52 ACICR, B G 035_014, Report compiled by P. Thomas for the year 1949, 7 January 1950.

53 ACICR, B G 035_018, Minutes of the meeting held between the representative of the *Volksbund Deutsche Kriegsgräberfürsorge e. V.* and the ICRC, 12 September 1949. If the *Volksbund Deutsche Kriegsgräberfürsorge* was not able to operate directly in France, the ICRC remained in close contact with it despite its 'hasty' denazification and a tendency to equate the fate of victims of Nazism with that of German soldiers. See David Livingstone, 'Remembering on Foreign Soil: The Activities of the German War Graves Commission', in Bill Niven and Chloe Paver (eds), *Memorialisation in Germany since 1945* (Basingstoke and New York: Palgrave Macmillan, 2010).

54 ACICR, B G 035_014, Note from the Paris Delegation to the ICRC, 3 March 1949.

55 ACICR, B G 035_014, Note from Graz to Thomas, 23 June 1949.

56 ACICR, G 8/51 XXVI, Note from the Paris Delegation to the ICRC, 10 November 1949.

57 *Ibid.*

58 ACICR, B G 035_014, Rapport (No. 6), de Mr Paul Thomas, délégués du CICR sur la situation des cimetières et des tombes allemandes de la guerre 1940–1945 en France, February 1950.

59 ACICR, B G 035_014, Rapport de Mr Paul Thomas, sur son activité dans le recensement et le regroupement des disparus militaires en France, 15 June 1950. In an article published in 2002, Luc Capdevila and Danièle Voldman noted that the Armed Forces Service estimated that in France 10 to 15 per cent of the soldiers who fell between 1939 and 1945 were still missing or unidentified. See: Luc Capdevila and Danièle. Voldman, 'Du numéro matricule au code génétique: la manipulation du corps des tués de la guerre enquête d'identité', *International Review of the Red Cross*, 84:848 (2022), 760.

276 *The long Second World War, 1931–1953*

60 ACICR, G 8/51 XXVII, Rapport de M. Paul Thomas, Délégué du CICR sur son activité dans le recensement et le regroupement des disparus militaires en France, Paris, 15 June 1950.

61 ACICR, B G 035_015, Information reported by E. de Weck in a note, 15 March 1949.

62 ACICR, B G 035_015, Note to the Paris Delegation, 28 April 1950.

63 Convention conclue entre le gouvernement de la République française et le gouvernement de la République fédérale d'Allemagne relative aux sépultures militaire de la guerre de 1939–1945, 23 October 1954.

64 Convention conclue entre le gouvernement de la République française et le gouvernement de la République fédérale d'Allemagne relative aux sépultures de guerre allemandes en territoire français, 19 July 1966.

65 Wieviorka, *La mémoire désunie*.

66 ACICR, D EUR France 1 – 0703, Note de la Division Juridique du CICR sur l'"Avant-projet de Convention internationale concernant la déclaration de décès des personnes disparues', 11 October 1948.

67 Rapport sur les travaux de la Conférence préliminaire des Sociétés nationales de la Croix-Rouge pour l'étude des Conventions et de divers problèmes ayant trait à la Croix-Rouge, *International Review of the Red Cross*, 28:335 (1946), 879–940.

# Index

The 1951 Refugee Convention 14

Agier, Michel 111
Aglan, Alya 5
*Agrupación de Guerrilleros
    Españoles* 189
Ajlec, Kornelija 110
Al-Arish 117
Alcantara, Rito 94
Alderidge, Frederick F. 121
Alderson, Nik 31
*Alerta en la frontera (Border
    Alert), film* 163, 167
Algeria 95, 183
Al-Khatabta 118
American Graves Registration
    Command 265
Alsace–Lorraine 180, 182,
    183, 262
American Association of Oral and
    Plastic Surgeons 240
American Bureau of Medical Aids
    to China 242
American Friends Service
    Committee 7, 178
American military 206, 209
American Negro Exposition 212
American Relief Administration 6
American Unitarian
    Association 178
Andean War 170
Andrews, Bridie 133

Annecy 264
anti-colonialism 59
ARC Arts and Skills 205, 221
Ardèche 263
Argelès 183
Argentina 155, 162, 169
*Art for War Veterans* 224–225
Asquith, Wendy 205
Aujoulat, Louis-Paul 70–71
Auslander, Leora 42
Ayos 2

Bado, Jean-Paul 61
Bailkin, Jordanna 112
Baldin, Damien 41
Barcarès 183
Barnes, Nicole 35, 133, 241
Barnett, Michael 3, 6
Barsky, Edward 188, 190
Bassett, Kendall 221
Baudendistel, Rainer 89–90
Baughan, Emily 88
Berlant, Lauren 40
Betts, Paul 257
Bieber, Florian 117
Biéchy, Mgr 96
Bierroff, Suzanne 249
Boer Wars 86–87
Bonnecase, Vincent 73–74
Borgwardt, Elizabeth 171
Boston School for Social Work 181
Branscombe, Martha 114

278           *Index*

Brazil 155, 162, 169
Brazzaville 45, 69, 72, 96
British cemeteries 256
Brooklyn Museum of
   Art 207
Brooks, Jane 43
Brown, Sydney 11, 90
Buchanan, Andrew 5
Burma 242

Cabanes, Bruno 257
Cameroon 45, 59, 72, 84, 96
Carden-Coyne, Ana 43, 205, 237
Central Institute of National
   Medicine (CINM) 131–135,
   137–138, 140–141, 144,
   147–148
*Centre de dépistage et de*
   *prophylaxie* 184
Centre for Burn and Cold Injury
   Treatment 243
Changchun city 243
Chee, Liz. P.Y. 236
Chengdu 137, 139, 141–142, 145,
   148, 242–245
Chiang Kai-shek 131, 241
Chicago 203, 212–213
*The Chicago Defender* 212
Chile 155, 157, 162, 169
China 5, 9, 11, 17, 20, 35,
   131–133, 135, 139,
   141–142, 147, 235–237,
   240–247, 249, 250–251
Chippaux, Claude 76
Chongqing 17, 131–132, 135, 137,
   139–140, 243
Chorley, Kenneth 224–225
civilian internees 41, 95–101
Colomb-Beschar 183
*Comité de Coordination pour*
   *l'Assistance dans les*
   *Camps* 181
Confino, Alon 257
Congo 96
Conklin, Alice 70
conscientious objectors 30–31

Convention on the Prevention and
   Punishment of the Crime of
   Genocide in 1948 14
*Craft Horizons* 203, 207–208,
   210, 212, 219
craft therapy 19, 202–208, 210,
   212–214, 221, 225–226
Crum, J. Howard 239
Cultural Revolution 250

D'Amico, Victor 221–222
Dakar 62, 68
Dampier, Helen 37
Dartmouth College 218, 220
Davila, Luis Robalino 158
Davis, John Staige 238, 240
De Gaulle, Charles 269
dentistry 184, 235, 238–240, 242,
   245, 251
dermatology 184
*Design* 203, 207, 213–214, 218
Dexter, Robert 180
Dinshaw, Carolyn 37
disability 247, 248
Divorne, Marguerite 101
Djelfa 183
Domergue-Cloarec, Danielle 61
Douzou, Laurent 32, 47
Drôme 263

Eckert, Andreas 86
Ecuador 8, 17, 154
Ecumenical Relief Council 185
El Oro 170–171
El Shatt 13, 16, 109–124
Eritrea 97
Ethiopia 10–11, 97
Eure 265
Everill, Bronwen 100
Executive Order 9981 212
Eyidi Bebey, Marcel 1–2

Farré, Sébastien 6, 205
Fassin, Didier 34
Fayet, Jean-François 205
Feldman, Ilana 111

# Index

Ferrière, Suzanne 98
FFI (Forces Françaises de l'Intérieur) 66, 186, 189, 191, 264
Field, Noel 181, 183, 185, 187
Finistère 265
First World War 6, 12, 43, 62–63, 65, 87, 92, 94, 156, 170, 180, 203, 236, 238, 240, 256, 257, 258, 259, 266, 269–270
Forbs, Rosaleen 42
Franco-German reconciliation 269–270
Frank, Robert 5
French Equatorial Africa (A.E.F.) 45, 59, 84
French Republic 258
French Resistance 14, 32, 67
Free French 33, 45–46, 59, 62
Frère Benoît 264, 268
Freud, Anna 35
Friga, Ann 218
Fuller, Pierre 36

G. I. Bill 219
Gaillard, Pierre 94
Garland de Prado, Enriqueta 8, 164
Gatrell, Peter 12, 111
refugeedom 111
Gauducheau, Alexandre 73–74
Gaulle, Charles de 96
Gautier van Berchem, Marguerite 94, 101
Gemie, Sharif 5
Geneva Conventions of 1949 14
German cemetery 259
Ghobrial, John-Paul A. 3
Gill, Rebecca 37
Gilles, Harold H. 238
Gilmore, Otto 122–123
Gómez Álvarez, María 164, 189
Gordon, Neve 89
Grasset, Edmond 97–99

Guénon, Paul 47
Guomindang (GMD) 131
Gurs 183
Guyon, Anthony 59, 66

Hamilton Des Quartiers, Dorothy 118, 120
Hartman, Saidiya 32, 38, 48, 49
Haute-Savoie 264
Hermann, Kurt 163
Herzfeld, Michael 35
homosociality 206
Hospital and Recreation Corps 203
*How to Make Objects of Wood* 226–227
Huaxi 241–246
Hughes, Bill 247

ICRC (International Committee of the Red Cross) 2, 7, 10–11, 13, 15–16, 20, 45, 84–101, 157, 159, 182, 256–267, 269–271
Central Prisoners of War Agency 16, 85, 91–96, 101, 270
Imperial War Grave Commission 256
International Association of Oral and Maxillofacial Surgeons (IAOMS) 235
International Brigades 178
International Conference on Oral and Maxillofacial Surgery (ICOMS) 235
International Refugee Organization (IRO) 270
internment camps 87, 178–179, 183
intimacy (definition of) 34
cultural intimacy 35, 109
Italo-Ethiopian War 3, 9–11, 15–16, 84–85, 87, 89
Ivy, Robert H. 241–242

280 *Index*

Jamot, Eugène 62, 68
Japan 9, 35, 131, 136, 138, 242
Jarvis, Christina 206
Jennings, Eric 63, 65, 84
Jewish Children's Aid Society 182, 187
Jiao Yitang 135–136
Jin Hankui 248
Joint Anti-Fascist Refugee Committee 188–190
Joint Relief Commission of the International Red Cross 182, 184
Joy, Charles R. 180–181
Junod, Henri-Philippe 97–98
Junod, Marcel 10, 90, 97

Kea, Salaria 11, 37
Kelly, Monroe 224–225
Kelly, Tobias 33
Knaff, Donna B. 206
Koerber, Robert 75
Korea 5
Korean War 10, 14, 20, 235–237, 242–248
Kosykh, C. F. 246
Kraus, Hertha 1–2

*L'Humanité* 263
*L'Ordre des Médecins* 185
Lachenal, Guillaume 60, 71–72
Laigret, Jean 68
Lambie, Thomas 90
Le Vernet 183
League of Nations 6–7, 9, 19, 157–158
League of Nations' Disarmament Section 181
League of Red Cross Societies 84, 182
League of the Red Cross Societies 87–88, 91
Lefrou, Gustave 64–65, 67
Lei, Sean Hsiang-lin 133
Léopold II 86

Les Milles 183–184
Lewis, Su Lin 45
Li Ziyou 137
Liang Qichao 136
Liberation 59–60, 66, 116, 179, 186–187, 262
Liebes, Dorothy 203
Lisbon 178, 180
Liss, Edward 204
Lowe, Lisa 40
Lowrie, Donald A. 181
Lumb, Mary W. 119
Lyon 263, 268

*Maison d'Enfants* 191
Mangin, Charles 60, 62–63
Mao Zedong 147–148
Marinkovic, Lepa 123
Marseille 18, 65, 179–186
Marseille city council 184
Marseille Clinic 18, 179, 182–183, 184, 186, 187
Marseille University Hospital 186
Martín-Moruno, Dolores 37
maxillofacial surgeons 235, 238, 240, 249, 251
maxillofacial surgery 20, 235–238, 240–242, 244–251
Mayenne 265
Mayer, André 77
Mazower, Mark 5, 12
McCarthyism 190–191
mental illness 215
Metropolitan Museum of Art 203, 204, 217
Michel, William 260
Middle East Relief and Refugee Administration (MERRA) 110, 117
Miller, Persis 93, 191
*Ministère des Anciens Combattants* 260–262, 264, 268
Miot, Claire 66
Montélimar camp 263
Moore, Claire 219–220

## Index

Moynier, Gustave 86
Muraz, Gaston 68
Museum of Modern Art (MoMA) 19, 203–205, 207, 221–227
Mussolini 180

Neill, Deborah 60
New Caledonia 45
New Hebrides 45
New York 203, 207, 210, 217–218, 221–223, 225, 227, 241
Noé 183, 188
Noel Field 182
North Africa 59, 84, 87, 92, 269
North Korea 20, 237, 243
Nuseirat 118
Nyassaland 99

O'Sullivan, Kevin 5–6
Odier, Lucie 98
Odría, Manuel 154
Office of the Coordinator of Inter-American Affairs (OIAA) 169
*Operación Reconquista de España* 189
orthopaedics 184
otorhinolaryngology 184
Ott, Katherine 205

paediatric 184
Pales, Léon 65, 74–75
Paulmann, Johannes 6
Pearson, Jessica 60, 71
*People's Daily* 250
People's Volunteer Army 243
Perrot, Emile 61
Perry Myers, Sara 206
Peru 8, 17, 154
Perugini, Nicola 89
photography 122
Pierre Bossier 259
Pignet, Maurice Charles Joseph 64
Piketty, Guillaume 257
Piller, Elisabeth 37

plastic surgery 238–245, 251
Poling, Virgil 218
prisoners of war (PoWs) 16, 20, 45, 85, 91–99, 156, 160–162, 181, 257–259, 261, 263, 266–267
professionalisation 8–9, 17, 145
PVA soldiers 243–244, 249

Qiu Weiliu 235
Quakers 1–2, 117
Quito 158, 162, 166

Rachamimov, Iris 41
Rankin, Monica 169–170
Récébédou 183, 188
Red Cross
  activism 9, 16
  actors 10
  colonial branches/sections 15, 16, 84–85, 95
  emblem 160
  Movement 10, 15–16, 85, 100, 158
  network 16
Red Cross and Red Crescent Societies
  American 96, 117, 202–203, 207, 210, 221–222, 225
  Belgian 96
  British 88–89, 99–100, 117–119
  Chinese 144
  Dutch 89
  Ecuadorian 158, 161
  Egyptian 89
  Ethiopian 89–91, 95
  Finnish 89
  French 96, 186
  Greek 117
  Norwegian 10, 89
  Peruvian 157, 161
  South African 87, 95, 97–99, 101
  Soviet Red Cross Alliance 91
  Swedish 89, 91
  Swiss 185

282 *Index*

Reinisch, Jessica 12
Resistance 18, 33, 42, 44, 46–48,
 178, 180, 182, 185, 192
Rhodesia 13, 99
Rhône 264
Ribi, Amalia 89
Rieucros 183
Rif War 86, 89
Rivesaltes 183–184
Rochester University
 Hospital 241
Rominger, Chris 43
Rouček, Joseph S. 11
Rowntree, Michael 30
Royal Society of Medicine in
 London 239
Ruyao, Song 243, 250

Saint-Julien-de-Crempse 266
Salisbury 99
Salvatici, Silvia 6
San Francisco 203
Sarraut, Albert 65
Saulnier-Boucher, Françoise 111
Save the Children 6–7, 88,
 117, 123
School for the American Craftsmen
 (SAC) 203
Schroer, Timothy L. 85
Schumann, Dirk 257
Séché, Alphonse 66
Second Sino Japanese War 9
Second World War 1, 18, 68, 133,
 171, 179, 181–182, 189,
 191–193, 236–237,
 239–240, 246, 251, 256
Senghor, Léopold Sedar 94
Senn, Geoffrey Cassian 97, 99
*Service de l'Etat civil et des
 recherches du Ministère des
 Anciens Combattants et
 Victimes de la Guerre* 260
Shanghai 133, 143, 148, 235,
 241–244
Sharp, Waitstill H. 180
Sicé, Adolphe 68, 72, 77

Sichuan 17, 132, 134, 139–140,
 142, 148
Sino Japanese War 3, 10–11, 17
*Sociedad Ecuatoriana de
 Transportes Aéreos*
 (SEDTA) 162
Somalia 97
Song Ruyao 8, 241–242, 244,
 246–247, 249–250
South Africa 13, 98
Soviet Union 4, 20, 71, 235–236,
 245–247, 251
Soviet-Finnish War 10
Spanish Civil War 3, 7, 9–11,
 159, 188
Spanish Republic 180
stomatology 235–236, 245, 247
Strasbourg 182
Szitanyi, Stephanie 206

Taithe, Bertrand 205
Tappert, Tara 204
Taylor, Francis Henry 204
Terrenoire, Elisabeth 33
Thomas, Paul 20, 262, 264,
 267–268
Thompson, Andrew 88
Tito, Josip 190
Tongji University 242
Torrubia, Josep 189
Toulouse 18, 164, 179,
 187–191
Truman, Harry S. 212
Tuskegee U.S. Veterans
 Hospital 212

U.S. Congress 190
*Unión Nacional Española* 189
Unitarian Service Committee (USC)
 18, 178–193
United Coalition and UN
 Peace enforcement
 operation 14
United Kingdom 4, 46, 92,
 109, 112, 119–120,
 122–123, 258

## Index

United Nations 7, 14, 60, 71–72, 77, 110, 112, 114, 243
United Nations Relief and Rehabilitation Administration (UNRRA) 110, 114–117, 119, 121–122
United States 1, 5–6, 8, 11, 19–20, 38, 40, 59, 67, 71, 90, 91, 109–110, 122–123, 154–155, 159, 162, 168–170, 172, 180–181, 183–184, 192, 202–203, 212–213, 235–238, 240– 243, 247, 251, 258
Ureta, General 161, 166–167
US federal National War Fund 187–188

Varsovie Hospital 18, 164, 179, 187–190
Vatican 7
Vaucel, Marcel 71–72
Vaughan, Megan 60
Vence 186
Vialard-Goudou, Jean 42
Vichy regime 11, 16, 45–46, 59, 85, 93, 96, 178–182
Vidal-Naquet, Clémentine 32, 47–48
Vieser, Herta K. 182

Waller, Willard 212
Wang Hanzhang 8, 246, 248
War Veterans Art Center 203, 221
Washington, DC 167
Webster, Richard 242
Wehrmachtsauskunftstelle 262
Weill, Joseph 182
Weimar Republic 239
Western medicine 17, 132–137, 139–141, 146
white privilege 206, 218
Whiting, Harold B. 218
Wilson, Ara 39
Wilson, Elizabeth 35
Wirz, Albert 86
Wood, Bryce 156
World Health Organization 19, 60, 68, 70
World Vision 13

YMCA 94, 181–182
Yu Yan 136
Yugoslavia 110, 115–117
partisans 116

Zhang Disheng 241–244
Zimmer, René 182–186, 193
Zuniga, Jean-Paul 3

EU authorised representative for GPSR:
Easy Access System Europe, Mustamäe tee 50,
10621 Tallinn, Estonia
gpsr.requests@easproject.com

www.ingramcontent.com/pod-product-compliance
Lightning Source LLC
LaVergne TN
LVHW020248020825
817679LV00004B/206